Advanced

HATHA YOGA

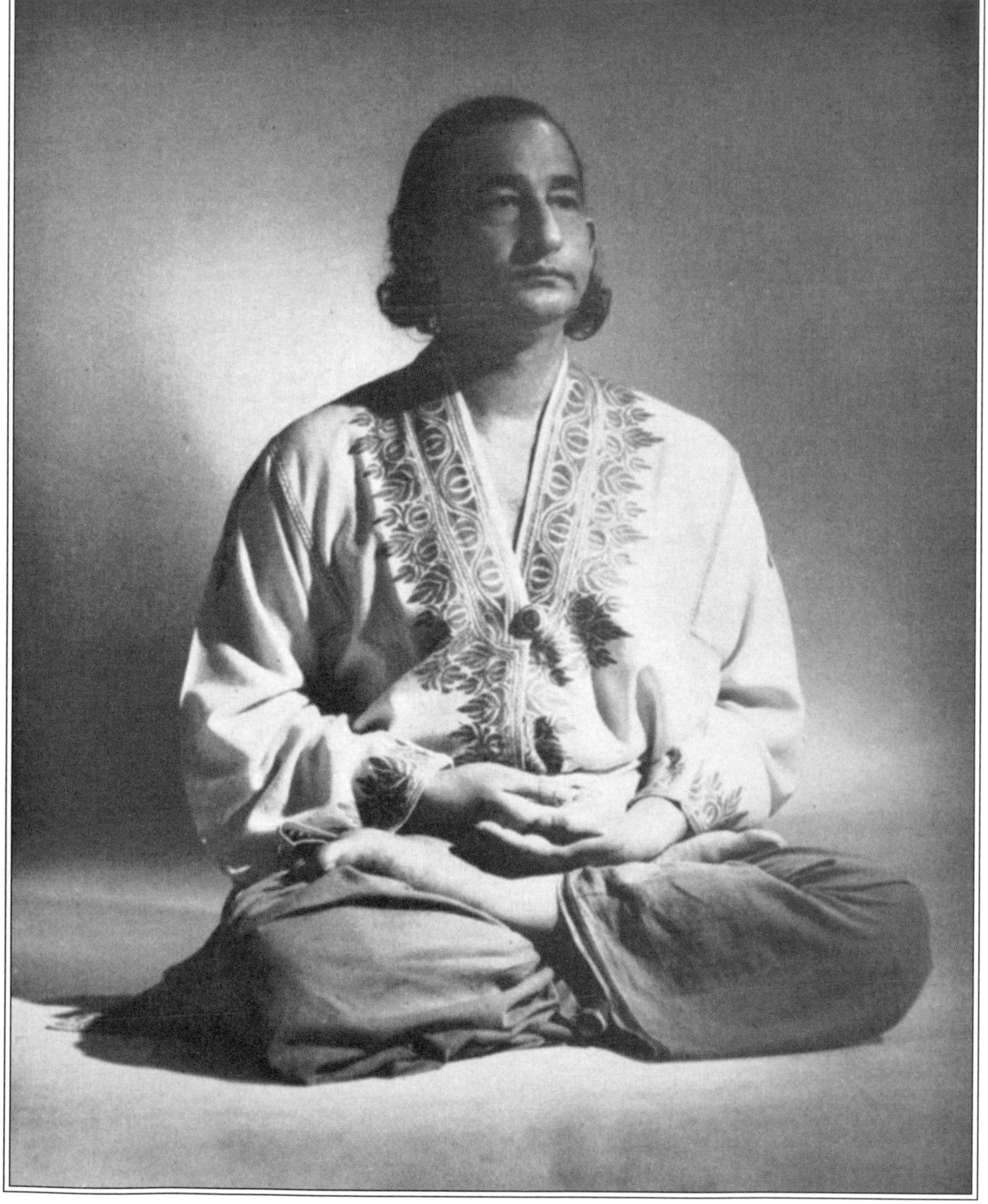

Shyam Sundar Goswami

Advanced HATHA YOGA

Classic Methods of Physical Education and Concentration

Shyam Sundar Goswami

Inner Traditions
Rochester, Vermont • Toronto, Canada

Inner Traditions
One Park Street
Rochester, Vermont 05767
www.InnerTraditions.com

Originally published in London in 1959 and 1963 by L. N. Fowler & Co., Ltd., under the title *Haṭha Yoga: An Advanced Method of Physical Education and Concentration*

Library of Congress Cataloging-in-Publication Data
Goswami, Shyam Sundar.
[Hatha-yoga]
Advanced hatha yoga : classic methods of physical education and concentration / Shyam Sundar Goswami.
p. cm.
Originally published under title: Hatha-yoga : an advanced method of physical education and concentration : London : L.N. Fowler, 1959.
Includes bibliographical references and index.
ISBN 978-1-59477-453-9 (pbk.) — ISBN 978-1-59477-696-0 (e-book)
1. Hatha yoga. I. Title.
RA781.7.G674 2012
613.7'046—dc23

2012017253

Printed and bound in the United States by P. A. Hutchison

10 9 8 7 6 5 4 3 2 1

Text design by Virginia Scott Bowman and layout by Priscilla Baker
This book was typeset in Garamond Premier Pro with Bodoni Antiqua, Gentle Sans, and Gill Sans used as display typefaces

For more information about Shyam Sundar Goswami and the Goswami Yoga Institute, please visit the institute's website at **www.goswamiyogainstitute.com**.

To the Lord Śiva

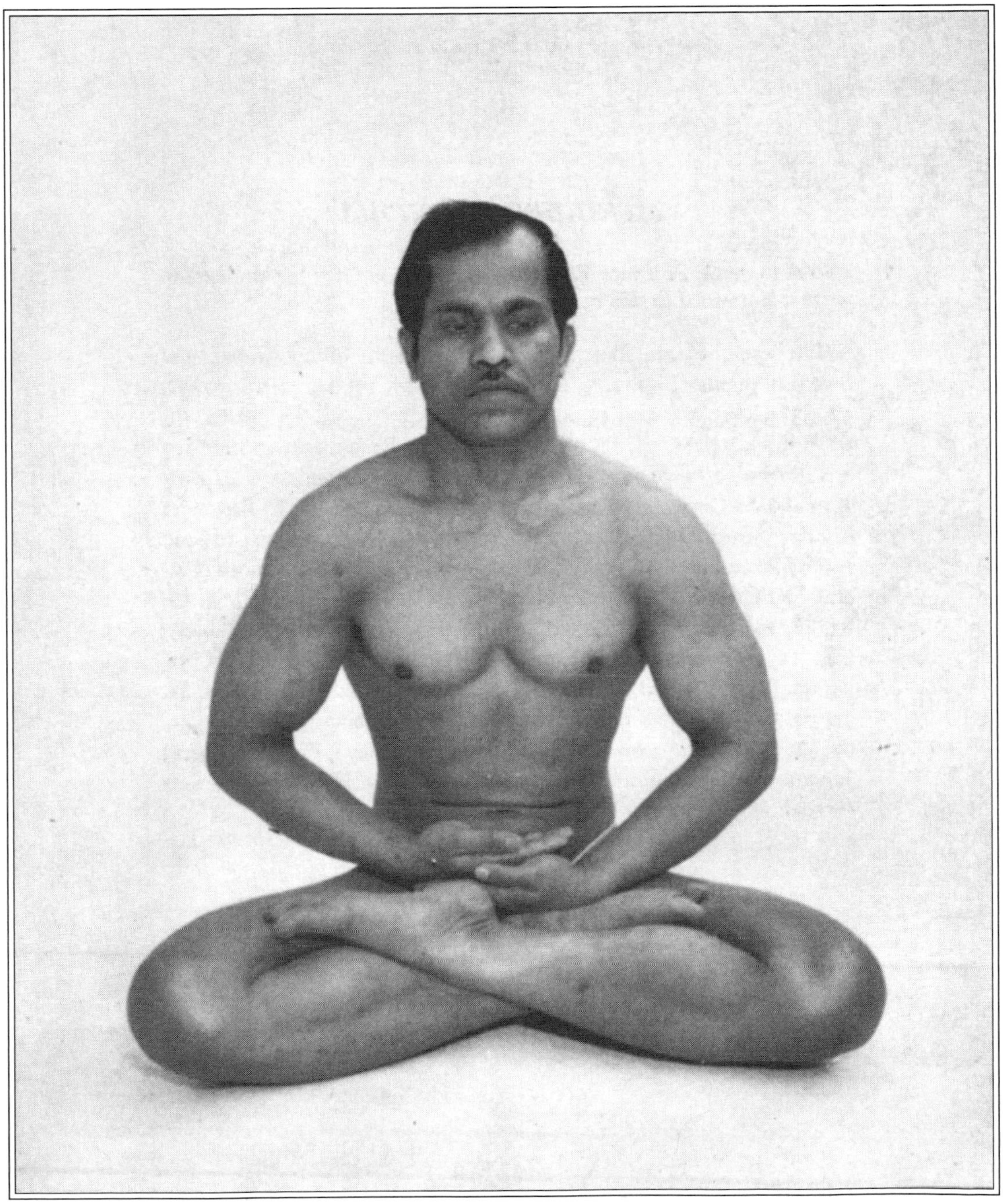

Śiva
Posed by Dinabandhu Pramanick

Contents

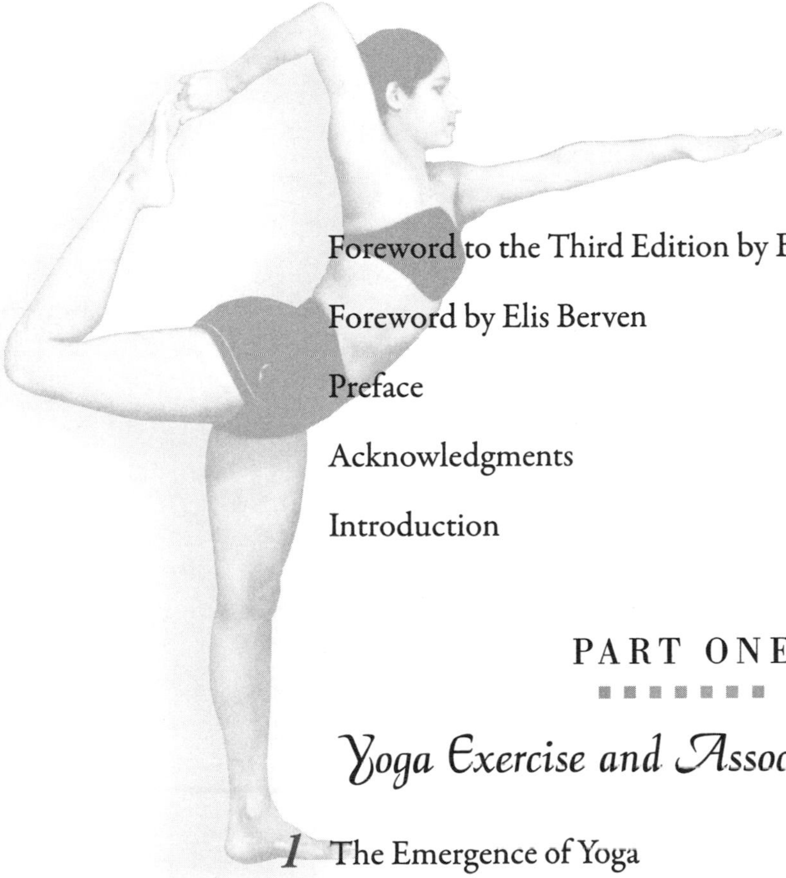

PART TWO

Technical Aspects of Yoga Exercise

PART THREE

Exercise Plans

Foreword to the Third Edition

Basile P. Catoméris

The author of this classic book is widely recognized by his peers as one of the major pioneers of contemporary Yoga.

> *[Sri S. S. Goswami is] the foremost exponent of Yoga in modern time.*
>
> Acharya Karunamoya Saraswati

> *The scientific and creative exposition of Haṭha Yoga in our time is due mostly to the work of two distinguished yogis, Yogi Madhavdas and Shyam Sundar Goswami. . . .*
>
> *[Sri Goswami's book] is modern, cogent and the most comprehensive, definitive treatment of Haṭha Yoga to be found in the Western world today. It is also the most completely illustrated book.*
>
> Sachindra Kumar Majumdar, author of *Introduction to Yoga Principles and Practices* (Pelham Books)

It is with feelings of immense gratitude, honor, and responsibility that I write this foreword to the third edition of Sri Shyam Sundar Goswami's book, *Haṭha Yoga*. In this new edition, now titled *Advanced Hatha Yoga,* special thanks are extended to Professor Göran Hedenstierna, Head of the Research Department of Clinical Physiology at the Uppsala University Hospital, Sweden.

I am very thankful for Inner Tradition's editorial team's constructive intiatives, in particular those of Laura Schlivek and Nancy Yeilding, whose meticulous editorial work has allowed most valuable improvements.

This long-overdue revision of *Haṭha Yoga* is set apart by the addition of a more comprehensive index and a revised chapter on *prāṇāyāma* (chapter 21), with elaborations taken from material originally intended to be part of Sri Shyam Sundar Goswami's ambitious, five-volume *Haṭha Yoga*—a project that only an enlightened Yoga master could undertake. It has not been deemed necessary to update the original chapter on diet (chapter 7) in the light of the many, often contradictory, theories and recommendations on nutrition.

Please note that for safety's sake certain exercises included in this manual require a competent instructor's supervision, while other advanced exercises, which are actually intended for spiritually oriented people, need a different level of supervision—that of a *guru,* or spiritual guide. When the personal instruction of a teacher is necessary, it has been noted in the exercise directions.

Sri S. S. Goswami was remarkable for his outstanding personal achievements and for having presented astounding demonstrations of yogic bodily control in many locations throughout the world. He also shared with thousands of pupils the timeless experiences and values inherited from his own spiritual achievements in both Haṭha Yoga and Laya Yoga—two rather different yogic disciplines. The "Lion of Bengal," as an admiring maharaja once liked to call him, was also an exceptional man of action, a yogi who dedicated about seventy years of his life exclusively to the regular practice, study, and investigation of the vast field of Yoga.

Dedicated to the Lord of Yoga, scientifically presented as a valuable bridge between India's ancestral spiritual legacy and searching Western civilization, Sri S. S. Goswami's methodically elaborated *Advanced Hatha Yoga* has been for many years, and will surely continue to be, an exclusive reference for future generations, and as such replace the old manual *Haṭha Yoga Pradipikā,* which—like two other major references, the *Gheraṇḍa Samhitā* and the *Śiva Samhitā*—is derived from very ancient texts. Sri S. S. Goswami's holistic teachings on the vast subject of Yoga, and in particular of the pragmatic philosophy of Haṭha Yoga, are actually a manifestation of the Bhagavad Gītā's triptych: knowledge, action, and love.

To all those who aspire to seriously undertake Haṭha Yoga, Sri S. S. Goswami recalls the necessity to first adopt the tenfold vitalizing and cleaning processes known as *yama* and *niyama*. This admonition is in harmony with the *Yoga Bhāshya Vivarana* 2.29, whose tenet is that *shanti*—poise or peace of mind—is needed to qualify for Haṭha Yoga's six further steps (*angas*). The ageless Haṭha Yoga is the most adapted to modern lifestyles among existing Ashtānga Yoga paths.

As a practical philosophy, Haṭha Yoga is particularly designed to fit typical representatives of the so-called Middle Way. It thus addresses those who stand with one foot in the frantic, centrifugal rhythm of social life and at the same time harbor genuine spiritual aspirations with the wish to enter into the evolutionary sphere of spiritual quest. Sri S. S. Goswami's classic *Advanced Hatha Yoga* is a precious cognitive tool for harmoniously combining these two lifestyles.

As a personal message, I should say that for many years I've personally enjoyed, and still enjoy, in the fall of my life, the most appreciable and durable benefits from the regular practice of Sri Goswami's efficient philosophy of Haṭha Yoga. How? Mostly by improved immunity and vitality, strength and endurance, determination, peace of mind, mental power, and—still more important—the privilege of a spiritual teacher's lasting inspiration.

The author has commented, in an unpublished manuscript, upon lesser-known principles of Haṭha Yoga. A substantial part of these and other valuable original teachings will be published in my forthcoming book titled *Foundations of Yoga* (Inner Traditions), along with one chapter dedicated to *cāraṇā*, one of the traditionally concealed methods, disclosed to the body of Yoga practitioners for the first time in the present book (see page 27).

Basile Catoméris, a dedicated disciple of Sri Shyam Sundar Goswami, went on to head the Goswami Institute in Sweden, where he taught Goswami's style of Yoga to hundreds of students from different parts of the world.

Foreword

Elis Berven

Yoga is a most ancient system of education, based on a higher philosophical knowledge and a spiritual conception of man, for the harmonious development of the body and mind. It recognizes the necessity of developing a healthy, vital, and well-controlled body for the attainment of a high order of mental life.

From his lifelong study and experience, Goswami has written a book on Haṭha Yoga in which he has been able to expound Yoga in a remarkable manner. Various forms of exercises have been presented in a systematic way. The book teaches how one can develop thc power of concentration, control one's mind, and build a healthy, strong, and beautiful body.

I hope the book will be very helpful for Western people and others who are interested in Yoga and desire to attain physical, mental, and spiritual development.

STOCKHOLM
JUNE 17, 1954

ELIS BERVEN was Professor Emeritus of Radiotherapy, Chief of Radiumhemmet, Stockholm, and Vice President for the European Section of Union Internationale Centre le Cancer.

Preface

During my visit a few years ago to London, Paris, Zurich, and other places in Europe, where I gave lectures on Yoga and demonstrations, I encountered an interest that was considerably greater than before the war, and I was repeatedly asked to give practical instructions in Yoga. Even medical men showed great interest and I had the opportunity to demonstrate before well-known surgeons and physicians the more advanced muscle control that is a part of Haṭha Yoga. Haṭha Yoga is not merely a means of acquiring a sound, strong, and vital body but also a reliable method of acquiring happiness and harmony and, above all, of developing the inner strength that enables a person to bear sorrow, pain, and failures with equanimity.

It has been my firm conviction that there exists a serious demand for a methodical and practical exposition of the Haṭha Yoga system, with a view to the acquisition of physical strength and mental harmony. I have been asked to meet this demand by people very much interested in this matter, by friends and pupils, and have finally decided to write a book based upon personal experiences and fundamental studies.

This book is mainly based upon original works on Yoga in Sanskrit, the majority of which are only available in the form of unpublished manuscripts, but it is also based upon instructions that have been conveyed from teacher to pupil throughout generations for thousands of years.

Through personal experience I have been able to ascertain for myself the practical value of Haṭha Yoga. From my very childhood I was physically undeveloped, weak, and susceptible to disease. Neither medicines nor ordinary dietetic measures helped. Physical exercises improved my physical condition to some extent but did not increase my power of resistance. I searched everywhere for a possibility to improve my poor health and thus came in contact with a remarkable man, named Kali Singha, who at that time was about 110 years old. He was the first who drew my attention to Haṭha Yoga, as a reliable means to give me what I needed. Singha was a dependable source, as he himself had practiced Haṭha Yoga under the tuition of a guru. For some time I became his pupil, when I was seventeen.

About this time K. Rammurti caused a great sensation in India by his demonstrations of supporting an elephant upon his chest. He claimed that his strength was due to Yoga exercises and especially to certain breathing exercises. My interest was greatly stimulated, and I decided to dedicate my time exclusively to the study of Yoga. As Kali Singha had died, I looked for a new teacher, and found him in my guru, the great yogin Balaka Bharati, who initiated me in Haṭha Yoga and taught me the fundamentals of this unique system. My continuous exercises led to a quick and very satisfactory physical improvement. My muscles increased in size and strength, and finally I could control their movements completely. When a muscle was contracted, it was so hard that no impression could be made on it even with a pair of iron tongs. The muscles of the throat could be contracted to such an extent that throttling with an iron chain pulled by twelve men had no effect. I became more and more hardened against heat and cold.

Most important of all, I developed a power of resistance, which spared me every kind of illness. I became a healthy man. I realized that a weakened body was an obstacle for the efficient expression and working of the mental powers and that a clean and healthy body was an important condition for clear thinking and concentration. Further, I realized that only a person who is harmonious and well balanced in body and mind can develop spiritual powers to a maximum degree.

In India, where Yoga is considered to be a method for the spiritual progress of humanity, by means of the right control of the body and mind, many institutions of more or less permanent character have sprung up. The pupils in these schools receive theoretical and practical instructions, adopt a new mode of life, and follow certain physical and moral rules. Their exercises become more and more difficult and, finally, they reach the highest stage of mental concentration. In this way Yoga has been imparted for thousands of years. It has thus been possible to collect experiences and make continuous observations to ascertain the effects of the methods on human subjects. According to my opinion, these methods must be considered to be much more reliable than any of the modern systems, which are based upon experiences and observations of a very short period of time.

In my school in Kolkata, I have personally taught the Yoga method for thirty-five years, with good results, to a great number of pupils of both genders, different ages, and different conditions of health. Some people think that Yoga exercises are not suitable for Western people. This has been contradicted by my own experience, which confirms that Western pupils have been able to master the yogic exercises equally as well as my Eastern pupils and to derive the same benefit. Some of them have reached a very high standard, as can be seen from the illustrations of many of the exercises in this book as performed by my Swedish pupils. The secret of success lies in determination, perseverance, and proper guidance.

Another question has been raised about whether Yoga practice is necessarily very time-consuming. This time factor may be considered from two points of view: the time devoted in each day or week to the exercise and the time required to get results. For ordinary busy people three to five hours a week are sufficient, and most of them will be able to devote this much time for their physical health and mental revitalization. But those who want to reach perfection have to devote much more time. This is not only true with Yoga, but also with athletics, sports, gymnastics, and, in fact, everything. We are not always conscious of how much time we waste every day on useless social pleasures and many other things. If we learn to economize time, it will not be difficult for us to spend the necessary time for rebuilding ourselves.

I would like to stress still another point—namely, that if the Yoga method seems to stand in contradiction to generally accepted views, it should not be discarded, for that reason, as being unscientific, useless, or even harmful. These methods, however strange and peculiar they may appear to the Western mind, have stood the test of time. Instead of throwing them aside as worthless, they should be studied and tested in clinical experiments that can be replicated for confirmation of the results, which I am sure will bring ultimate conviction of their worth.

Certain ideas and interpretations in this book may not be familiar to the way of thinking of many Western people, so I suggest that the reader first try to assimilate them by reading it carefully and thinking them over. I have tried my best to make the book as clear and palatable as possible, but still many readers may think that it is a highly specialized work. I know definitely that it is useless to deal with the subject more superficially simply to make it acceptable to the reader. Shallow knowledge will not help here. The reader must be ready to welcome new thoughts, because this is the only way of self-expansion. After clear understanding of these ideas is gained, that knowledge can be translated into action by practicing the exercises and following other instructions contained in the book.

I sincerely believe that, with a normalized and controlled body and a vitalized and concentrated mind, attained through the practice of Yoga, life will appear more beauteous and charming, more lovable and enjoyable. Life will be worth living.

Acknowledgments

I wish to thank Professor Elis Berven, Stockholm, for his kindness in writing a foreword to this book.

The exercises are illustrated by photographs of my Indian and Swedish pupils:

Dinabandhu Pramanick
Figs. 12.1, 12.5, 12.6, 12.7, 12.9, 12.15, 12.16, 12.17, 12.19, 12.21a, 12.22, 12.26, 12.31, 12.32, 13.1, 13.2, 14.1, 14.2, 14.4, 14.10, 14.11, 14.12, 14.13, 14.14, 14.15, 14.17, 14.18, 14.21, 14.25, 15.1, 15.2, 15.3, 15.4, 16.1, 16.4, 16.5, 16.6, 16.7, 16.9, 17.1, 17.2, 17.6, 17.7, 17.8, 18.8, 18.9, 19.1, 19.2, and 19.3

Kamalaksha Goswami (Kolkata)
Fig. 12.4

Brajendra Sundar Goswami (Kolkata)
Figs. 12.8, 12.14, 12.30, and 18.15

Renu Ghosh (Kolkata)
Figs. 12.10, 12.12, 12.23, 15.9, 15.11, 18.1, 18.5, 19.4, and 20.2

Leela Ghosh (Kolkata)
Figs. 12.29 and 20.4

Parvati Devi (Karin Schalander, Stockholm)
Figs. 12.24, 12.25, 12.27, 12.28, 14.3, 14.5, 14.6, 14.7, 14.9, 14.16, 14.23, 14.24, 14.26, 17.3, 17.4, 17.5, 18.2, 20.1, and 20.3

Kerstin Aldin (Stockholm)
Fig. 12.11

Olle Söderblom (Stockholm)
Figs. 12.2, 12.3, 12.13, 12.18, 12.20, 14.20, 14.22, 15.10, 18.3, 18.4, 18.7, and 18.16

Vishuddhananda Giri (Basile Catoméris, France)
Figs. 14.8, 16.2, 16.3, 18.10, 18.11, and 18.12

Arne Lundgren (Stockholm)
Figs. 12.21b, 14.19, 15.5, 15.6, 15.7, 15.8, and 18.6

Bertil Johansson (Stockholm)
Fig. 16.8

Henrik Levkowetz (Oslo)
Figs. 18.13 and 18.14

I wish to thank them all.

Introduction

In Yoga a motionless, changeless, eternal principle has been recognized. From the yogic point of view, recognition of an intellectual verbosity, philosophical speculation, or psychological curiosity is not considered very important. Rather, the recognition valued by Yoga is entirely based on spiritual realization of the changeless principle, experienced as the ultimate reality. This realization is only possible when the subject-object experiences are transformed into a homogeneous pattern. The process involved is technically known as *samādhi* (super concentration).

Consciousness at the human level is split into subjective and objective forms upon which rest the world experiences. By careful analysis we find that the subjective aspect of consciousness is composed of two component parts: I + my = I-my feeling. The main part is the "I" without "my." This means pure "I" without any trace of relation to objective consciousness. But at the common level it is almost impossible to isolate "I" from "my" and objects.

The subject apparently projects itself beyond its boundaries up to its objects. The projections are not without passion: they are fully saturated with desires, and the whole experience results in one of the three kinds of reaction: the experience of pleasure, the experience of pain, or a temporary inertia combined with bewilderment when there is excessive pleasure or pain. Everything together is the world experience.

Desires arise in the subject and link it with objects. At the back of desire is interest. The subject feels interested in those objects that will give it enjoyment. How does the subject know that certain objects will give it enjoyment? The answer may be that the subject has prior experience. But how did the first experience come? The reply is usually given by stating that the whole phenomenon is "without beginning." The example of a seed tree is often cited in this connection. However, this interpretation is inadequate.

The first interest in objects is not due to any previous experience of the subject. It has been embedded in the subject and therefore it has no beginning. It is beyond cause and effect. Both the subject and the objects are born at the same moment, and before any experience of enjoyment due to contact with the object, the subject shows clear interest for objects. This interest is, so to speak, a memory of some blissful experience that the subject had before it was born. This means that consciousness beyond the subject-object phenomenon is in its own real form, which is bliss. This is Supreme Consciousness, which is being-consciousness-bliss. Without the recognition of Supreme Consciousness as the ultimate reality, the static background of all motional phenomena, the behavior of the subject cannot be rationally explained.

The cosmic phenomenon is the manifested Will of the unlimited, the indestructible quiescent Supreme Consciousness—a Will having the creative potency capable of being expressed fully. This is why the Will is called Śakti. Śakti is the massive concentrated energy that is in the nature of consciousness and associated with bliss and at the same time capable of being expressed as creation. A dichotomy in the consciousness appears due to the influence of Māyā, an aspect of Śakti in her creative mood.

An object at the gross level is a compound of five *mahābhūtas* (essentials), which is matter. In isolation from the compound, each of the *mahābhūtas* is a form of nonmaterial subtle energy ultimately derived from still subtler and most concentrated forms of nonmaterial energy called *tanmātras*. Objects being dematerialized by the sensory processes are represented in the consciousness as heterogeneous images revolving around the "I." The constant molding of the objective aspect of consciousness into images that are of the sensory pattern is called *vṛitti*. It is the distracted state of the mind. When it is transformed into the single-intent state by the processes of *dhāraṇā* (elementary concentration), *dhyāna* (unbroken concentration), and *samādhi* (super concentration), a brighter form of mental life is evolved and gradually the mind is transformed into an extraordinary state in which, ultimately, the complete elimination of *vṛitti* occurs. It is a state that is beyond the knowledge of the known, a state of realization of the Unknown, a state of realization that is beyond realization. It is the state of *asamprajñāta samādhi*.

According to Haṭha Yoga, physical as well as mental factors are involved in concentration. Physical and mental need to function together harmoniously, along with a third factor: that of *prāṇa*, the kinetic principle. When the movement potential of *prāṇa* operates at the *mahābhūtas* level, it expresses what is known as the phenomenon of life.

It is not a wise plan to live mostly in one aspect of life, ignoring the rest. A brilliant expression of mind in a sickly and devitalized body may appear very impressive, or a superbly developed body with a meager mental life may be quite charming. However, such a mode of living will ultimately go wrong and break down. The mind and body are out of balance. To find out the correct balance is the starting point of Haṭha Yoga. *Prāṇa* is the balance beam on which the body and the mind can be properly balanced. But in our everyday life the prāṇic line is not straight as it should be, and this is why there is such a lack of harmony. When the pranic line is made straight, the problem is solved.

The functioning of the body as well as of the mind is entirely dependent on *prāṇa*. All the organic movements of the living body, from the minutest to the grossest, are the expression of extraphysical subtler pranic movements. Haṭha Yoga aims at gaining full control over the gross movements with a view to transforming the centrifugal forces operating in them into centripetal force. In this process of transformation, the mind is released, step by step, from physical influence; its distraction changes into single-intentness. The control process starts with the musculo-diaphragmatic movements, because it is easier to approach the other movements through them.

At the physical level, *prāṇa* becomes the energy-acquiring and energy-consuming principles of the body. At the mental level, *prāṇa* becomes the subtle forces of activation and inhibition; it causes distraction and infatuation as well as temporary calmness of the mind. Unless these forces and principles are harmonized, an imbalance is established in the organism, making the body devitalized, weak, and short-lived, and the mind restless, dull, and dark.

The process of harmonization is termed Nāḍī Śuddhi. It consists of two parts: gross and subtle. The gross process includes six purificatory acts, plus posture exercise, special posture and control exercise, and contraction exercise; the right application of these aspects of the gross process purifies and vitalizes the body, making it fit for the practice of the subtle process. The subtle process is a special form of breath-control exercise (*prāṇāyāma*) by which Nāḍī Śuddhi is attained. After this a student may go deeper into breath control as advocated in Haṭha Yoga or can adopt Mantra Yoga or Laya Yoga for developing concentration.

By the practice of breath control (*prāṇāyāma*) various extraordinary powers are attained. The writer had an opportunity to witness the phenomenal physical strength exhibited by his Haṭha Yoga guru (teacher), Balaka Bharati. One day the yogin broke a very large trunk of a living tree in an attempt to pull it out after a team of six strong men had unsuccessfully tried to do so. He also had other super powers. One day I picked up a very hot copper pot without knowing it was hot. It was so hot that it immediately slipped from my hand, and I was feeling intense pain and feared blistering. The yogin was there, and as soon as he saw this, he immediately came near me and put his hand on my burnt palm. To my utter surprise, the pain at once disappeared and there was no blister formation. While making oblations, he used to hold a very hot earthen pot in which charcoal was burning on the bare palm of his left hand for more than half an hour without any burns or pain. An accomplished yogin can walk barefooted on fire. The writer's pupil Dinabandhu Pramanick demonstrated fire walking.

At the highest stage of breath control the human body rises upward above the ground and floats in the air. A yogin named Sisala of Madras kept himself suspended in the air, assuming the Lotus Posture, without any support except for resting his right hand lightly on a rolled deer hide that projected horizontally from a vertically placed brass rod fixed on a wooden stool. The yogin used to stay in this position for a long time with his eyes closed.

Another levitation act was shown by a yogin named Suhbayah Pallavar of Tinnevelly. He remained suspended horizontally in the air for about four minutes, without any support except for resting his hand lightly on top of a cloth-covered stick. Then the yogin began to descend from the top to the bottom of the stick; within five minutes he had covered a distance of about three feet, still remaining in the horizontal position. The yogin was in a trance and in a state of rigor mortis. He was so stiff that four or five men could not bend his limbs. After the act was over, he was massaged and subjected to a cold pouring bath. Then he returned to his normal state. This is, of course, a comparatively advanced form of levitation.

Breath control develops such extraordinary control over the vital organs that their normal functions may be altered and even suspended. The stopping of the heart and pulse and the suspension of breathing for a long period have been demonstrated. A condition of latent life—which is an impossible form of existence for man at a common level—has also been demonstrated.

In 1837, the great Haṭha Yoga master Haridāsa gave a demonstration of how he could remain buried underground for forty days. Present at his burial were Maharaja Ranjit Sing, the ruler of the Punjab, his court, and a number of English and French gentlemen, among whom were medical men. General Ventura of Paris and Colonel Sir C. M. Wade, the political agent of the British Government, were also present. The yogin assumed the Lotus Posture, with his nostrils and the external acoustic meatus blocked by wax. He also closed the rima glottidis by retroverting his tongue. This means he adopted the Khecarī Mudrā. He was then wrapped in linen and placed in a wooden box on which a strong lock was put by the Maharaja, and the Maharaja's seal was put on several parts of the box. The box was then buried. Barley was sown on the ground the space was enclosed with a wall and it was guarded by sentinels. On the fortieth day, the box was brought up and opened and the yogin was found in the same sitting posture he had assumed at the commencement. The body of the yogin was examined by Dr. McGregor, Residency Surgeon, and Dr. Murray. There was no pulsation at the wrist, no signs of animation. Then he was resuscitated by his pupils. Another thing to be noted was that he had been shaven on the day of his burial, but at his exhumation it was found that no hair had grown at all on his cheeks.

Vital endurance is greatly increased by the practice of Yoga. In Benares, Bhaskarananda Sarasvati kept his bare body exposed day and night to the intense heat of summer and cold of winter. The yogins also attain great age. The great yogin Tailanga Swami lived 280 years. Lokanatha Brahmachari lived 166 years.

Apart from the attainment of spiritual development and super powers, Haṭha Yoga is an advanced method of physical education. Through the right application of its various processes and exercises, we can attain a body that is vital, healthy, clean, strong, enduring, well controlled, and symmetrically developed, and a mind that is imaginative, determinative, forceful, chaste, calm, and happy. We can raise human efficiency to a higher level by the practice of Yoga. Yoga is for saints and spiritual pupils. It is also for worldly men and women. Yoga should be applied in everyday life and in every phase of life to hasten human advancement toward health, happiness, harmony, and peace.

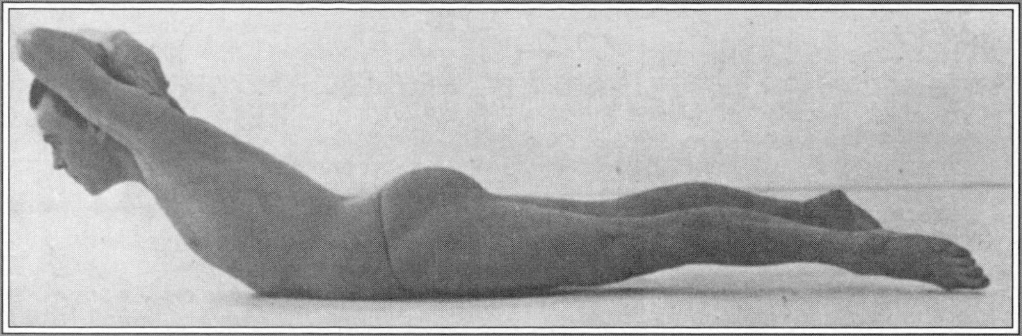

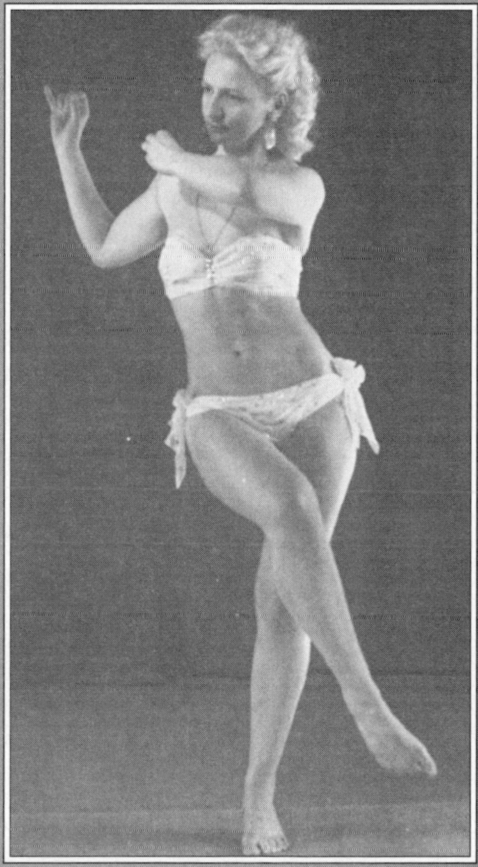

PART ONE

YOGA EXERCISE AND ASSOCIATED FACTORS

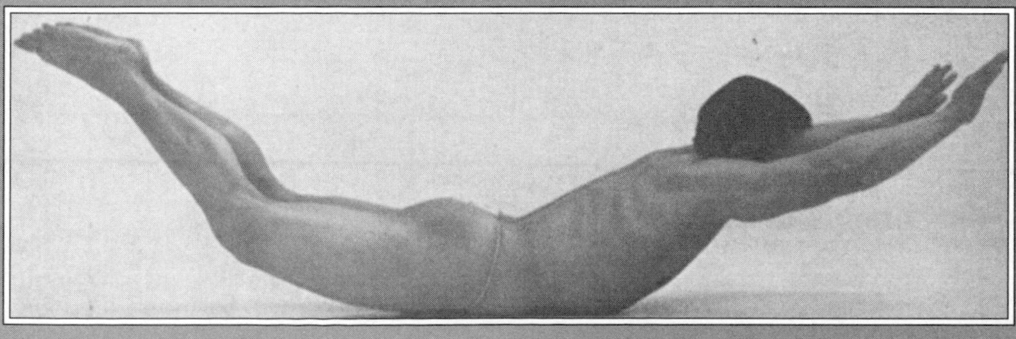

1

The Emergence of Yoga

Muscle, in motion as well as in repose, has played a most important role in human development—a focus of forces operating through an organism, whose structural and functional complexity is the most perplexing in nature—in a gradual unfoldment through which the marvelous possibilities and probabilities lying within have begun to be actual. But muscle had a very long history before it reached the human level. Its functioning, which is expressed as movement at all levels and in all ages, is associated with the gross manifestation of the dynamic aspect of the life principle.

Education through muscle movement has been an intrinsic part of life of those organisms endowed with it. This education is intimately associated with survival and progressive development. The earliest pattern of human physical education, shaped in the Paleolithic Age, was the outcome of natural habit. Humans naturally attained a vigorous form of physical life, which proved suitable for the gradual unfoldment of mental life.

The tables below present three groupings of the principal human physical education activities, as developed in different parts of the world. Stage 1 represents those activities thought to have been acquired first; stage 2, those acquired later. The third grouping is of advanced activities, acquired when human nervous and mental life had appreciably progressed.

Yoga as a Means for Attaining Spiritual Goals

At a certain stage of the growth of the mental life of human beings a new demand was created, and, in meeting it, muscle had to take a different role. This was the purposeful motionless attitude of the body, requiring the static transformation of the dynamic muscle. The specialty and superiority of human beings lies less in external growth than in mental life. They survived, not because of physical strength, but because of their high order of mental life. Even at a very early stage humans began to use their brains. A transformation of human life in which mental growth is arrested is a biological degradation of the human organism and has less survival value.

HUMAN PHYSICAL EDUCATION ACTIVITIES: STAGE 1

	Walking	Running	Jumping	Throwing
Paleolithic	Walking	Running	Jumping	Stone-throwing; perhaps crude javelin-throwing
Neolithic	"	"	"	Stone-throwing; javelin-throwing
Sumerian (3200–2187 BCE)	"	"	"	Mace-throwing; javelin-throwing; throwing a curved weapon like Indian *kharga*
Egyptian (3000–1090 BCE)	"	"	Jumping; hop, step anc jump	Ball-throwing; knife-throwing; javelin-throwing
Indian (3000–500 BCE)	"	"	Jumping	Ball-throwing; javelin-throwing; discus-throwing; club-throwing; stone-throwing
Cretan (2100–1200 BCE)	"	"	"	Stone-throwing; javelin-throwing
Chinese (1557–256 BCE)	"	"	"	Javelin-throwing
Assyrian (745–626 BCE)	"	"	"	Javelin-throwing
Persian (708–330 BCE)	"	"	"	Javelin-throwing; equitative javelin-throwing
Greek (700–400 BCE)	"	"	Jumping: running-high and running-broad; standing-high and standing-broad	Javelin-throwing; discus-throwing
Roman (509 BCE–CE 180)	"	"	Jumping	Stone-throwing; javelin-throwing; discus-throwing (later times)
Age of chivalry in Europe (tenth to fourteenth centuries CE)	"	"	"	Putting stone; javelin-throwing
European (sixteenth century CE)	"	"	Jumping, high and broad	Putting stone; throwing the bar; javelin-throwing
European (eighteenth century CE)	"	"	Jumping, high and broad, across ditches; pole vaulting	Putting stone; javelin-throwing; throwing a wooden discus; throwing at a target
European (nineteenth century CE)	"	"	"	"
Modern	"	Running; relay; cross-country run	Jumping, high and broad; standing, high and broad; hop, step, and jump; pole vault; hurdles	16 lb. shot putt; 16 lb. hammer-throwing; discus-throwing; javelin-throwing; 56 lb. weight-throwing

HUMAN PHYSICAL EDUCATION ACTIVITIES: STAGE 2

	Climbing	Lifting	Swimming	Combat activities		
				Grappling	*Striking*	
					(a) With hand	(b) With club
Palaeolithic	Tree	Lifting	Swimming	Grappling	Striking	Club
Neolithic	"	"	"	"	"	Club, spear, dagger
Sumerian (3200–2187 BCE)	Tree, pole, rope, and wall	Mace-lifting	"	Wrestling	Boxing	Spear and dagger
Egyptian (3000–1090 BCE)		Weightlifting	"	"		Mace, club, sword, dagger, spear, stick, neboot
Indian (3000–500 BCE)		"	"	"	"	Club, spear, sword, dagger
Cretan (2100–1200 BCE)			"	"	"	Spear, sword
Chinese (1557–256 BCE)		Weightlifting (later times)	"	Chinese wrestling (similar to *pankration*)		Battle-ax, lance
Assyrian (745–626 BCE)	Tree		"		"	Mace, ax, spear, sword
Persian (708–330 BCE)			"			Spear, sword
Greek (700–400 BCE)		Weightlifting	"	Wrestling and *pankration*	"	Spear, sword
Roman (509 BCE–CE 180)			"	Wrestling	"	Spear, sword
Age of chivalry in Europe (tenth to fourteenth centuries CE)	Rope, pole, ladder, wall		"	"	"	
European (sixteenth century CE)	Rope, tree, mast, wall	"	"	"	"	
European (eighteenth century CE)	Rope, mast, and wall	"	"	"	"	
European (nineteenth century CE)	"	"	"	"	"	
Modern	Ladder and rope	"	"	"	"	

ADVANCED PHYSICAL EDUCATION ACTIVITIES

	Dancing	Archery	Rowing	Fencing		Sports and games
Paleolithic	Dancing perhaps from Aurignacian Period	Archery perhaps from Aurignacian or Magdalenian Period				
Neolithic	Dancing	Archery	Perhaps rudimentary rowing	Perhaps rudimentary fencing		
Sumerian (3200–2187 BCE)	"	"	Rowing			
Egyptian (3000–1090 BCE)	"	"	"	Fencing	Tumbling	Ball games, hoop game
Indian (3000–500 BCE)	"	"	"	"	"	Ball games
Cretan (2100–1200 BCE)	"	"	"	"	"	
Chinese (1557–256 BCE)	"	"	"			Football
Assyrian (745–626 BCE)	"	Foot and equitative archery	"	"		
Persian (708–330 BCE)		"	"	"		
Greek (700–400 BCE)	"	"	"	"	"	A kind of hockey; a ball game resembling handball; perhaps rudimentary rugby football; various games
Roman (509 BCE–CE 180)	"	Foot and equitative archery (not much)	"	"		Ball games; various games
Age of chivalry in Europe (tenth to fourteenth centuries)	"	Foot and equitative archery	"	"		Golf, cricket, football
European (sixteenth century CE)	"	"	"			Tennis, ball games, pitching quoits
European (eighteenth century CE)	"	"	"	"		Skating, coasting, rugby football
European (nineteenth century CE)	"	"	"	"	"	Skittles, skating, golf, hockey, bowling, cricket, quoits, tennis, rugby football, association football, curling, and so on
Modern	"	"	"	"	"	Modern sports and games

A condition of existence in which the mental life shrinks is more dangerous than that which brings about physical degeneracy. In fact, physical development alone cannot prevent human decay if the mental side is neglected.

He who tries to concentrate on something makes his body or certain parts of his body stationary. When a cat is about to jump on its prey, it first makes its body very still. When you want to look at some finer things or hear some sound from a greater distance, you keep your body stationary for the moment. Motion is antagonistic to concentration. In a crude way, this has been demonstrated in animals, but it has been fully developed in human beings. Our specialty does not lie in our constant movements, though adequate movements are necessary for life. With the gradual unfoldment of our mental life we experienced that the nonmotion state of the body was absolutely necessary for developing concentration. According to Yoga, our motions, executed by our muscles, are important insofar as they maintain our body in a state most suitable for the manifestation of our mental life—a mental life in which concentration predominates. This is the starting point of Yoga.

At a lower plane the mind is dark and dull. At this plane, ignorance, miscomprehension, inattention, and delusion predominate. It is degraded to almost an animal level. An active mental life is the seat of desires and drives, longing and greed, restlessness and uncontrolled actions. In a high order of mental life brilliant thinking and constructive imagination blend with the increased power of concentration and control, and the whole mental life is illuminated with spiritual light. Our smallness or greatness, darkness or brightness, selfishness or self-sacrifice, narrowness or broadness—all depend on the order of our mental life. Our body is merely an instrument through which our mental life—our greed and sensuality or our sacrifice and love—is expressed. This does not mean that the body is of no importance. We should not forget that we are also animals, with animal hungers. But in a higher order of mental life these hungers do not go beyond the normal human limit but remain under our control. In a dark and unrestrained mental life they appear in vicious forms and give an ugly picture of the person. However, Yoga makes it possible for us to attain a high order of mental life, backed by a body that is healthy, strong, symmetrical, and obedient to our mind, in which concentration reaches its peak.

Each human being is a grand center of manifestation of the power arising from and lying within the eternal and unknown reality in an inseparable form, something like waves that are inseparable from the ocean. Our eternal principle—our absolute form, which is in reality one with the nonmanifested: immovable, immutable, eternal, inconceivable, and unspecifiable—is masked, so we appear to be moving, changeable, limited, perishable, conceivable, and specifiable. Yoga, as it is revealed to those who have attained illuminative life, is the realization of absorption into and identification with the eternal reality. And the means to its attainment is also Yoga. Yoga is not merely a system, a method, or a group of processes. It is a spiritual state, christened as *Yoga,* in which the eternal principle of humanity is revealed. Spiritually this is the highest aim and grandest human achievement, in which supreme knowledge is immersed in eternal bliss.

Two ideas, one conveying the sense of union and the other concentration, are component parts of the word *Yoga*. These ideas in connection with Yoga originated in the early Vedic period (early Chalcolithic Age) in India. It was revealed to the sages that through the spiritual processes of union and concentration a person can reach the Unknown. The rishi (seer) says in the *Ṛigveda*: "The limited human consciousness becomes illuminated in the Supreme Consciousness which is the greatest of all and all-knowing after their union." The word *union* is used here in the spiritual sense to mean "the expansion of the restricted consciousness into the stage of Supreme Consciousness," that is, the transformation of the limited into the unlimited. The first phase of union is effected through the mind in concentration. It is clearly expressed in the *Ṛigveda*. *Yajurveda* also says: "We unite our mind with the Supreme Consciousness, having infinite power by our own concentration for liberation."

Thus, a clear idea of the Supreme Consciousness was formed and the importance of concentrating the mind on appropriate objects was realized in the early Vedic period. Seers of that early age knew that the body was perishable, mind oscillating, and passion strong. They also knew that the invisible reality pervades all created things and also extends far beyond the material world; the face of the real is hidden by a golden vase; and the Supreme Consciousness is omnipresent, omnipotent, and omniscient, with no body, no disease, no birth, and no beginning. They realized that concentration was necessary for liberation and for knowing the Unknown, and that it could be developed by systematic efforts in that direction.

The conception and practice of concentration exercises are possible only for those who are endowed with a high order of mental life, glowing with intellectual eminence and backed by spiritual strength. In the Vedas, the fundamentals of Yoga were expressed in a language that we may call spiritual language, difficult to understand by those who are not specially taught by the masters. In the post-Vedic period attempts were made to remove the mask and present Yoga in a more understandable way.

The secret of remaining nonmoving in the moving thought-world has been disclosed in Yoga. The final phase of the spiritual union is attained when a yogin reaches the stage of nonmentalization, which in the yogic terminology is called *asamprajñāta samādhi* (supreme concentration). In *asamprajñāta samādhi* the complete elimination of all *vṛittis* (the moldings of consciousness into the form of an object, either external or internal) occurs. It is stated in the *Agni-purāṇa* that Yoga, which is spiritual union, is attainable when the *vṛittis* are completely eliminated. This definition of Yoga, originating in the Vedic period, remained unmodified in the post-Vedic period and has been accepted by yogins of all ages.

Patañjali's definition of Yoga is essentially based on the above-mentioned older conception of Yoga, but expressed in a language in which the concentration factor is more clearly defined. Patañjali says: "Yoga is that state in which the mind ceases to function as *vṛittis*" (*Patañjala Yoga-sūtra*).

Concentration Stage by Stage

In the ordinary state of existence, consciousness is constantly being molded into objects based on a sensory pattern. The molding is effected either directly through the senses of perception, the *jñanindriyas,* by the application of the knowledge of relationship (inference), through spoken or written statements (direct or indirect communication), from the development of certain ideas expressed in words without corresponding objects in reality (higher thinking), through wrong representation by the senses (misconception), or from the reproduction of previously cognized objects (memory). Ordinarily the moldings are of mixed character. This is the state of *vṛittis* of the mind. It is the common form of mind, a form in which it is recognized as such.

The extra-*vṛitti* state of the mind is ordinarily unknown. Only in sleep does the conscious principle cease to function; then there is no expression of consciousness and its molding into various forms. This coiling of consciousness is an aspect of the mind in which other forms of molding remain in a potential form. Or, in other words, the nonexpression of consciousness is the grand latent period of the state of mind. We can therefore divide the state of mind into two: latent state in which the activities of the mind cease for the recuperation of power necessary to maintain the active state, and the active state in which the conscious activities are manifested. For the acquirement of Yoga the elimination of both latent and active states of the mind is the sine qua non. This elimination is termed *nirodha*.

Pratyāhāra (Sensory Control)

The organs of the senses (*jñanindriyas*) are the mind's faculties for the respective perception of smell, taste, colors and forms, touch sensations, and sound. These five are the general patterns of knowing external objects. When they function at a common level they operate through physical organs, called external sense organs. The five conative senses (speech, prehension, locomotion, organic activities, and reproduction) are called *karmendriyas*.

A countless number of sensations or impressions of external objects are constantly being received through the gates of sense organs. These sensations are manifold and nonspecific in character. This nonspecificity is then transformed into a specific sensation by a power of the mind called *manas* through its functions of attention, selection, and synthesis. When *manas* is controlled, the other five faculties do not operate and become disconnected from the external sense organs. This sense-withdrawal produces a sensory void. Through this process, known as *pratyāhāra* (sensory control), the formation of sensory images in the mind is prevented, thus creating a most suitable mental state for concentration.

Dhāraṇā (Elementary Concentration)

The elimination of *vṛittis* is the highest state of concentration, which is attainable only through a systematized method. The characteristic of the mind is to take an image and keep it for a brief period. Then it leaves that image and takes another, and then another, and so on. Ordinarily the mind tends to take different images, one after another, without retaining any of them for a long time. The process in which the mind is educated to take a chosen image and refresh it again and again at successive intervals without taking new ones is called *dhāraṇā* (elementary concentration). *Dhāraṇā* is just like identical drops of water being released one by one from a vessel full of water. When a chosen image appears in the mind again and again in the same way it is called *dhāraṇā*.

An easy method of developing *dhāraṇā* is *mantra japa*. *Mantra* is "the sound pattern of power," which manifests as mind and matter. With the help of *mantra* we can reach the power level that is beyond the manifested mind-matter level, and at that stage power is revealed as radiant energy gradually transforming into an inner consciousness. *Japa* is the technical term used to mean "the production of a particular manifested sound form represented by a *mantra* in a specific way and at specified intervals, one after another," which is continued until a certain number is finished. With the help of *mantra, dhāraṇā* can be comparatively easily mastered. When the *mantra* is said mentally, the mind is molded into a new image composed of two parts, form and sound. The first image stays in the mind during the period of saying the *mantra*. Then there is a brief interval—a void—before it is said the second time. In this way the saying of *mantra* goes on with brief intervals between. The working on *mantra* is so arranged that this void period is rightly adjusted to the intervening period, that is, the period between the throwing out of an image and the taking of a new one by the mind. In this way *dhāraṇā* is acquired with the help of *mantra*. This process has been fully dealt with in Mantra Yoga.

Mind operating on the extraphysical plane is able to acquire knowledge of external objects without the usual means through the sense organs. Knowledge can be acquired pre- and supersensorially at a higher stage of concentration.

Dhyāna (Unbroken Concentration)

The next stage of concentration is *dhyāna* (unbroken concentration). When an interrupted flow of an image (*dhāraṇā*) is transformed into a continuous flow of that image, it is called *dhyāna*. Again take the illustration of the falling of water, as it is released drop by drop from a vessel full of water. If the control mechanism is removed, then the flow of water will be continuous, without any break, in one stream instead of falling down in drops. *Dhāraṇā* develops into *dhyāna*. Here the image is continuous. Now the mind has been educated not to throw away a particular image but retain it.

Samprajñāta Samādhi (Super Concentration with Super Knowledge)

Dhyāna ripens into *samādhi,* the final stage of the process of concentration. *Samādhi* again is subdivided into *samprajñāta* and *asamprajñāta*. *Samprajñāta* is that form of *samādhi* in which the realization of four forms of object occurs stage by stage: *vitarka* (deliberation), *vicāra* (reflection), *ānanda* (joy), and *asmitā* (pure I-feeling).

Vitarka Samādhi

The image of a material object is the result of the combined actions of the senses operating through the sense organs. All of our senses act together, though each of them plays its specific role. The outcome of their combined actions is the knowledge of a particular object, which is a compound of five fundamental forms of nonmaterial energy. Of course, all objects do not contain these energies in the same proportions. This is the cause of differences in objects.

In an ordinary state, it is not possible to isolate one form of energy from the rest, as they are in compound forms. In the state of *vitarka samādhi* the power of isolation is developed. In this state we are able to "know" one particular form of energy isolated from the rest. When a form of energy is completely isolated from the other four and is "seen," a new form of knowledge appears, which reveals an unknown aspect of the material object: the "essential," known as *mahābhūta,* which constitutes the particular form of a sense object. This gives an entirely different outlook on the external world. The compound image of an object vanishes and instead a newly developed isolated "image" of only one predominating essential floats. This is the presensory type of knowledge of a sense object.

In the state of *vitarka samādhi,* the mixed form, that is, the image we get of a sense object, vanishes and the isolated form of a particular essential appears. At this stage the whole world appears as if it is made only of one particular essential.

Vicāra Samādhi

The essential constituting the sense object can be reduced to a still finer "form" in the shape of the most concentrated force being expressed as the "thatness" or *tanmātra* of that essential. The *tanmātras,* like *mahābhūtas,* are five in number. The realization of the *tanmātras* occurs in the *vicāra samādhi.* The distinctive characteristic of an essential is lost at this state.

When the image of a particular essential is concentrated upon in *vitarka samādhi,* it will appear in place of the image of a sense object and it will appear as vast. Now if concentration is applied on a minute portion of the vast essential, it will appear also as vast. Again, concentration should be practiced on the minute part of that appearing as vast and this minute part will reappear as vast. In this way, by repeated applications of concentration a stage will be reached when the power of receiving the finest state of the essential—the "thatness"—will be fully developed. This is the stage of the *vicāra samādhi.*

The realization that is attained in *vitarka* and *vicāra samādhi* consists of two stages. In the first stage the realized phenomenon can be brought into the intellectual level and expressed through words. In the last stage the realized phenomenon cannot be given an intellectual form and consequently remains beyond language. The first stage of *vitarka* and *vicāra* is called *savitarka* and *savicāra,* respectively, and the last stage *nirvitarka* and *nirvicāra,* respectively.

Ānanda Samādhi

At this stage of *samādhi* mind is able to go beyond the pain-pleasure phenomena. Now senses become actionless and the power of the mind relating to them becomes calm. A yogin can successfully practice *ānanda samādhi* when his mind is able to go to the ultra-*tanmātra* stage. In this *samādhi* a realization of a divine being occurs through the most intensified and concentrated flow of sublime love. It is inseparably associated with bliss without any tinge of pain or sorrow. This is the stage of *ānanda samādhi.*

Asmitā Samādhi

At this stage the realization of "I"-less consciousness occurs. "I"-ness that is associated with objects disappears and along with it images of all things completely vanish. What remains now is deindividualized consciousness. This is the last stage of the *samprajñāta samādhi.*

Asamprajñāta Samādhi (Supreme Concentration)

The last stage of concentration is the *asamprajñāta samādhi.* In this stage deindividualized consciousness merges in Supreme Consciousness. Consciousness as it is known is an inseparable aspect of the mind. It is the common state of human existence, giving rise to a dualistic experience. This is the knowledge of the "known." By the systematic practice of the processes of concentration the mind ascends from the state of *vṛitti* to the extra-*vṛitti* state. At the last stage, that is, at the stage of *asamprajñāta samādhi,* the complete elimination of *vṛittis* occurs. This is the stage of Yoga—of the realization of the Unknown, of the realization of the Supreme Consciousness, which is actually a realization beyond realization.

Summary

The mental images acquired by the mind are influenced by the practice of concentration. The changes in mental images in the different states of consciousness may be summarized as follows:

1. Ordinary state: constantly changing sensory images in the mind
2. *Pratyāhāra:* the formation of sensory images in the mind is prevented
3. *Dhāraṇā* state: interrupted flow of one image (sensory in origin) in the mind

4. *Dhyāna* state: continuous flow of one image (sensory, extrasensory, and supersensory) without any break
5. *Vitarka samādhi* state: image of one *mahābhūta* or "essential" isolated from the rest (presensory)
6. *Vicāra samādhi* state: image of one *tanmātra* or "thatness" (presensory)
7. *Ānanda samādhi* state: an experience of super consciousness with uninterrupted bliss (nonsensory)
8. *Asmitā samādhi* state: realization of deindividualized consciousness (nonsensory)
9. *Asamprajñāta samādhi* state: characterized by the absence of the subjective and objective aspects of consciousness and the transformation of deindividualized consciousness into Supreme Consciousness

Concentration Exercises

Now we have a clear picture of the whole process of concentration in Yoga. It consists of four main exercises already stated: *pratyāhāra* (sensory control), *dhāraṇā* (elementary concentration), *dhyāna* (unbroken concentration), and *samādhi* (super concentration). *Samādhi* is again subdivided into *samprajñāta* (super concentration with super knowledge) and *asamprajñāta* (supreme concentration). Concentration exercises are the higher form of Yoga exercises; they form a most important part of Ashtangha Yoga (the eightfold Yoga), the earliest systematic form, as well as Mantra, Laya, Haṭha, and Rāja Yogas, later elaborations that each stress different aspects.

Concentration exercises have been fully developed in Rāja Yoga, with the four stages of *vitarka, vicāra, ānanda,* and *asmitā.* Rāja Yoga has also shown that *samprajñāta* can be ultimately developed into *asamprajñāta,* the last stage of *samādhi.* This is the chief characteristic feature of Rāja Yoga. The other three major forms of Yoga—Mantra, Laya, and Haṭha—only lead to *samprajñāta samādhi.*

Motionless Attitude of the Body

Concentration demands that the whole body should be kept motionless. Deeper concentration is incompatible with the body in motion. This is the beginning of what in Yoga is called *āsana* (posture).

Posture, as defined by Patañjali, is an attitude in which the body can be kept motionless yet at the same time produces a feeling of ease. For the practice of concentration, the motionless attitude of the body is to be maintained. One of the chief characteristic features of posture is the folded leg. A most intense type of human activity is exhibited in running. Motion is intensified in speed, and speed is best expressed in running. The speed work is principally executed by the leg muscles. Therefore the legs are apparatuses of intense activity. The energy of the body in motion in the form of extreme speed manifests through the legs. All the vital organs of the body—respiratory, circulatory, glandular, and nervous—take part and cooperate with the muscular system. In a word, the whole body functions in a specific way to support the action executed by the legs. This is very important for physical life, as these activities are associated with the development of vital vigor and organic strength. But this state of the body is not suitable at the time when the mind is in a contemplative state.

For intense concentration we need to restrain the trend of the body toward such intense action. In Yoga, an attempt has been made to prevent as much as possible the escape of energy manifesting as intense activity. That fosters the ability of the will to cooperate fully in mental concentration, by voluntarily making the instruments of this intense action inoperative. This is most successfully effected by assuming a folded-leg posture. Therefore in Yoga a motionless attitude with folded legs is considered the most suitable posture for concentration, and experience shows that it is so.

Another important feature of posture is to maintain the trunk erect. The importance of erect posture during concentration was realized very early, and it became an essential part of posture. In this new human position the brain and the muscles could cooperate to support concentration. A highly developed mental life and cerebral development are intimately related to an erect posture, with which the functioning of the fundamental musculature is associated.

In addition to folding the legs, the arms—instruments for performing complex movements and exhibiting strength—are also made motionless. Their motionlessness and relaxation help further in concentration. This is accomplished by assuming Dhyāna Mudrā, in which the hands are placed one upon the other, palms upward, at the center of the body, or by assuming Jñāna Mudrā, in which the arms are stretched and the hands are placed on the knees with the tips of the index finger and the thumb touching each other.

As the folded-leg, erect trunk, motionless attitude is to be maintained for a long period for the practice of concentration, it should also be easy. The earliest pattern of the motionless folded-leg posture seems to be what is called Pleasant Posture (Sukhāsana), in which the folded right leg is placed on the folded left one. The word *sukha,* which is found in *Ṛigveda,* means "easy." That form of folded-leg posture that has been termed Pleasant Posture is the easiest of all postures. It developed into Auspicious Posture, in which the right foot is inserted into the space between the left thigh and shank and the left foot into the space between the right thigh and shank. The next stage of development is what is known as Accomplished Posture, in which the left heel is set against the perineum and the right heel against the pubic bone just above the genitals. The Even Posture (Samāsana) is the result of the modification of the Auspicious and Accomplished Postures.

Then an important development occurred in the folded-leg posture with an introduction of crossed leg with foot-lock. The first stage was reached in Hero Posture, in which one foot is placed on the opposite groin. Finally it developed into the well-known Lotus Posture, in which the right foot is placed on the left groin and the left foot on the right groin. These are the principal concentration postures of Yoga. Discomfort and pain are usually associated with posture. They should be conquered by practice and then the posture will prove most suitable for concentration.

The development of the concentration postures took place in the early Vedic Age. The yogins in that period could not reach the higher stage of concentration without perfecting the concentration postures. Many of the names given to these postures are found in the Vedas. The Auspicious Posture (Svastikāsana) is derived from *svasti,* which means "success or prosperity" (*Ṛigveda*); it was symbolized as a special cross mark called *svastika,* which denoted success in an endeavor in the Chalcolithic Age in India. From *sidh,* which means to be successful (*Ṛigveda*), came Accomplished Posture (Siddhāsana), that is, a posture that leads to success in concentration. *Vīra,* from which came Hero Posture (Vīrāsana), means "a hero" (*Ṛigveda*), who is able to go deep into concentration in a difficult posture.

The word *kamala,* found in the *Atharvaveda* and *Taittirīya-saṁhitā,* means the characteristic red color of the lotus flower. This color is the symbol of the creative energy operating within a person. Brahma, or the creative aspect of the Supreme Consciousness, is represented by the red color and is seated in Kamalāsana (Lotus Posture). This is also mentioned in the Bhagavad Gītā. This creative energy usually expresses as the world consciousness representing the picture of the oscillating mind. The arousing, conveying, and controlling of this great energy are required at the higher stage of concentration. The most suitable posture for this purpose is Kamalāsana. In later periods Kamalāsana was also called Padmāsana, which means the same thing.

The folded-leg concentration postures were so popular in the Chalcolithic Age in India that they were portrayed in seals such as those discovered at Mohenjo-daro. The Lotus Posture was introduced into Egypt, and it formed a part of the Egyptian gymnastic dance during the Old Kingdom (about 3000 to 2475 BCE).

The concentration postures formed an essential part of the eightfold Yoga and also of the Mantra Yoga, Laya Yoga, Haṭha Yoga, and Rāja Yoga. Gradually other postures for concentration were developed. In Haṭha Yoga, in addition to the development of the folded-leg postures into more difficult postures, a system of posture exercise was evolved.

Breath Control in Concentration

In a folded-leg concentration posture, the legs and arms are in an attitude of rest and the trunk is erect and steady. When the posture is mastered, the body remains still, free from pain and discomfort, and relaxed. One becomes more or less unconscious of the body. Only the feeling of breathing movements is experienced. The body is now quite still except that faint breathing movements go on.

In a healthy state we are generally unconscious of our breathing, except in running or when doing other heavy forms of exercise. In a concentration posture—when the body is still and the mind is inwardly directed—we become conscious of breathing. We experience that not only are the up and down movements of respiration going on regularly, but also that breathing causes a feeling of heaviness. We are conscious of an action, feeling that we are not quite inactive even in the stationary position of the body. The breathing movements prove a hindrance to concentration. But if we can manage to go a bit deeper in concentration, breathing begins to be slower.

Breathing is an indicator of the action level of our body. The energy demands of the body are met by respiration. When the body is at rest, the volume per minute of lung ventilation is minimum. Action causes an increase in the volume per minute of lung ventilation, and the increase is in proportion to the intensity of action. The increased pulmonary ventilation is effected by an increase both in rate and depth. In speed exercise, especially fast running, the maximum increase of lung ventilation occurs.

The state of the body accompanying increased pulmonary ventilation is unfavorable for concentration. The greater the increase, the less suitable is the condition for concentration. By assuming the folded-leg concentration posture the action level of the body is minimum, and so the lung ventilation is minimum. This is a most favorable condition to start concentration. When the mind becomes comparatively calm in this posture, even the minimum breathing movements prove unfavorable for deep concentration. However, with the intensification of concentration, the rate and the depth of breathing begin to go below the normal level. As concentration becomes deeper and deeper, breathing becomes slower and slower, and at a certain stage of concentration, it is almost stopped. If concentration goes still deeper, breathing actually stops.

The observation of the intimate relation of breathing to concentration resulted in the development of *prāṇāyāma,* the well-known breath-control system of Yoga. The breath-control system is essentially concerned with regulating breathing in such a way as to make it helpful for concentration. It was observed that at the suspension point concentration was the deepest. This is why breath suspension (*kumbhaka*) became the principal part of breath control, and inhalation (*pūraka*) and exhalation (*recaka*) were so regulated as to be helpful in developing breath suspension. Moreover, willpower—upon which concentration depends so much—was found to be intimately related to breath suspension. Willpower is brought into play to the maximum degree and developed at a certain stage of breath suspension.

Breath control is the fourth limb of the eightfold Yoga (the eight limbs are: *yama, niyama, āsana, prāṇāyāma, pratyāhāra, dhāraṇā, dhyāna,* and *samādhi*). It seems that there existed some form of breath control before it became a part of Yoga. It was, perhaps, associated with religion in the Stone Age. Most probably the intellectual Stone Age priests somehow felt the utility of breath control in connection with prayer and concentration and practiced it in some shape. This archaic breath regulation was gradually transformed into breath control in the Chalcolithic age: in the time of *Ṛigveda* a system of breath culture was practiced; the importance of the purification, development, and control of breath-power was recognized (*Śuklayajurveda*); the long-slow type of breath control with breath suspension was practiced (*Atharvaveda*).

Breath control gradually grew in importance, and improved techniques were developed. Controlled inhalation and exhalation became an important factor in breath control (*Aitareya Brāhmaṇa*). The three phases of breath control—controlled inhalation, exhalation, and breath suspension—were practiced with *mantra* (*Aitareya Brāhmaṇa*). Breath suspension was practiced with *mantra* (*Śatapatha Brāhmaṇa*). The length of the *mantra* was regulated according to the breath power. An interrelation between the mind and the breath was recognized (*Śatapatha Brāhmaṇa*). It was further recognized that mind played an important role in controlling breath (*Kauṣītaki Brāhmaṇa*).

In the post-Vedic period, *dhyāna* (unbroken concentration) and breath control became major parts of Yoga. The breath-control part, called Saguna Yoga, became a system consisting of five limbs and twenty-four kinds of breath-control exercises (Mahābhārata). It was practiced with and without *mantras.* Breath control with *mantras* was called *sabīja* and without *mantras nirbīja* (Mahābhārata).

The importance of breath control in mind control was demonstrated. According to Yājñavalkya, mind is purified by breath control (*Garuḍa-purāṇa*). It is said that the Lord Brahma controlled his mind through the control of breath (*Bhāgavata-purāṇa*). The purification of the breath, senses, and mind is absolutely necessary for the successful practice of mental concentration, and this purification is best effected through breath control (*Bhāgavata-purāṇa*). This is why rishis (sages of ancient India) regularly practiced breath control. It was their preparatory exercise for *samādhi* (*Śiva-purāṇa*). The Lord Kṛiṣṇa himself practiced breath control (Mahābhārata).

Yama and *Niyama*

Yama (self-restraint) and *niyama* (self-regulation), the first two limbs of the eightfold Yoga, each have five aspects. *Yama* consists of abstinence from injury (*ahimsā*), truthfulness (*satya*), abstinence from theft (*asteya*), sexual control in thoughts, emotion, and action (*brahmacarya*), and abstinence from acceptance of gifts (*aparigraha*). *Niyama* consists of cleanliness (*śauca*), contentment (*santoṣa*), asceticism (*tapas*), study (*svādhyāya*), and meditation on God (*īśvarapraṇidhāna*). *Yama* and *niyama* are actually a mode of life in which discipline has been imposed to protect the student of Yoga from physical, moral, and spiritual decay. The power to overcome hunger, thirst, sleep, and sexual impulses is developed and the person begins to be conscious of our spiritual existence.

The fabric of our everyday thought is mainly woven with greed and sensuality. This makes us narrow and selfish, creating a life in which we live for ourselves, for the satisfaction of our longings. A pleasure-seeking and comfort-loving bent of mind decreases our willpower and vital endurance to a very great extent. We become prisoners in a self-woven thought-web. We need an awakening, a right understanding of our real state. For this study has been prescribed.

As students of Yoga we try to replace our ordinary thought-world with a new one through *yama* and *niyama*. We seriously undertake to build this newer pattern of thoughts and to remold our emotions and actions according to this pattern. To strengthen our willpower and build up our vital endurance we need asceticism. To conquer greed we need to be educated by the practice of nonavarice and nonstealing. Through nonavarice we learn to renounce everything except those things that are really necessary for healthful existence. Nonstealing teaches us to conquer excessive longings for wealth. Through the practice of sexual continence we learn how to build a pattern of thought capable of piercing the sensual curtain and apprehending the inner beauty of the members of the opposite sex, and of oneself too, where the fire of lust does not kindle.

Such a way of life results in an inner feeling of contentment never experienced before. Cleanliness becomes our habit. Our behavior toward others now becomes regulated by harmlessness and truthfulness. The vacuum that has been created within by the elimination of thoughts centered on mundane pleasures is now filled with devotion to God. By imposing upon ourselves the spiritual disciplines of *yama* and *niyama* we can elude the deleterious influence of the mode of life that we are living and create a condition for physical and moral uplift and spiritual progress.

The rudimentary forms of certain practices of *yama* and *niyama* were originated as early as the Stone Ages. Early Stone Age humans had to endure the heat of the sun, the cold of the winter, wind, rain, and snow. They frequently had to go without food and sleep. These vital habits helped to mold their mind, nervous system, internal organs, and muscles into a pattern that was helpful for survival and physical and mental development. The germ of austerity lay in the natural mode of existence.

With the changes of living conditions, when humans were no longer forced to struggle as much against the rigors of the seasons and a lack of food and sleep, they tried to maintain these virile habits voluntarily. In an early civilization of India these most ancient natural habits were given a spiritual character and termed as *tapasyā* (asceticism). This took the form of exposing oneself in the hot season to five fires, four from the four quarters, the fifth being the sun above, of plunging the body into cold water in the winter, staying in the rain without any clothing, fasting completely by drinking only water, or by staying on a restricted diet, and bearing various other hardships. These biologically important practices were gradually incorporated into Yoga.

Cleanliness in its nonartificial form was the normal habit of early humans. They kept themselves clean, externally as well as internally, by fasting, eating natural foods, living outdoors, constant physical exercise, and exposing their bodies to air, sun, rain, and cold. An elaborate method of external and internal baths was developed from this natural practice.

Early humans believed that sexual privation was virtuous and a promoter of strength, endurance, and courage. They tried to develop these crucially important qualities through the practice of continence, which was linked to a belief in the existence of an unknown, invisible, and all-powerful being and an attempt to please him. Civilization brought with it more sexual opportunities and more suitable conditions for fanning the flame of lust. Then the importance of sexual regulation was keenly felt and insisted on through physical education, moral teachings, and religion. The ancient practice, christened *brahmacarya* (sexual continence), was widely practiced by great men in the Vedic period. It was regarded as the promoter of long life (*Atharvaveda*) and became an intrinsic part of Yoga.

The Role of Haṭha Yoga

Haṭha Yoga, which expounded the physical basis of concentration, emerged from the elaboration of certain practices of the eightfold Yoga, especially posture, breath control, cleanliness, and sexual continence. Posture, breath control, and cleanliness were transformed into distinct subsystems. The vital flow that supplies the necessary strength of the mind to manifest its desires to a point of satisfaction needs to be under control to create the most suitable mental atmosphere for the growth of concentration. The Lord Śiva, the first *guru* (teacher) of Haṭha Yoga, therefore says that its practice is necessary for success in Rāja Yoga, which essentially consists of concentration with all its stages.

Haṭha Yoga, in fact, is a systematic method of education, which aims at the purification, rebuilding, vitalization, and control of the body to enable it to successfully undertake breath control. Breath control ultimately causes the molding of the body into the pattern most suitable for molding the mind into a form in which it is able to undergo the stages of *dhāraṇā, dhyāna,* and *samādhi*. The word *haṭha* consists of two letters *ha* and *ṭha*. *Ha* signifies the sun and *ṭha* the moon. The sun is the symbol of the expression of energy and the moon is that of the conservation of the same. Two grand processes are constantly at work in our bodies, one in which the energy is spent and the other in which the energy is acquired and conserved. The energy-consuming force is manifested by the sun principle and the energy-building force by the moon principle. Haṭha Yoga is that form of Yoga in which concentration is acquired through the normalization and union of these two principles by breath control.

Posture exercise, control exercise, contraction exercise, purificatory acts, and other processes were employed to bring about this normalization, embracing all the processes and tissues of the entire body. Under this ideal physical condition, breath control becomes really effective and leads ultimately to the acquisition of a state of mind in which concentration is properly developed. This is Haṭha Yoga, and breath control is its principal process.

There are many indications that Haṭha Yoga was in practice in the Vedic period. One of the seals discovered at Mohenjo-daro portrays a three-faced human figure, surrounded by animals and wearing a horned headdress, seated in a folded-leg posture with heels touching each other and close to the body and arms extended downward with hands resting on knees. There are two more seals from Mohenjo-daro presenting the same folded-leg posture. In one the figure is three-faced and in another it has one face. This folded-leg posture is an important posture of Haṭha Yoga named Happy Posture (Bhadrāsana). The word *bhadra* occurs in the *Ṛigveda* and other Vedas and means "happy." The name means that the posture is designed to give happiness. It is a development of Accomplished Posture. In Accomplished Posture the left heel is set against the perineum, whereas in Happy Posture both heels are set against the perineum. This posture is an excellent pelvic exercise. An advanced Haṭha Yoga student uses it also as a concentration posture.

Moreover, the figure, which is surrounded by animals, has its eyes fixed on the tip of the nose. In Yoga this is called Nāsāgra-dṛiṣṭi (Nasal Gaze). The nasal gaze is a form of Trāṭaka (Gazing), an important practice of Haṭha Yoga. It is an excellent eye exercise and is very helpful for concentration. A steatite male head of the same era also has been discovered at Mohenjo-daro with its eyes concentrated on the tip of the nose.

The *Sāmaveda* says that breath gives health and long life. It means that by the right regulation of the respiration through an appropriate process, health and long life are attained. This process is, of course, breath control. It is clearly stated in the *Atharvaveda* that breathing, when properly regulated, lengthens life. There is also the clear instruction to avoid respiratory abuses that are antagonistic to breath control. This secondary aspect of breath control, which is connected with the health of the body, is associated with Haṭha Yoga. It shows that already in the Vedic period breath control was practiced not only in connection with concentration but also with building health.

Yoga Exercise

Haṭha Yoga teaches that the relatively new role of muscles—the static transformation of the dynamic muscles, which is the basis of the development of the contemplative aspect of human existence—becomes most effective when the dynamic functioning is not ignored but rightly utilized. Haṭha Yoga aims at having the maximum result in concentration through the motionlessness of the body without sacrificing the organic soundness of the body, which can only be maintained through muscle movement.

Yoga exercise thus developed in two directions—concentration exercise based on static bodily attitudes and dynamic exercise based on motion. Haṭha Yoga has demonstrated that these two types are not really antagonistic to each other but twin functionings of the organized whole, one cooperating with the other to support the achievement of a higher order of mental life while maintaining a vigorous form of physical life. Yoga exercise is essentially based on the delicate static-dynamic balance of the body.

In concentration exercise the body is made motionless, respiration controlled, and mind concentrated. In dynamic exercise muscles are energetically brought into play, regulated respiratory movements are executed, and the mind is concentrated on muscles and their movements. At the height of its development the dynamic form consisted of breath-control exercise (*prāṇāyāma*), control exercise (*ṣaṭ karman* and *mudrā*), contraction exercise (*cāraṇā*), and posture exercise (*āsana* and *mudrā*). These are the main divisions. There are also subdivisions.

Breath control and posture, therefore, have two aspects—concentration, which is primary, and health, which is secondary. The concentration aspect of breath control and posture has been adopted in all systems of Yoga, but the health aspect is specially dealt with in Haṭha Yoga.

Breath Control Stage by Stage

For physical education purposes breath-control exercise is utilized mainly to educate the respiratory muscles, lungs, heart, blood vessels, and the nervous system, thus enabling them to function more efficiently, and to develop the power of control over them. Respiratory exercise may be grouped under short-quick breath-control exercise, long-slow breath-control exercise, and breath-suspension exercise.

The earliest form of breath control seems to be what is known as the long-slow type with breath suspension. In the long-slow type of breath control, inhalation and exhalation are made longer and consequently slower, enabling them to be properly adjusted to breath suspension. This type of breath control seems to have commenced with inhalation through both nostrils to be followed by breath suspension and then exhalation through both nostrils. When the breath suspension is done without strain, it is called Sahaja Kumbhaka (Easy Breath Suspension). This form of breath control can be practiced while the body is maintained in a motionless state or while walking.

From Easy Breath Suspension another easy form gradually developed: Ujjāyī (Both-Nostrils Breath Control). It consists of inhalation through both nostrils with partially closed glottis, breath suspension, and exhalation through the left nostril with partially closed glottis. The exhalation also can be done through both nostrils. The front abdominal wall can be slightly controlled or kept relaxed. Special locking processes are not incorporated in the easy types of breath control. That is why they can be practiced not only in a sitting posture, but while standing as well as walking. Gadā Kumbhaka (Right-Nostril Exhalation Breath Control) also developed from Easy Breath Suspension. It consists of inhalation through both nostrils, breath suspension, and exhalation through the right nostril.

Instead of making a long, continuous inhalation, an interrupted inhalation with breath suspension between was also practiced. The interrupted inhalation consists of a series of inhalations, each followed by suspension. It is like inhalation–suspension–inhalation–suspension, and so on. Interrupted exhalation with suspension between was also practiced. From interrupted inhalation and exhalation breath control, the short-quick type of breath control developed. The two main short-quick types of breath control are Kapālabhātī (Abdominal Short-Quick Breathing) and Bhastrikā (Thoracic Short-Quick Breathing). In Abdominal Short-Quick Breathing exhalation and inhalation continue one after another without any break and without any rest in between until a round is completed. In Thoracic Short-Quick Breathing quick exhalation and inhalation are also performed without any pause until a round is completed. The speed rate in either of the exercises is from 60 to 120 breaths or more per minute.

Thoracic Short-Quick Breathing has been utilized in prolonging breath suspension. This short-quick respiratory exercise creates a suitable condition for gaining greater control over suspension. This is why the long-slow type also forms a part of this breath control. The long-slow type with breath suspension is to follow immediately after the completion of the short-quick type. The long-slow type consists of inhalation through right nostril, suspension, and exhalation through left nostril.

The Development of Sahita

At the intermediate stages an attempt was made to restrain the flow of breath in inhalation and exhalation and to prolong breath suspension. The flow of breath in inhalation and exhalation is controlled by partially closing the nostrils. It is called Apakarṣa Kumbhaka (Diminutive Breath Control). This restricted process prolongs inhalation and exhalation. When breath suspension was carried to the limit, it was called Utkarṣa Kumbhaka (Advanced Breath Control).

The well-known Sahita (Alternate-Nostril Breath Control with Breath Suspension) was developed from the combination of the Right-Nostril and Left-Nostril Inhalation Breath Control in which the principles of Diminutive and Advanced Breath Control were incorporated. Sahita consists of inhalation through the left nostril, while closing the right nostril with the right thumb, breath suspension, by closing both nostrils with the thumb and little and ring fingers, and exhalation through the right nostril, while closing the left one by the right ring and little fingers. In this manner again one should inhale through the right nostril, suspend, and exhale through the left nostril. In this breath control, inhalation, exhalation, and suspension are measured in a definite manner. The period of breath suspension is four times that of inhalation and the period of exhalation is twice that of inhalation, resulting in a ratio of 1–4–2.

As a part of this type of breath control, the Chin Lock (Jālandhara Bandha), Abdominal Retraction (Uḍḍīyāna Bandha), and Anal Lock (Mūla Bandha) were introduced. At the end of inhalation, the Chin Lock is done, and during breath suspension Abdominal Retraction and Anal Lock are done. At the end of the suspension all three are released. In the Chin Lock (Jālandhara Bandha), the chin is tucked tightly against the top of the sternum (breast bone). For the perfection of the Chin Lock two special exercises were introduced. They are Meru Cālana (Cervical Exercise) and Mani Cālana (Trunk-Cervical Exercise). For invigorating the whole body the exercise called Cakrī Bhanda (Wheel-Forming Lock) was practiced.

Over the course of time, *mantra* and concentration factors were added to Sahita Breath Control. When it is done in conjunction with *mantra* and mental concentration, it is called Sagarbha, and when it is done without them it is called Nigarbha. The *mantras* used may be the shortest *bīja mantra* (one conjunct letter) or a many-lettered *mantra,* as for example the *gāyatrī* (with sixty-two conjunct letters). The elementary Sagarbha Sahita Breath Control has been utilized as an advanced Nāḍī Śuddhi process, termed Bhūta Śuddhi breath control. After exercise and before concentration, the practice of Audāsīnyasthiti (Conscious Relaxation) was prescribed. The other auxiliary factors were fasting, frugal diet, baths, and massage.

At the last stage of Sahita Breath Control the power of levitation is acquired. Now more and more control over animation is gained and ultimately it is suspended. There is no inhalation and exhalation. Sahita Breath Control ultimately ends in the state of *kevala kumbhaka* (natural breath suspension). At this stage the outwardly directed flow of the mind is fully controlled and concentration reaches the *samādhi* state.

A modified form of Sahita Breath Control was developed in which breath suspension was eliminated. It is called Vāta-Krama Kapālabhātī (Alternate Nasal Breathing). This is a respiratory purificatory exercise. It consists of inhalation through left nostril, exhalation through right, then inhalation through right, and exhalation through left.

Other Developments

To increase the power of concentration, Bhrāmarī and Mūrcchā Breath Control were also developed. In Bhrāmarī Prāṇāyāma (Sound-Producing Breath Control) inhalation, suspension, and exhalation are done with special techniques resulting in the production of various kinds of inner sounds, culminating in what is known as *anāhata* (sound produced without striking, an extraphysical divine sound), in which the mind becomes completely absorbed. In Mūrcchā Prāṇāyāma (Mental Absorption–Causing Breath Control), inhalation is done with increased force; a pressure is applied to the brain during suspension and is then released, thus producing a condition in which deep concentration develops.

Inhalation was also done through the mouth, in a crow-beaked fashion, as if to draw in water through a pipe. The air was exhaled either through the mouth or nostrils. From this form of breathing Śītalī Prāṇāyāma (Lingual Breath Control) and Sītkārī Prāṇāyāma (Dental Breath Control) were developed. In lingual breath control, inhalation is done through the rolled tongue, then suspension and exhalation through both nostrils. Dental breath control consists of inhalation through the locked teeth with "seeth" sound, suspension, and exhalation through nostrils, or inhalation through the wide opened mouth and nostrils, and exhalation through the mouth with the "seeth" sound.

One-Nostril Inhalation

Then one-nostril inhalation through either the right or the left nostril was developed, in which inhalation was followed by breath suspension. One-nostril inhalation developed into Sūrya Kumbhaka (Right-Nostril Inhalation Breath Control)—in which inhalation through the right nostril is followed by breath suspension and exhalation through the left nostril—and Candra Kumbhaka (Left-Nostril Inhalation Breath Control)—in which inhalation is done through the left nostril, followed by breath suspension and finally exhalation through the right nostril.

From Sūrya Kumbhaka (Right-Nostril Inhalation Breath Control) arose Sūrya-Bhedana Prāṇāyāma (Right-Nostril Breath Control). It consists of inhalation through the right nostril, breath suspension, and exhalation through the left nostril. The difference between Right-Nostril Inhalation Breath Control and Right-Nostril Breath Control is that in the latter the locks have been incorporated and the duration of inhalation, suspension, and exhalation is regulated in a definite order.

Khecarī Mudrā

The most advanced process of prolonging breath suspension is Khecarī Mudrā. Khecarī essentially consists of the closing of the rima glottidis with the retroverted tongue. This completely closes the air passage and applies pressure in the region with the tip of the retroverted tongue. This process controls the strong impulse to breathe in and lengthens the period of breath suspension. For this purpose the tongue is first made soft and elongated by the process of milking, stretching, and cutting. Milking is the pulling of the tongue wrapped with a fine wet cloth. It is also stretched in all directions to make it supple. Finally, the frenum linguae is gradually cut with a suitable instrument according to a particular method. In this way the tongue should be fit for the work.

Khecarī consists of the following stages: first stage—Anal Lock; second stage—inhalation and breath suspension; third stage—Chin Lock; fourth stage—closing of the rima glottidis by the retroverted tongue.

Nāḍī Śuddhi

Nāḍī Śuddhi—the process of harmonizing the body's activating and inhibitory forces as well as energy-acquiring and energy-consuming principles—is a most important aspect of Haṭha Yoga, because it is related to the development of breath suspension power. A student with a clean and healthy body and peaceful and contemplative mind, disciplined with *yama* and *niyama,* temperate in eating and other habits of living, and who has mastered postures, is fit for the practice of Nāḍī Śuddhi. When the internal purificatory state is established, vital vigor is increased, alimentary functioning becomes normalized, bodily fat decreases to a normal limit, muscles are toned, the body becomes healthy, light, and charming, and the eyes become clear. The necessity of sleep decreases and greater control over the sex urge is attained. And, above all, the power to suspend breath for a prolonged period is gained.

In Nāḍī Śuddhi, an internal contraction process is applied in conjunction with breath control to prolong breath suspension. The first step of the process consists of the Chin Lock, Abdominal Retraction, and Anal Lock. When these three are performed rightly and forcefully, an internal condition is created within the body in which prolonged breath suspension becomes possible. But special bodily preparations are necessary for their successful application. For this purpose the *ṣaṭ karman* (six purifications) have been prescribed in Haṭha Yoga. In fact, Nāḍī Śuddhi has been classified into two: Samanu and Nirmanu. Samanu is done by breath control and Nirmanu by purifications.

Control Exercise (*Ṣaṭ Karman* and *Mudrā*)

Respiratory and abdominal efficiency and a clean and empty alimentary canal are absolutely necessary for the fruitful application of the internal contraction process to get control over breath. At an advanced stage, breath suspension is greatly helped when the ability to direct the flow of air from the lungs into the alimentary canal is developed. For this purpose the alimentary canal should be kept in a perfectly clean condition. This is done by the system of internal cleansing known in Haṭha Yoga as *ṣaṭ karman* (six purifications), which can be subdivided into two: extensive and abbreviated. The abbreviated system consists of:

1. Gastric Cloth-Cleansing (Vāsa Dhautī): cleans the alimentary canal
2. Colonic Auto-Lavage (Jala Vasti): cleans the alimentary canal
3. Nasal Thread-Cleansing (Sūtra Neti): cleans the nasal cavities and upper section of the throat
4. Straight Muscle Exercise (Naulī or Laulikī): develops the strength of and control over the abdominal muscles, so they can play their role fully in the internal contraction process
5. Abdominal Short-Quick Breathing (Kapālabhātī): purifies and strengthens the lungs
6. Gazing (Trāṭaka): purifies and strengthens the eyes, closely related to concentration

Cleansing the Alimentary Canal

In Gastric Cloth-Cleansing, a long narrow piece of fine cloth soaked in clean water is swallowed gradually, then gently withdrawn. Colonic Auto-Lavage consists of drawing water into the colon through the rectum without any instrumental aid. In addition to these two ways of purifying the alimentary canal, a few other advanced processes are included in the extensive system of internal cleansing: Alimentary Canal Auto-Lavage (Vāri Sāra), Alimentary Canal Auto-Air Bath (Vāta Sāra), Colonic Auto-Air Bath (Śuṣka Vasti), and Gastric Auto-Lavage (Vamana Dhautī).

Alimentary Canal Auto-Lavage consists of drinking water and then passing it from the stomach to the colon via the small intestine and finally discharging it with the intestinal contents out of the body without the help of any instrument. In this way the whole alimentary canal is adequately washed with water from the esophagus to the rectum. No instrumental aid is necessary this process.

Alimentary Canal Auto-Air Bath consists of swallowing air and then passing it from the stomach to the colon via the small intestine and expelling it through rectum from the body without any mechanical aid.

Colonic Auto-Air Bath is another special method of introducing air into the colon for purificatory purpose. It consists of sucking atmospheric air through the rectum into the colon without instrumentation.

Gastric Auto-Lavage is very helpful in washing out any excess gas and mucus accumulated in the stomach. It is a process of drinking water and then vomiting it completely.

The advanced Plāvanī (Floating Breath Control) is based on Alimentary Canal Auto-Air Bath and Colonic Auto-Air Bath. The foul air should first be eliminated from the colon and then it should be filled with pure external air by Colonic Auto-Air Bath. Then the stomach and the small intestine should be filled with the pure external air by Alimentary Canal Auto-Air Bath.

Muscle Control

That muscle state of the body in which one can apply maximum strength in internal contraction during breath control is to be developed. An exercise method, the chief characteristic of which is the conscious application of the mind to the muscles with a view to mold a particular pattern of movements in which the controlling factor predominates, was developed in Yoga. The large as well as small muscles were approached and controlled. It appears that the main cause of the development of control exercise was in relation to breath control. The internal contraction process utilized for prolonging breath suspension and the alimentary purificatory process, which is absolutely necessary for breath control, are both based on control exercise.

Control exercise seems to have started with abdominal control. The first stage of abdominal control was to alter the slight retraction and distension of the front abdominal wall that automatically occurs during respiration. It was changed into a voluntary powerful retraction in Agnisāra (Adominal Retraction and Release), in which, during the exhalation breath suspension, the abdomen is retracted as much as possible and then quickly released, without any intervals between the movements. The retraction movement reached its highest degree in Uḍḍīyāna Bandha (Abdominal Retraction). Abdominal Retraction consists of drawing the abdomen inward and upward to the maximum degree during the exhalation breath suspension. Agnisāra (Abdominal Retraction and Release) is included in the purificatory acts whereas Abdominal Retraction is a control exercise.

The automatic slight distension of the abdomen occurring during breathing is changed into a voluntary maximum abdominal distension in the exercise known as Tunda Cālana (Abdominal Control Exercise), an important contraction exercise. Abdominal Control Exercise consists of three movements: voluntary distension of the upper abdomen, voluntary distension of the lower abdomen, and downward wave-motions of the abdomen.

Abdominal control reached its highest level in the Straight Muscle Exercise known as Naulī or Laulikī, an important exercise belonging to purificatory acts. The "straight muscle" referred to is the rectus abdominis, each of a pair of long flat muscles at the front of the abdomen, which join the sternum to the pubis. The Straight Muscle Exercise consists of five main movements: the central isolation of the rectus abdominis, the right isolation of the rectus abdominis, the left isolation of the rectus abdominis, the right and left turning of the rectus abdominis, and the rolling of the rectus abdominis. The Straight Muscle Exercise is closely related to the advanced control exercises of Colonic Auto-Lavage, Colonic Auto-Air Bath, Alimentary Canal Auto-Lavage, and Alimentary Canal Auto-Air Bath.

Along with the abdominal control, pelvic control was developed, mainly in relation to breath control. The first stage of pelvic control exercise was to strengthen and gain control over the anal region. Two exercises were developed in this connection. The first is Aśvinī Mudrā (Anal Exercise) consisting of alternate contraction and relaxation of the anus. The second one is Mūla Bandha (Anal Lock), an important control exercise in which the anal contraction is retained. The anal canal needs to be kept in a clean condition by local cleansing with water. For this purpose anal cleansing was introduced. It is included in the purificatory acts. Anal Lock is practiced alone and later on in combination with Abdominal Retraction, Straight Muscle Exercise, and various posture exercises.

The control factor reached a very high stage of development in the well-known Vajrolī Mudrā (Gonadal Control Exercise), which is mainly designed to attain maximum sex efficiency and control. It is only for advanced male students. It consists of several stages. At the final stage urethral control is attained, culminating in the development of the power to suck fluids upward into the bladder through the urethra without any instrumental aid. At the last stage the atmospheric air can be sucked inside through the urethra without instrumentation.

Contraction Exercise (*Cāraṇā*)

The system of contraction exercise called *cāraṇā-kriyā* was developed in Haṭha Yoga to voluntarily contract, strengthen, and control the muscles of the body. It was specially developed in connection with Nāḍī Śuddhi. It is based on the natural and simple types of movements that human muscles are capable of: flexion and extension; forward, backward, and lateral bending; twisting; abduction and adduction; and rotation. The application of voluntary contraction and control not only contributes to better development of the muscles, it also secures greater control over them and develops the power of concentration of the mind.

Contraction exercise is divided into two groups: principal and secondary. The principal group consists of contraction and control of neck, abdomen, arms, thighs, legs, and feet. The secondary group consists of contraction and control of muscles connected with the wrists and other joints of the body.

The following is an abbreviated process of contraction system:

1. Neck motion, consisting of flexion, extension, lateral bending, and rotation of the head, with voluntary contraction, and controlled movements of platysma and sternocleidomastoid.
2. Abdominal motion, consisting of (a) flexion, extension, lateral flexion, and rotation of the trunk, and (b) hip flexion, with voluntary contraction, and controlled movements of the rectus abdominis and obliquus externus abdominis.
3. Pectoral (upper) limb motion, consisting of (a) upward, downward, forward, and backward movements of the shoulder-girdle, (b) flexion, extension, abduction, adduction, rotation, and circumduction of the arm, (c) flexion, extension, pronation, and supination of the forearm, (d) flexion, extension, abduction, and circumduction of the hand, and (e) flexion and extension of the fingers, with voluntary contraction, and controlled movements of the pectoralis major, serratus anterior, latissimus dorsi, shoulder blades, trapezius, deltoid, biceps, triceps, and flexors and extensors of the forearm.
4. Pelvic (lower) limb motion, consisting of (a) flexion, extension, abduction, adduction, rotation, and circumduction of the thigh, (b) flexion and extension of the leg, (c) flexion and extension of the foot, and (d) flexion, extension, abduction, and adduction of the toes, with voluntary contraction, and controlled movements of the thigh and calf muscles.

Posture Exercise (*Āsana*)

The term *āsana* was originally given to the concentration posture—the third great limb of the most ancient eightfold Yoga. *Āsana* as posture exercise was developed from the motionless concentration posture in Haṭha Yoga. In addition, many of the elements of posture exercise were derived from ancient Indian dancing, which was a mixture of gestural, locomotor, gymnastic, and mimetic types of movements. Dancing movements were influenced by the imitation of movements and postures of animals. However, gesture—an attitude or a movement expressive of a person's feelings—was the backbone of ancient dancing. The locomotor movements of walking, running, and jumping in modified forms were parts of the gestural dance. To these movements, the simpler type of natural movements consisting of various movements of the head, trunk, arms, and legs were also added. These nonlocomotor simpler movements were gradually transformed into more difficult gymnastic movements.

The elimination of the most ancient locomotor activities from posture exercise gave it a new character, indicating its divergence from the old type of human muscular exercise. As we have seen, at a certain stage of development the most ancient habit of continuous exercise had to be modified. Mental concentration and thinking required the suspension of activities. The result was the incorporation of a motionless attitude of the body, favoring repose and relaxation. In Yoga the motionlessness of the body has been carried to the maximum limit for deep concentration.

However, this interruption of ceaseless activities needed to be compensated by a more concentrative type of exercise requiring more systematic muscular endeavor and greater control over movements in order to meet the body's actual need of exercise. It was achieved in Yoga through the use of the fundamental musculature—the oldest in the history of muscle—in a most systematized, economical, and fruitful manner. The limb muscles were made to cooperate fully with the spinal musculature to make the movements vigorous and more effective. This pattern of exercise is termed posture exercise (*āsana*). The development of posture exercises took two main courses, according to their source: one from Accomplished Posture and another from Lotus Posture.

Postures Developed from Accomplished Posture

From Accomplished Posture (fig. 20.1) a number of heel-perineal, heel-anal, and heel-abdominal postures arose. An important development was Happy Posture (fig. 15.9), in which the heels, right to the right side and left to the left side, are set against the perineum, with the soles together and toes extending toward the front. This turned into the Posterior-Heel-Perineal Posture, with the joined soles and toes extended backward and the heels placed against the perineum. When the heels were placed contrariwise against the perineum, the right heel to the left and the left one to the right side of the perineum, it became Lion Posture.

The Accomplished Posture itself was modified as follows: the left heel is placed at the root of the genitals instead of against the perineum, and the right heel is placed above the left one. This is also called Liberated Posture. Another such modification is simply the adoption of the reverse leg position, that is, the right heel pressing the perineum and the left heel against the pubic bone and just above the genitals. In the third modification the anterior folding of the legs is changed into posterior folding and the feet are placed by the sides of the anus. These two forms of Accomplished Posture are also called Adamantine Posture.

When the posture is so modified as to place the feet in a manner in which the heels are set against the anus, it is called Tortoise Posture. There is yet another modification in which the heels of the joined soles are placed against the pubic bone and just above the genitals. It is also called Guarded Posture. The Guarded Posture itself took another form, in which the anus is placed on the joined heels.

Two important posture exercises were developed from Accomplished Posture by the introduction of new arrangements of the feet. One is Frog Posture, in which the posterior leg-folding assumed in Adamantine Posture is maintained but carried to the back and the toes of the right foot touch those of the left. The other is the extremely difficult Abdominal Pressing Posture, in which a kneeling position is assumed and the upper part of the feet (instead of the soles) are joined together from the ankle to the toes and the fibular sides of the feet are placed against the abdomen.

Leg-stretch postures were developed from Accomplished Posture. The first development was Great Trunk-Bend Posture, in which the heel of one leg is set against the perineum as in Accomplished Posture and the other leg is extended, the body is bent in the direction of the extended leg, and the big toe of the extended leg is held with the hands. It is especially intended for breath control. The next development was the Head-Knee Posture (fig. 12.16), in which the head is bent on the knee of the extended leg while one holds the toes of the same leg with the hands. Finally, Spinal-Stretch Posture (fig. 12.15) was developed, in which both legs were fully extended, the toes were held with the hands, and the head was bent on the knees.

Arm-leg and foot-head postures were also developed from the heel-perineum element of Accomplished Posture. Arm-Head Posture (fig. 15.2) is the typical arm-leg posture in which the heel of one leg is placed against the perineum and the other leg is placed across the upper part of the arm of the same side. Similarly, Single Foot-Head Posture (fig. 15.3) is an example of a foot-head posture, in which one leg is placed across the back of the neck, while the heel of the other leg is set against the perineum. Arm-Leg Posture (fig. 16.6) and Foot-Head Posture were transformed into Four-Point Posture (fig. 16.4) and Double Foot-Head Posture (fig. 15.4) respectively. In both of these postures the heel-perineum factor was eliminated because of the changed position of the legs. These two postures were further transformed into Single Arm-Stand Posture (fig. 18.14) and Standing Single Foot-Head Posture (fig. 18.6), in which the leg-raised factor was retained but the heel-perineal factor was eliminated because of the necessity of standing on one leg. Still further transformation of these two postures was effected in their combination with the head-knee postures in which the leg-raised factor was retained and the other leg was kept extended, the toes were held with the hands and the head was bent on the knee (fig. 18.2). They are called Wing Posture (fig. 18.3) and Bent-Head Wing Posture (fig. 18.4).

Single Foot-Head Posture and Double Foot-Head Posture were further transformed into Pillow Posture (fig. 14.19) and Noose Posture (fig. 15.8) respectively when they were executed in the supine position. The main factor in the Pillow Posture is the single foot-neck lock and in the Noose Posture the double foot-neck lock.

Spinal-Stretch Posture (fig. 12.15) became transformed into Forward Head-Bend Posture (fig. 12.17), in which the legs are placed apart, the toe-hold is maintained, and the head is bent on the floor. It was further changed into Sideward Head-Bend Posture, in which the toe-hold was eliminated and the head was bent sideward to the floor. Both Spinal-Stretch Posture and Forward Head-Bend Posture were also practiced without toe-hold. The forward trunk bend factor of Spinal-Stretch Posture was carried in greater range in Foot-Hand Posture (fig. 12.21a).

From Spinal-Stretch Posture developed the raised-leg postures while sitting with the legs extended. The most important development was Knee-Touching Spine Posture (fig. 14.18), in which the legs are raised toward the head and the head is bent to the knees. At the final stage it became Pillar Posture (fig. 15.7), in which the legs are raised vertically and straight to a point. In modified forms one leg is raised both in Raised-Leg Head-Knee Posture and Pillar Posture. Another important exercise developed from Spinal-Stretch Posture is Risen Right-Angle Posture (fig. 14.21), in which the buttock and the extended legs are raised off the floor.

Adamantine Posture became Supine Adamantine Posture with the trunk bent backward to the floor. When the hips are raised and the body stands on the knees and toes it is called Kneeling Posture. When the head is bent backward to the floor from Kneeling Posture, it is called Bent-Head Adamantine Posture (fig. 12.11). When the backward bend is partly done with hand support it is called Camel Posture. The backward trunk-bend factor is carried to a greater degree in Back Posture, in which the trunk is bent backward from the standing position and the ankles are held with the hands. The backward trunk-bend is carried still further in Wheel Posture (fig. 12.14). When the trunk is only bent backward horizontally it is called Modified Wheel Posture (fig. 12.12).

In supine position the backward trunk-bend is done in Raised Bow Posture (fig. 12.10). In prone position also a number of backward trunk-bend postures were developed. The most important are Cobra Posture (fig. 12.1), Bow Posture (fig. 12.5), Locust Posture (fig. 12.4), and Swing Posture (fig. 12.7). In prone position the backward trunk-bend is carried to the limit in King-Cobra Posture (fig. 12.8). In the inverse body position the backward trunk-bend is made in Modified Scorpion Posture and is carried to the limit in Scorpion Posture (fig. 18.15).

A number of forward trunk-bend postures were developed from Adamantine Posture. When the body is bent forward with the arms extended and the forehead and the hands touching the floor it is called Modified Tortoise Posture. The same movement is also executed from Kneeling Posture. The forward trunk-bend is made with the head touching the floor in close contact with the knees and the heels held with the hands in Rabbit Posture.

In supine position the forward trunk-bend became trunk flexion and leg-raising became hip flexion and pelvis-raising. There was also the combination of the trunk-hip flexion. The main trunk flexion postures are Spine Posture and its variations. The hip flexion postures are Risen Leg Posture (fig. 14.14), Sideward Leg-Motion Posture (fig. 14.15), and some others. Plow Posture (fig. 14.9) is a typical pelvis-raising posture. The examples of the trunk-hip flexion postures are Head-Knee Spine Posture (fig. 14.17) and Knee-Touching Spine Posture (fig. 14.18).

Postures Developed from Lotus Posture

Another main line of development of posture exercise was from the Lotus Posture. Lotus Posture with the crossed arms in front became Chest Posture. Lotus Posture with the crossed arms behind the back and a toe-hold became Toe-Hold Lotus Posture (fig. 20.4). It became Mountain Posture (fig. 18.8) with the body standing on the knees. Risen Lotus Posture (fig. 16.1) and Great Piercing Act (Mahāveda) were developed from Lotus Posture in which the body is lifted off the ground while supported on the hands. When the arms were introduced into the spaces formed between the legs and thighs and the body was raised off the ground, supporting it on the hands, it became Cock Posture (fig. 16.2). The further development is Supine Tortoise Posture, in which the arms-between-legs-thighs factor of the Cock Posture is maintained, but the knees are raised from the ground and the neck is held with the hands. When this posture is done in sitting position with the body resting on the buttocks and holding the ears instead of the neck with the hands, it is called Fetus Posture.

The Lotus Posture in supine position becomes Fish Posture (fig. 12.32). When the head and the trunk are raised off the ground while the body is in supine position with Lotus Posture, it is called Balance Posture. In supine position with Lotus Posture, when the legs, hips, and trunk are raised, it becomes Risen Back Posture (fig. 14.12). When the knees are carried toward the head and placed on the floor beyond the head, it becomes Lotus-Plow Posture (fig. 14.13). Lotus Posture has also been combined with Peacock Posture (fig. 18.9). The combination is called Rolling Posture (fig. 18.11). When Lotus Posture is done in the inverse body position while the head rests on the floor, it becomes Inverse Lotus Posture (fig. 19.4).

Certain important postures were developed from the one-foot-on-thigh factor of Lotus Posture. The most important is Spinal-Twist Posture (fig. 12.29), in which one foot is placed on the hip joint and the other leg, with the knee raised erect, is placed by the side of the knee of the opposite leg and the trunk is twisted to the limit. When the one-foot-on-thigh factor is eliminated and the heel-perineum factor of Accomplished Posture is adopted, it becomes Modified Spinal-Twist Posture (fig. 12.26). When it is done with the ankle hold it is called Ankle-Hold Modified Spinal-Twist Posture (figs. 12.27, 12.28). The one-foot-on-thigh and the heel-perineum factors have been combined in Great Binding Posture.

A number of postures were developed in which the trunk-twist factor of Spinal-Twist Posture was retained but the one-foot-on-thigh factor was eliminated. In Twist Posture (fig. 12.25) the trunk-twist is made in a sitting posture with legs extended in front and far apart. In Hip-Bend Posture (fig. 12.23) the trunk-twist is done in standing position.

The lateral trunk-flexion was also introduced in posture exercise along with other trunk-bending movements. In Angle Posture the lateral trunk-bend is done with the leg of the bending side bent at the knee. In Half-Moon Posture (fig. 12.22) the body is bent from the hip laterally with straight legs. The lateral flexion is thus carried still further in Hip-Bend Posture and to the highest limit in Moon Posture (fig. 12.24), in which the body is bent to the limit without bending the legs.

A number of posture exercises were developed to counteract the harmful effects of the prolonged static contraction of the muscles of the pelvic limbs and the interruption of circulation in those parts due to prolonged static sitting postures required in concentration. Those are thigh and leg postures. These postures are essentially based on Squat Posture. When the body is straightened from this posture and lowered again, it is called Thigh Posture (fig. 17.1). When it is done with one leg, it is called One-Legged Squat Posture. Rising on toes with both legs in Squat Posture is known as Toe Posture (fig. 17.7). When the rising on toes with one leg is done, it is called One-Legged Toe Posture.

The prolonged inactivity of the pectoral limbs was similarly counteracted by certain posture exercises. In Four-Point Posture (fig. 16.4) the body is held horizontally on the extended arms and stretched legs and lowered and raised alternately. In Three-Footed Posture (fig. 16.5) the body is supported on one extended arm and stretched legs and lowered and raised alternately. In Arm-Leg Posture (fig. 16.6) the body is supported on one extended arm and one stretched leg and alternately lowered and raised. In Arm Posture (fig. 16.8) the head is lowered to the hand of the supporting arm in Squat Posture.

For the development of the power of concentration certain inverse body postures were developed. These postures proved to be restful, relaxing, and suitable for concentration when they were perfected. The most important are the Head Posture (fig. 19.3), in which the body stands on the head, the whole body from head to foot being inverted, and the Inversion Posture (fig. 19.1), in which the posterior part of the head, neck, and scapular region lie on the floor. The functional activities of the internal organs are profoundly influenced by these postures. The evil effect of the biped position is counteracted and a better-balanced condition is created. Other inverse body postures were developed in Haṭha Yoga mainly for physical education purposes. The most important among them are Shoulder-Stand Posture (fig. 19.2) and Arm-Stand Posture (fig. 18.13) and its varieties. In Shoulder-Stand Posture the body stands at a right angle with the neck, which lies horizontally on the ground. In Arm-Stand Posture (fig. 18.13) the body stands on the stretched arms or on one arm in the Single Arm-Stand Posture variation (fig. 18.14).

In the inverse body postures balance is an important factor. To develop balance, balance posture exercise was developed in Haṭha Yoga. One of the important postures is Eagle Posture (fig. 18.1), in which the body is supported by one leg, with the other leg encircling it. Another important posture is Knee-Heel Posture (fig. 18.5), in which the body is supported by one leg, with the foot of the other leg placed on the groin of the standing leg. In Heron Posture the body is balanced on the stretched arms in a squatting position. The body is balanced horizontally on the forearms in Peacock Posture (fig. 18.9). This posture was essentially developed in connection with colonic auto-cleansing and the anorectal control associated with it. In Crab Posture (fig. 18.10) the body is similarly balanced, but on one hand only.

2

Fundamentals of Yoga Exercise

In Yoga the meaning of exercise has been extended and its application broadened, as the body has increasingly been looked upon in a more comprehensive manner. Yoga is based on a broader conception of human goals, activities, meaning in this world, everything. According to Yoga the material body, which is a compound of tissues, is the last stage of the body—an elaboration of the internal body necessary for full human expression on the earth plane.

Static-Dynamic Aspects of Human Beings

From the history of the body we understand that the human being is related to two fundamental factors: the static and the dynamic. The dynamic aspect encompasses all our changes, motions, limit, world-consciousness, and world experiences. In all stages of our dynamic existence there is always a static background. In that lies our eternal nonmoving indestructible principle, conscious radiant energy in a quiescent state. Conscious radiant energy in the nonmanifested state is one and the same as Supreme Consciousness. When consciousness in the form of radiant energy becomes dynamic, it is Śakti. There is no separate entity. When a stress comes, when the radiant energy is about to manifest, it appears as something else; something dynamic is forced on the static state.

Our dynamic aspect is expressed in action and our static aspect is realizable through mental concentration. In the lowest order of mental life the contemplative side is almost completely hidden and the active side is either semiparalyzed or uncontrolled. In the higher order, the contemplative side is well developed and the dynamic side is fully controlled. From the yogic point of view exercise is intimately related to both motion and concentration.

Exercise Defined

When exercise is considered in relation to the physical body, it is a systematized method of movements of muscles done purposefully for the development of the material body. But in Yoga, exercise is used in a broader sense. Exercise as it is understood in Yoga aims not merely at the material body isolated from the rest of the human being, nor the mind similarly isolated, but at the full development of the whole person, which culminates in the attainment of the spiritual goal. This is why it is called *sādhana,* "the path or means of accomplishment."

Exercise in Yoga consists of purificatory exercises (*ṣaṭ karman*), posture exercise (*āsana*), control exercise, contraction exercise, breath-control exercise (*prāṇāyāma*), sensory-control exercise (*pratyāhāra),* and concentration exercise (*dhāraṇā, dhyāna,* and *samādhi*). When these factors are applied rightly, the body is purified, strengthened, controlled, and refined, and the mind becomes calm and concentrated. Purificatory exercise, posture exercise, control exercise, and contraction exercise are related mainly to the body, breath control to both body and mind, and sensory-control, *dhāraṇā, dhyāna,* and *samādhi* to the mind. These factors have been tried for thousands of years and have proved successful in millions of cases. To make the exercise most successful, all these factors should be applied simultaneously and harmoniously. This, in short, is the whole picture of exercise in Yoga.

Exercise, therefore, is a process, or a combination of processes, so designed as to effect our gradual unfoldment from the narrow stage of consciousness, to ultimately reach our static existence in which the "whole" is realized. In the whole process our dynamic function is so regulated as to be helpful in this endeavor. In this unfoldment both the body and the mind play their parts. Through the process of exercise the body and mind are molded into a pattern most suitable for functioning dynamically as well as statically. By the influence of the exercise the body helps the mind in concentration and the mind helps the body in its firmness, refinement, and control.

It is also possible to divide exercise into two categories: concentration exercise and muscular-respiratory-neural exercise. Concentration exercise is for developing the power of mental concentration to reveal a new world of power, knowledge, and bliss. It culminates in realization of our eternal nondestructive principle. It consists of the processes of *pratyāhāra, dhāraṇā, dhyāna,* and *samādhi.* The muscular-respiratory-neural exercise is to educate the body in a manner that is most suitable for concentration. The education of the body mainly consists of two parts: the purification, vitalization, strengthening, and controlling of the body, and the development of motionlessness. According to Yoga this is physical education and it is intimately related to concentration. Yoga physical education consists of posture exercise, control exercise, contraction exercise, purificatory exercise, and breath-control exercise.

The Pattern of Body Aimed at in Yoga

Yoga physical education with its various processes aims at developing the body into a certain pattern that is most suitable for the attainment of motionlessness, calmness, and concentration. For our convenience this type of body can be considered from two perspectives: external, which is related to its appearance, that is, size, shape, and bulk; and internal, which is related to the functional efficiency of the body as a whole. We can call the first the growth factor and the second the efficiency factor. The growth factor is subordinate to the efficiency factor.

The efficiency factor is a compound of several important factors. The first of these is health. Health is not mere freedom from disease, though that is the first step to health. Health is a positive factor, an essential factor of efficiency. In a state of health not only do all the organs of the body function noninterruptedly and in a most coordinated way, but the natural disease-resisting power of the body is at the maximum stage of development and there is a feeling of joy, power, and courage. This state of the body is what is meant in Yoga by *ārogya*. The normal and easy functioning of the body associated with health has been termed *svacchanda-deha*.

Associated with health are four factors: loveliness, youthfulness, a sweet smell in the body, and vitality. The really healthy body is vital, youthful, lovely, and fragrant. In such a body premature senility does not appear, and youthful appearance and vigor are prolonged. Life is extended. This is the picture of health in Yoga. Moreover, such a healthy body is always fit and the source of great energy, capable of making strenuous and continued exertion. The body becomes muscularly strong, nimble, and firm. This is the efficiency factor. Such a body is not lean and ugly. It is in a well-nourished condition and at the same time free from excess fat. The abdominal region is specially maintained free from fat. It is not only muscularly well developed but symmetrically built up, and it therefore looks beautiful.

Moreover, the body is fit for concentration. It is habitually erect and well-controlled, and can be made motionless when required. This type of body is termed *deva deha* in Yoga.

Fundamental Posture in Yoga

A motionless attitude of the body that is characterized by the elimination of all voluntary movements becomes really helpful if a condition is created in which the functional activities of all the vital organs are diminished to a point at which deep concentration is possible without any disturbance in the body. Two factors are most important in this connection—easy and uninterrupted respiration and circulation. The feeling of ease that appears after the posture is perfected and controlled and upon which concentration so much depends is intimately associated with these respiratory and circulatory conditions. This means that the diaphragm and the heart will be in a position in which they will be able to function most efficiently and without any obstruction, and there will be no unnecessary pressure or drag on the great blood vessels.

In a motionless state of the body easy respiration mainly depends upon the right position of the diaphragm in the thorax. In this attitude venous circulation is not helped by muscular movements, but rather it depends mainly upon the diaphragmatic pump and the tonic contraction of the abdominal muscles.

The habitual posture of the chest is a most important factor that governs the position of the diaphragm. The position of the chest at the end of normal exhalation is regarded as the rest position. Normally from this position the diaphragm descends in inhalation and ascends during exhalation, returning to the resting position at the end of exhalation. The diaphragmatic motion is greatly increased in forced respiration.

In a drooped chest the diaphragm is displaced downward and remains there in an inhalation position. The origin and insertion of the diaphragm are also brought closer together, resulting in its inefficient function. The chest may change its shape and become narrow at the ninth rib. Under these conditions the diaphragmatic movements in normal respiration are decreased. This respiratory condition is unsuitable for deep concentration. When the diaphragm assumes a low position in the thorax, the heart and aorta are also dragged downward. This is an unfavorable condition for the efficient functioning of the heart, especially when the body is motionless.

The diaphragm plays an important role in venous circulation by exercising a pumping action on the inferior vena cava. If the normal range of movement of the diaphragm is diminished due to its lower position, the diaphragmatic pump becomes very ineffective. This may also cause splanchnic congestion. This interference in the venous flow toward the heart and consequent congestion are very unfavorable for deep concentration. Adequate circulation in the brain should be maintained with ease during concentration. Therefore, no condition that affects circulation in any way should be created. The nerves supplying the heart and diaphragm may be impacted and in some way may interfere with the nerve action.

The low position of the diaphragm causes a downward pressure on and a slight displacement of the abdominal organs. This results in the relaxation and protrusion of the abdominal wall. If this abdominal condition is habitually maintained, the tone and strength of the abdominal muscles are diminished. The pelvic organs are also pressed downward by the pressure of the displaced abdominal organs. It may be noted here that the abdominal organs have no particular positions and their range of mobility is great. They are constantly changing their positions and in this way their functional activities are normally carried out. This means that they must have enough room in the abdomen for their full mobility. If the diaphragm is habitually in a low position, it decreases the abdominal cavity, causes unnecessary pressure on the abdominal viscera, and forces them to assume certain positions not normally designed for them.

In a normal state the upper part of the abdominal cavity is larger than the lower part, and this affords plenty of room for the full mobility of the viscera. In a faulty spinal posture the shape of the abdominal cavity changes. The upper part becomes narrower with the abdominal wall unnecessarily relaxed, stretched, and protuberant. A change of the abdominal shape may accompany a change in the thoracic cavity in which it becomes narrower and longer, with the diaphragm assuming a low position. Under this condition the blood and nerve supply to the viscera may be disturbed.

Weakness of the abdominal muscles, especially the transversus abdominis, results in the protuberance of the anterior abdominal wall. The condition of the relaxed protuberant abdominal wall becomes worse when fat accumulates there, as, for example, in obesity. This abdominal fat accumulation results in an increase of the normal spinal curves because of the change of the line of gravity. The fatty abdomen and the increased intra-abdominal fat cause disturbances in normal respiration, especially when an erect posture is assumed.

When the chest droops downward, the origins and insertions of the abdominal muscles are brought closer together and consequently they become functionally less efficient. When the chest is held high the abdominal muscles are in the correct position to provide support for the viscera, compress the abdomen, and hold the pelvis up in front.

Incorrect positions of the vertebrae due to incorrect posture may put pressure upon the spinal nerves and blood vessels, thus interfering with the normal activities of those organs and parts supplied by them. Certain ligaments and muscles associated with the vertebral column may be overstretched while others may be abnormally shortened. If this state is continued for a long period, their functional efficiency is impaired and the normal range of motion is reduced or otherwise altered. Even the shape of bone may be changed in extreme cases.

Such unfavorable thoracic and abdominal conditions are to a very great extent due to a habitually incorrect trunk position in which the normal anterior convex curves of the cervical and lumbar spines and the forward concave curve of the dorsal spine are increased. In an increased lordotic position of the lumbar spine the weight of the body is largely transferred to the posterior part of the intervertebral discs and the articular facets and capsules may be crowded together and may also cause the narrowing of the size of the intervertebral foramina. The spinous processes may come close together and may even impinge on one another. The transverse processes and the cervical spine are also affected by bad posture. In an increased anterior concavity of the dorsal spine the weight of the body is mostly transferred to the front part of the vertebral bodies. The articular facets are pulled apart.

The most important spinal extensor muscles are the sacrospinalis group (erector spinae). These muscles normally keep the vertebral column in a straight position. If the habitual position of the trunk is incorrect, with the normal spinal curves exaggerated, the positions of the origins and insertions of the erector spinae muscles are altered, which makes them functionally less effective. Their postural tone and strength are decreased.

The spinal extensor muscles are also helped by the abdominal muscles. The abdominal muscles function in a most effective manner when the pelvis is held up in front by them. Weakness of the rectus abdominis increases the anterior convexity of the lumbar spine. Weakness of the external oblique muscle causes either lumbar lordosis or an anterior pelvic displacement.

When the vertebral column is held straight, the ribs are straight and the thorax is fixed high. A normal development of the chest and other trunk muscles is also absolutely necessary for maintaining the thorax in a proper position. If these muscles are weak, the thorax will fall downward and will be in an exhalation position. This will cause an interference with normal respiration. On the other hand, if a barrel-shaped and highly arched chest is developed by wrong application of strength exercise, the thorax will be placed in an inhalation position, which will also interfere with normal respiration.

Two points have been emphasized in Yoga in connection with the motionless attitude: erect trunk posture and proper muscular development, especially the development of the extensor muscles of the spine and thoracic and abdominal muscles. These two factors create the most suitable condition in the body when a concentration posture is assumed. In the erect posture the trunk is held straight, back flat, chest up, abdomen slightly in, head up and chin in. The folded legs are helpful in keeping the trunk erect in a sitting position. The exaggerated erect posture, with hollow back, chest too high, and shoulders back, is also faulty and should be avoided. The erect posture should be easy, with all the muscles in a relaxed state. The sense awareness of correct posture can be developed by practice and should also be maintained while standing as well as when working in a sitting or standing position.

Proper exercise is absolutely necessary for the development of the muscles. Posture exercise has been intended for this purpose. Posture exercise is subdivided into static posture exercise and dynamic posture exercise. The right combination of the two forms produces the most satisfactory results.

Static Posture Exercise

Muscles may remain in a state of contraction or a state of relaxation. Contraction may be subdivided into postural contraction and phasic contraction. Postural contraction is the sustained contraction of a group of muscles, which serves to maintain a static posture but does not result in movement. When muscular contraction results in movements, it is called phasic contraction. All muscles of the body exhibit both postural and phasic contractions. In postural contraction a small number of fibers are involved at a time, producing what is called muscle tone or postural tone, which is responsible for maintaining a posture. Postural tone is most pronounced in the extensor muscles, which keep the body erect against the force of gravity.

When a movement is exhibited by a group of muscles, the postural tone of the muscles antagonistic to them is temporarily reduced. However, the body is always maintained in a posture suitable to the type of movements being executed at any given time. In a certain type of movement, as for example strength exercise, a certain posture is constantly being maintained until the exercise is over. In strength movement of arms or neck, the trunk and legs are kept in static postures. In locomotor movements, the trunk posture is maintained. On the other hand, there are movements in which the posture of the body is constantly being changed, such as dancing or wrestling. This we may call dynamic or moving posture.

In a state of general relaxation of the body, the postural tone probably decreases. However, even when the body is completely relaxed, that amount of postural contraction that is necessary to maintain the body in a posture remains. In a lying position with complete relaxation the total postural tone is the minimum. In a sitting posture with complete relaxation the postural tone is greater, because the trunk is kept erect by the postural contraction of the extensor muscles of the vertebral column. There are degrees of relaxation. The power of complete relaxation is predominantly a mental phenomenon, which can be developed by education.

When mental control over muscle is sufficiently developed, the power of volitionally contracting one, two, three, or four muscles, located in different parts of the body, or the simultaneous contraction of all the muscles of the body, as well as the power of conscious relaxation of one or more muscles or all the muscles (except certain muscles) is gained. At an advanced stage the power of complete relaxation is attained.

Static posture exercise is a form of muscle education in which the body is made to assume a desired pattern of posture, which is accompanied by certain circulatory, respiratory, glandular, and nervous changes. It results in increased vitality, health, and efficiency of the body and the creation of a most favorable condition of the body for mental calmness and increased power of control and concentration. According to the position of the body, postures may be divided into three groups: horizontal, vertical, and inverse. Through different postures the trunk, the neck, and the pectoral and pelvic limbs are involved, enabling the entire body to be exercised statically.

Static posture exercise consists of three stages: preliminary, comfort (or static), and discomfort.

In the preliminary stage the body is brought to a desired particular posture by the movements of the appropriate muscles. It is the stage of movement.

At the comfort stage the particular posture that has been assumed is maintained for a certain period of time. This stage lasts as long as the feeling of comfort is not interrupted.

As soon as discomfort is experienced, the third stage—the stage of discomfort—is reached.

The series of movements executed in the preliminary stage to attain a desired body posture are secondary. These are not repeated but stopped as soon as the desired posture is attained. Preliminary muscle training through movement exercise is, of course, absolutely necessary for the attainment of efficiency for the postures. However, the important part of the exercise is the static aspect of the exercise in the second stage. If the posture is assumed in a right manner and the muscles are properly trained beforehand for the postures, there will be a feeling of comfort at the second stage.

When a posture is perfected and well controlled, certain muscles will be in a state of contraction (of the phasic type), certain other muscles will be in a state of postural contraction, and the rest of the muscles will be in a state of relaxation. In this condition the activity and the expenditure of energy are considerably reduced. Ease experienced at this stage is indicative of the right circulatory, respiratory, nervous, and other adjustments in the body and the uninterrupted functioning of the body as a whole. It is a condition of the body in which better health is promoted and a balance between body and mind is established. The motionlessness of the body now becomes most helpful in concentration. When a state of comfort (or ease) is created in different static postures of the body, a higher level of vital vigor is attained. Haṭha Yoga aims not only at developing perfect health but also at creating, through different motionless attitudes of the body, a state of mind that is most suitable for greater power of concentration.

The third stage begins when the toleration point is reached. At first a feeling of discomfort is experienced, which gradually becomes more and more intensified and finally turns into a positive feeling of pain. The pain ultimately becomes so intense that to maintain thc posture is almost impossible. By regular practice the appearance of the pain phase of the third stage may be deferred; in addition, the power of toleration of pain is amazingly increased. The vital endurance and the natural disease-resisting power of the body are increased if the posture is retained at the pain phase, up to a certain time limit. When it is carried still further, a stage is reached which is especially favorable for the development of willpower. But finally a point comes when it becomes intolerable. At this point the posture should be discontinued.

Only advanced students are advised to continue the pain phase up to the vital endurance and willpower stages. Beginners should discontinue a posture when discomfort is experienced. Then, step by step, the duration of the comfort stage should be increased. After reaching a certain time limit, students can then begin to accustom themselves to endure discomfort experienced at the beginning of the third stage. Then, gradually, they can go to the endurance and pain points.

After the discontinuance of a posture and the assumption of a relaxation posture, the feeling of discomfort and pain will disappear. But if the posture is continued and the body begins to tremble, it is a sign that the dose has been too much, a clear indication the time limit should be regulated accordingly.

Those students who are undergoing static posture exercise for merely physical education purposes may remain physically relaxed and mentally calm during the maintenance of the static posture. But those who are willing to utilize it for higher purposes are advised to practice concentration during this time, after sufficient control over the posture is gained. The following forms of concentration are suggested:

1. Concentration on breathing
2. Breathing with *mantra*
3. *Mantra japa*
4. *Mantra japa* with concentration

5. Concentration
6. Breathing with *mantra japa* and concentration

For the attainment of success in static posture exercise, the body should be well prepared by dynamic posture exercise. Muscles should be made strong, enduring, flexible, and well controlled, and the full mobility of the joints should be secured. This physical preparation is absolutely necessary for the execution of static posture in a most effective way.

Dynamic Posture Exercise

In dynamic posture exercise certain groups of muscles are allowed to act in such a way that a particular pattern of movements is made in which either the trunk, abdomen, neck, pectoral limbs, or pelvic limbs, or more than one part of the body are involved. According to their specific role the muscles involved in the activities may be divided into three groups:

1. Principal muscles, which are directly involved in the desired movement
2. Auxiliary muscles, which help the principal muscles
3. Postural muscles, which are involved in maintaining the posture suitable for the movement

The actions of the first two groups are of the phasic type, and that of the third is of the postural type. The movement may be local or more extensive in character. In the local type of movement many other muscles of the body may be completely uninvolved. In the extensive type practically the whole body may be involved. However, the idle muscles in a particular pattern of movement need to be kept relaxed. Therefore, in a dynamic posture exercise the body is simultaneously educated in motion, posture, and relaxation. Here motion is the principal factor and the other factors are subordinate but important.

The movement factor of posture exercise is intrinsically related to the fundamental muscle groups. Developmentally, the earliest patterns of movements were those executed by the spinal musculature. They were associated with locomotion. At a higher stage of biological development the locomotion aspect of spinal movements was transferred to limb musculature, and the spinal movements became nonlocomotive in nature. The elimination of locomotor movements, however, did not lessen the importance of the spinal musculature. Free from locomotion, the movement potential of the spinal musculature was expressed in a way essential to higher forms of life. The spinal musculature developed into three main forms: spinal, abdominal, and thoracic-diaphragmatic (respiratory). The spinal muscles became the most important postural muscles in maintaining the trunk erect (in humans) and were also concerned in trunk movements. The abdominal muscles functioned in three ways—in supporting the abdominal viscera, in respiration, and in trunk movements.

The spinal, abdominal, and respiratory muscles function as fundamental muscles in mammals including humans. The fundamental musculature is involved in all movements including the movements of the limbs. At the human stage the pectoral limbs, free from the task of locomotion, have become a most important apparatus for exhibiting complex movements requiring great skill. Locomotor activities have been handed over to the pelvic limb muscles. They are also postural muscles, which support the body in a standing position. Both the pectoral and pelvic limb muscles function in intimate relation to and in cooperation with the fundamental musculature. Only in this manner are their movements vigorous and most effective. A brief study of the different kinds of movements is necessary for the right understanding of the dynamic posture exercise.

Types of Muscular Movements

Muscular movements may be divided into two main types: locomotor and nonlocomotor. Movements that cause the body to move from one place to another are locomotor movements. These movements are executed principally by the muscles of the pelvic limbs. There are three main forms of locomotor movements—walking, running, and jumping. According to the rates of progression, the locomotor movements are classified into speed exercise and endurance exercise. When maximum or very great speed in progression is involved, it is called speed exercise. When the same movements are carried on at a reduced speed to such a degree as to enable a person to continue activity for a prolonged period, it is called endurance exercise.

Combined speed-endurance exercise includes walking, jogging, running at slow and moderate speeds, sprint, broad jump, high jump, and mountain climbing. It is involved in various outdoor sports and games.

The nonlocomotor type of movement is that in which the body as a whole or some of its parts are involved without resulting in progression. This type of movement is essentially based on simple forms of movements, such as flexion, extension, lateral bending, rotation, circumduction, abduction, adduction, pronation, and supination. More extensive and complex forms of movements have been elaborated from the simpler forms.

When the simpler movements are combined and executed in a manner as to effect a desired pattern of movement through a desired group or groups of muscles and in which the degree of contraction is regulated, it is called strength exercise. The regulation results in either a light contraction in which only a small number of muscle fibers are brought into play, a moderate contraction involving a larger number of fibers, or a very powerful contraction involving a very great number of fibers.

Strength exercise may be classified under the following:

1. Light Contraction Exercise
   a) Noninstrumental
   b) Instrumental

   Light contraction exercise prepares the body for more advanced exercise.
2. Voluntary Full Contraction Exercise
   a) Noninstrumental
   b) Instrumental

   Voluntary full contraction exercise has greater developmental value and is useful to gain control over muscles.
3. Body Resistance Exercise
   a) Noninstrumental
   b) Instrumental

   Body resistance exercise is useful for development.
4. Weightlifting Exercise

   Weightlifting exercise is very suitable for the development of bulk and strength of muscles.

If weightlifting is combined with voluntary full contraction exercise and body resistance exercise, very satisfactory results in muscle size, muscle shapeliness, and muscle separation may be obtained. Weightlifting becomes more effective when it is combined with wrestling, which is itself an advanced strength exercise.

Psychoneural Exercise

Psychoneural exercise includes all movements requiring great skill and control. They may be locomotor or nonlocomotor, instrumental or noninstrumental. Psychoneural exercise trains the higher brain centers. It develops mental concentration, attention, control, coordination, and alertness. It enables the individual to perform various complex movements gracefully. It economizes the expenditure of energy. It shortens the latent period. It trains the memory and develops presence of mind, capacity of quick action, and other mental attributes. For physical education purposes the psychoneural exercise should be applied in relation to the fundamental musculature.

Posture Movements of Yoga

Posture movements are a systematized form of nonlocomotor type of movements, based essentially on the strength form of exercise in which elements of psychoneural exercise are included. By developing and fully utilizing the postural and movement potentials of the fundamental musculature, which is intimately related to organic development, posture movements play their role in the attainment and maintenance of a high standard of health and efficiency, which is equally necessary for a vigorous form of physical life and a higher order of mental life.

The effectiveness of posture movements greatly depends on two main principles: adoption of appropriate posture and a range of movements based on a graded system. An appropriate position of the body should be assumed at every stage of movement, otherwise correct execution of movement is not possible. To make the movements really effective, they should be executed in a graduated manner. At the final stage, the movements are carried out to their fullest extent, causing full contraction or full stretching of the muscles involved. There are certain posture exercises in which the movements are carried out to a moderate degree, while in other postures they are carried out to the fullest extent. In this way one posture may be converted into another posture. By assuming appropriate postures, light contraction is converted into medium contraction and finally into full contraction. Body resistance also works on a graduated principle in different postures. No instrument is used in posture exercise. Only appropriate posture patterns and associated movements with varying degrees of contraction are the guiding factors.

As the fundamental musculature, on which posture exercise is essentially based, has ultimately taken three forms—spinal, abdominal, and thoracic-diaphragmatic—so posture exercise has been developed into spinal, abdominal, and thoracic-diaphragmatic (or *prāṇāyāmic*) postures. The latter are static postures suitable for the practice of breath control in which the controlled movements of thoracic-diaphragmatic muscles are involved. The limb muscles have been utilized to effect the spinal or abdominal posture movements most effectively. These are the fundamental posture exercises. Accessory posture exercises have also been developed for the limb muscles. These may be considered as supplementary to the fundamental posture exercise.

For the most satisfactory results posture exercise should be combined with breath control, which is especially related to the development of the thoracic-diaphragmatic part of the fundamental musculature; contraction exercise for full contraction and control of muscles; and purificatory exercise for internal purification and control of the body.

3

Developmental Aspects of Yoga Exercise

Growth and development are inherent properties of the living body. Growth is an increase in the mass of the body, an increase in the length, thickness, and weight of the body or a part of it. Development is the gradual unfolding of the powers of the body. Growth and development are closely associated with each other.

Muscular Growth

Muscles are the organs over which we have the greatest command and which obey our will. We can influence the whole organism through this unique instrument, if it is properly cultured. Muscle is the central means through which the organic and nervous systems are approached and influenced. With the growth and development of muscle is linked the development of the alimentary, respiratory, circulatory, eliminative, glandular, and nervous systems. To a great extent the functioning of all the vital organs is adjusted to the demand of the muscles. Muscle has played a great role in molding the organic, nervous, and mental apparatuses into a pattern most suitable for human physical and mental development. The state of the muscle expresses in a clear language the state of the whole organism. The growth level of muscle is a clear index of the efficiency level of the whole body.

Growth is not merely associated with the changes in bulk and weight of the tissues. Morphological transformation is also closely related to the functional efficiency of the tissues and organs. The extension of the circulatory and nervous systems, the formation of new capillaries and nerve paths, and other internal changes indicate the far-reaching effects of muscular growth. Through the proper use and culturing of the muscles we can touch the fundamentals of life. Muscular growth helps in the attainment of organic and nervous health and efficiency, along with intellectual, moral, and spiritual powers.

It should be clearly borne in mind that a high standard of muscular growth cannot be attained

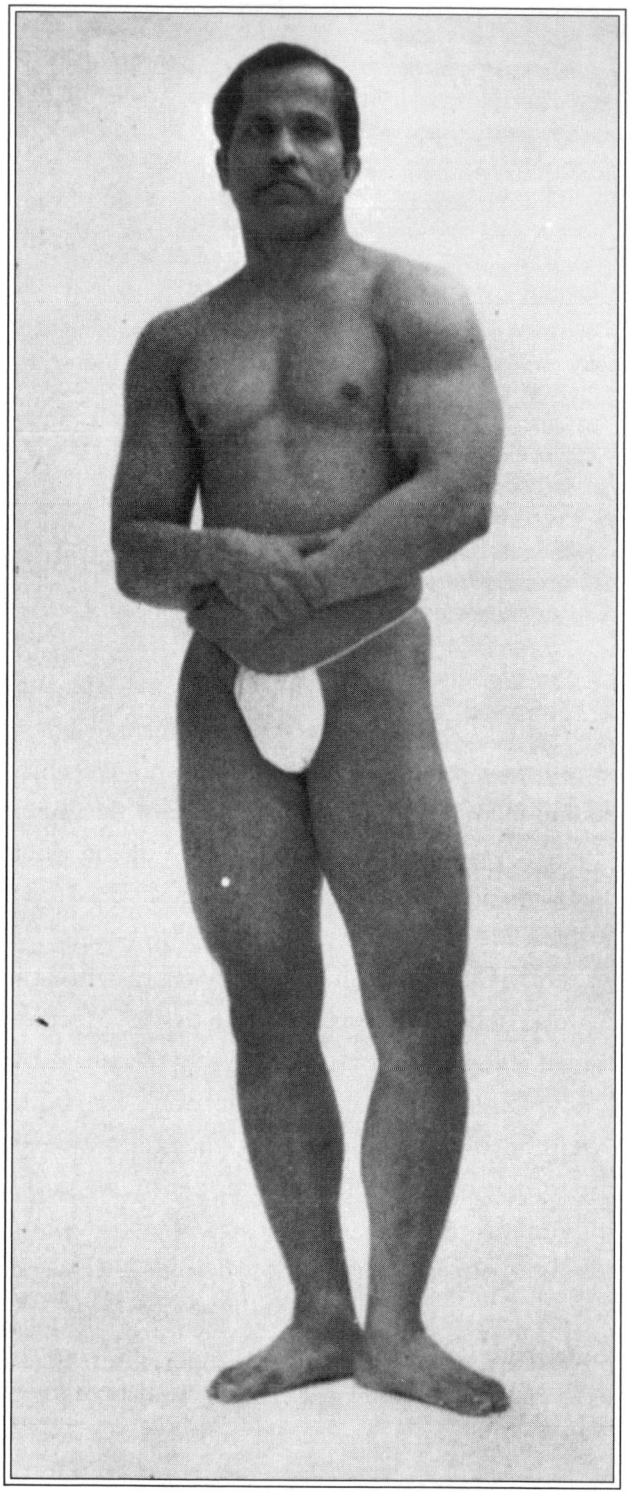

Fig. 3.1. Beauty and power in relaxation.
Posed by Dinabandhu Pramanick

unless suitable exercise is undertaken. The exercise should, of course, be combined with the right diet. The proper blending of exercise and diet is absolutely necessary in preventing undesirable fat accumulation and promoting actual muscular growth. When exercise is insufficient and the food intake is heavy, there is less increase of muscle tissues and more increase of fat. Even when exercise is heavy, if the amount of food eaten exceeds the actual needs of the body, the surplus will be deposited as fat. An increased amount of subcutaneous fat can occur along with the actual growth of muscles, making them look larger than their actual size. This is why many exceptionally strong men, who have not controlled their food intake, become overweight in spite of getting plenty of exercise.

Yoga exercise aims at attaining the degree of muscular growth that is absolutely necessary for building and maintaining maximum organic efficiency. The unnecessarily lean body is not the normal body and is not a beautiful body. We can, of course, shape the body on a more slender pattern without lowering vital vigor by regulating exercise and diet. But the level of growth should not be allowed to drop below normal requirements. On the other hand, we can attain muscular growth over and above the health needs of the body. But in attaining this "extra" growth, if the health of the body is disturbed, it becomes most undesirable. If we adopt unnatural and wrong methods in an attempt to attain rapid and excessive muscular growth, our object will be defeated.

Nutritional supplements are often employed in attaining extra muscular growth. By this means the body may be unnecessarily burdened with deposits of undesirable substances. This condition causes blood impurities, decreases vitality, and forces the body to develop disease in order to quickly eliminate the accumulated morbid material. In Yoga organic strength, endurance, agility, speed, and general physical fitness are not sacrificed for bulk.

Muscular Development

Muscular development means the gradual unfoldment of power lying dormant in muscle. A well-developed muscle is able to exhibit increased power. Muscular power in all forms is essential for living healthfully, working vigorously, and thinking efficiently. The ability to do work accurately, continue work for a prolonged period, and endure the work without any unhealthy impact on the organism are associated with muscular development. Muscular power is a chief element in a dynamic personality.

Muscular development does not always occur in proportion to muscular growth. Exercise is the main factor in muscular development. Diet occupies a secondary position. Exercise can be so regulated as to develop mainly the size of the muscles. However, the development of muscular power is not wholly independent of muscular growth. The size of a muscle is particularly dependent upon the form of power the muscle has to manifest. The form of power to be developed depends upon the nature of exercise performed; along with the development of that power the type and size of muscles most suitable for exhibiting that power are developed.

Muscular power may be divided into four: strength, speed, endurance, and skill.

Strength is that power of the muscle by which the external resistance applied to it is overcome by its powerful contraction. The strength of a muscle depends upon its cross-section area. Strength is best exhibited in weightlifting.

Speed is that power of muscle by which a series of movements are executed in the shortest

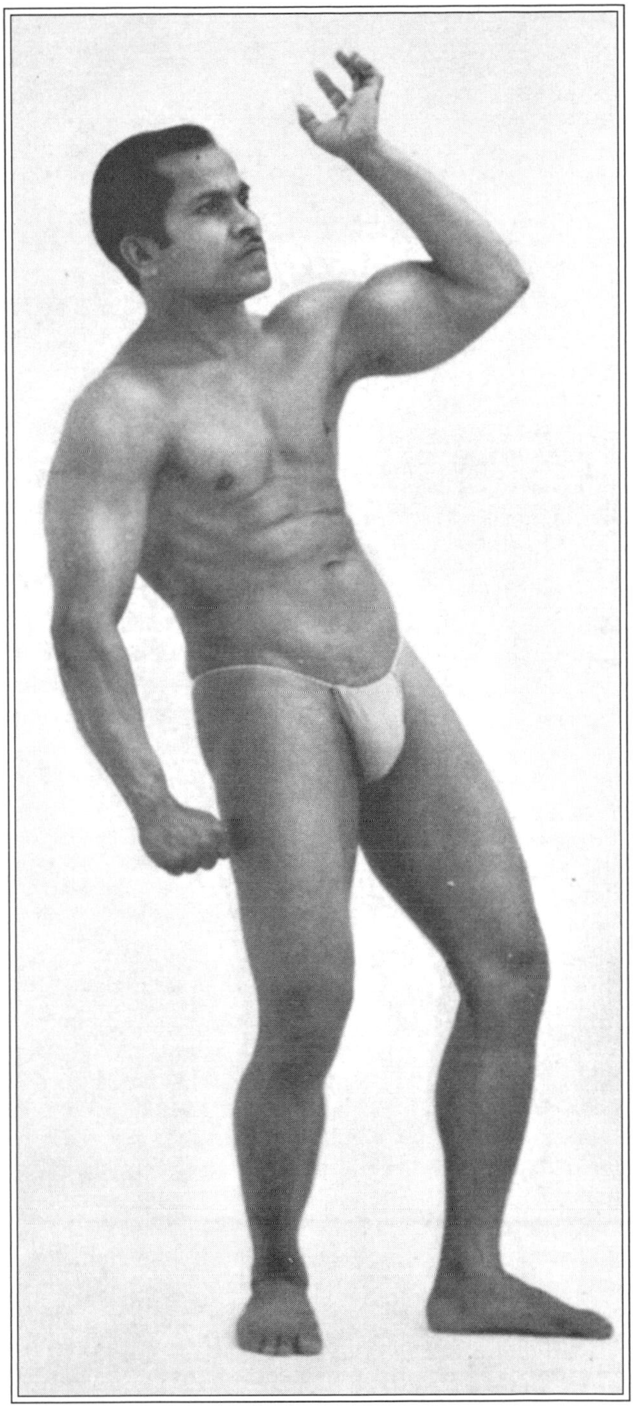

Fig. 3.2. An imitation of the Lord Kṛiṣṇa holding the Govardhana rock—a most symmetrically developed body. Posed by Dinabandhu Pramanick

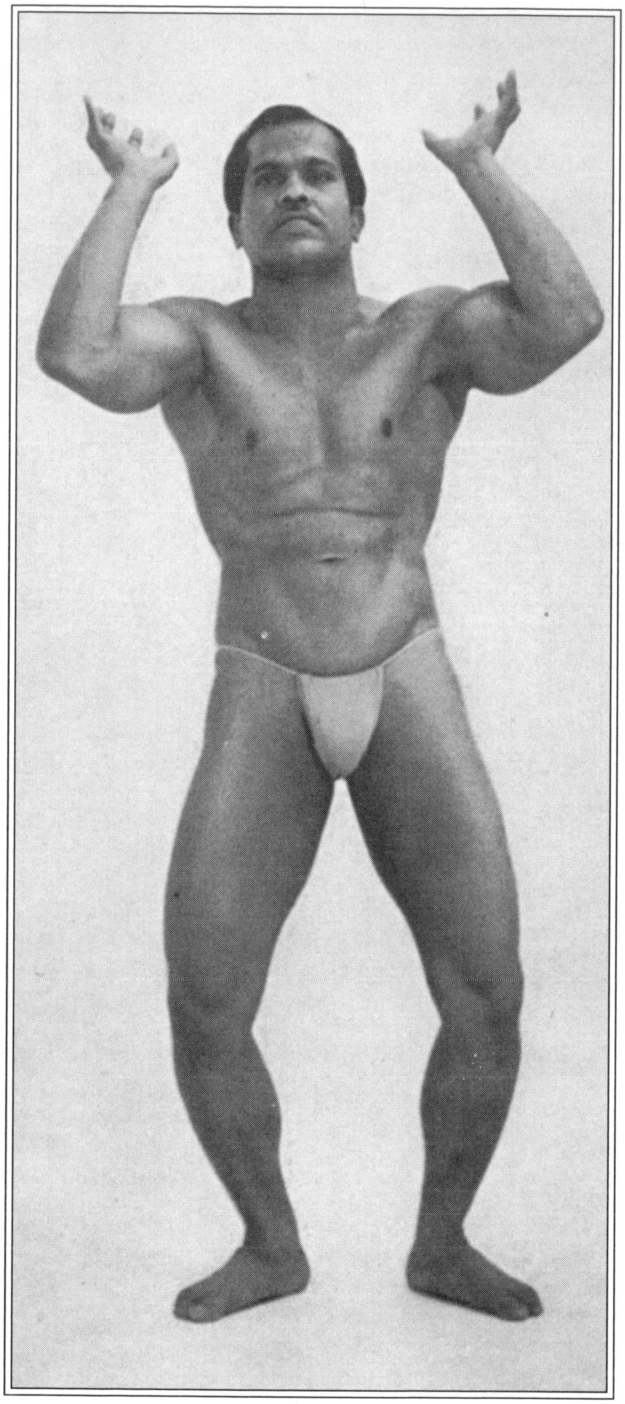

Fig. 3.3. An imitation of Mahavira carrying the Gandhamadana rock. Posed by Dinabandhu Pramanick

space of time by overcoming muscle viscosity. Sprinting is an example of extreme speed, and sprinters usually have a lower viscosity of muscle.

Endurance is that power of muscle by which movements are carried on for a prolonged period. The typical example of endurance is a marathon run.

Skill is associated with the ability of muscle to perform ordinary movements easily and economically, and more complicated movements accurately, efficiently, gracefully, and easily. Skill is especially involved in various sports and complex muscular movements.

The development of muscular strength, speed, endurance, and skill is not so much for the purpose of exhibition. These muscular achievements are closely related to organic and nervous development and are very useful in social and national life. Strength gives a feeling of well-being and power, develops self-confidence and fearlessness, and excites the desire for work. Strength and the feeling of strength are inseparable parts of health. When health begins to decline, strength also begins to ebb. This lack of strength impacts the body as well as the mind. Correct posture, which is necessary for nervous and organic health, depends to a great extent upon the strength and tone of muscles. Speed and endurance are specially connected with the development of organic vigor. Skill is necessary in all the activities of daily life if they are to be performed with ease, grace, and power. When skill is not properly developed, unnecessary nervous energy is expended, unnecessary muscles are used, movements are done more clumsily, more strain results, and there is less enjoyment of the activity.

In a particular type of movement either one or

more factors may predominate. In sprinting speed predominates and in long-distance running endurance prevails. In lifting heavy weights, especially of the slow type, strength predominates. In quick lifts, such as snatch or swing, strength is backed by speed. In wrestling strength, speed, endurance, and skill are involved.

Specialized Development of Physical Power

Is it possible to develop all forms of power simultaneously to a high standard? Many facts are involved in this matter. We know that neither a sprinter nor a marathoner can overpower a wrestler or defeat a weightlifter. Similarly, neither a wrestler nor a lifter is expected to outrun a sprinter or run a marathon race. Can we conclude from these facts that a wrestler does not possess speed and endurance or that a weightlifter is incapable of exhibiting speed and endurance? A wrestler exhibits not only wonderful skill, but great speed and alertness when executing various holds. Long continuous wrestling and the performance of 4,000 squats and 2,000 push-ups at a time by a wrestler are great feats of endurance. It is not possible for a runner to perform these. A weightlifter exhibits his power of endurance by lifting heavy weights for a prolonged period, and both strength and speed in quick lifts. A sprinter exhibits his speed in locomotion and a wrestler in other forms of motion.

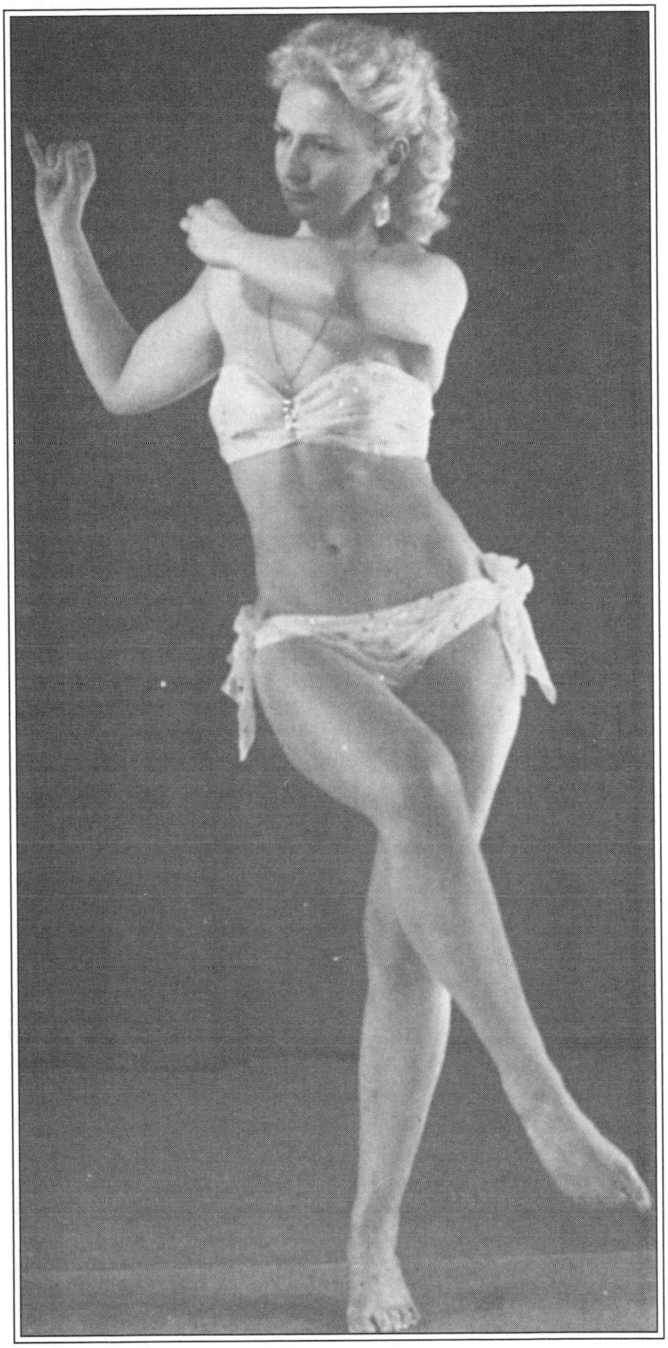

Fig. 3.4. Kṛṣṇa with His divine flute—beauty in form and grace in motion. Posed by Parvati Devi (Karin Schalander)

These observations seem to indicate that the body is able to exhibit a high degree of a particular form of power in a particular way, when specially trained for it. In other directions the same person's performances may be only mediocre. A particular type of exercise molds the muscles and nervous and organic apparatuses in a way that is most suitable for exhibiting that particular power in a particular manner. So, when the muscles are trained for speed in locomotion, records in sprinting are created. Similarly, when the muscles are trained by weight-lifting, the person is able to lift very heavy barbells or dumbbells. Further, if the muscles are trained to overcome resistance in some particular manner, it does not necessarily mean that the same person will be able to overcome resistance in other directions in which the muscles have not been trained. Similarly, skill improves only in relation to a particular form of activity in which the person is trained. Skill in one activity does not necessarily improve skill in other activities for which there has been no training.

A very high standard of development of physical power is a matter of specialization. A specialized achievement either in strength, speed, or endurance

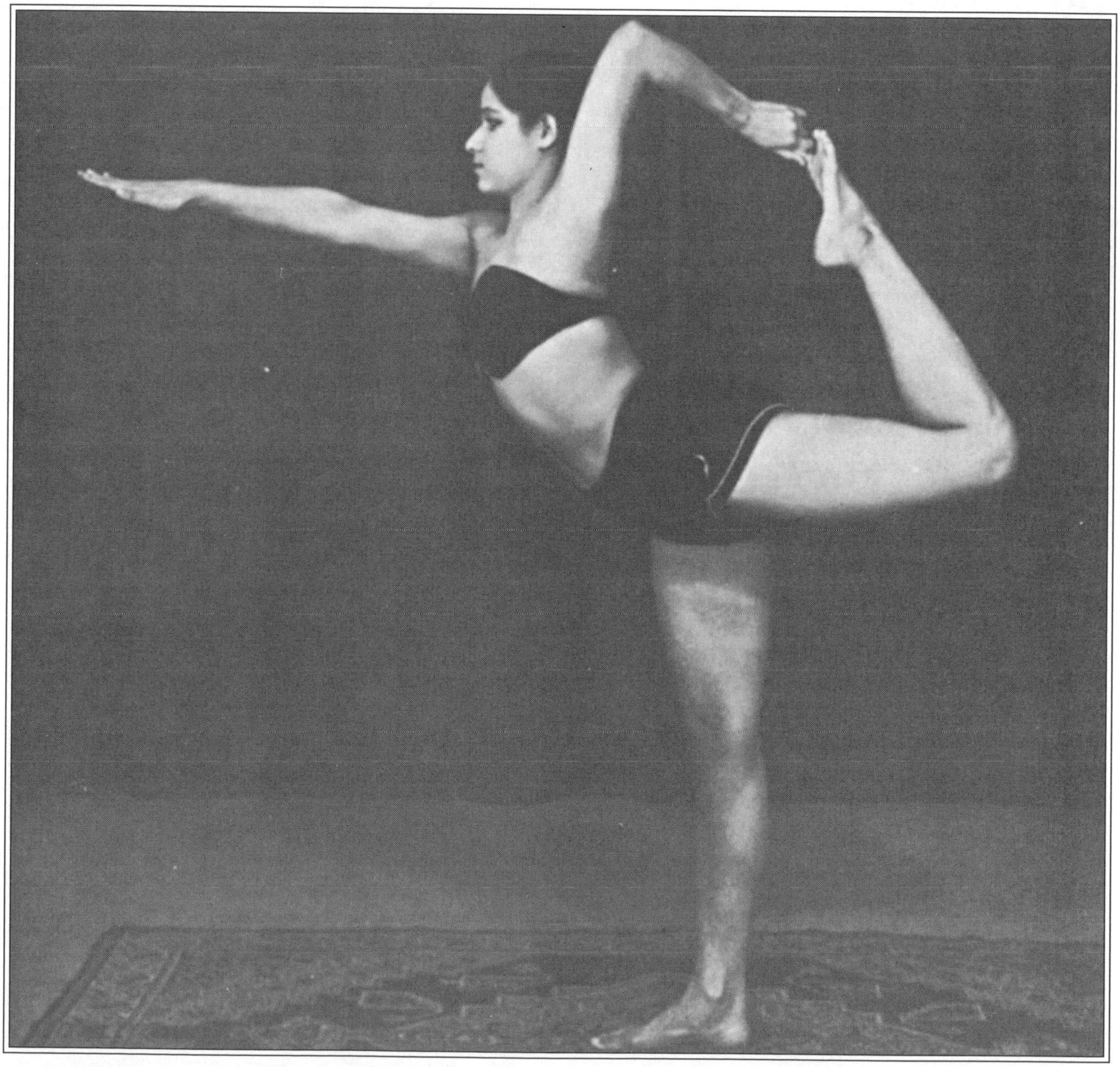

Fig. 3.5. Feminine beauty in a Yoga posture. Posed by Renu Ghosh

requires specialized training. It seems that for specialization all resources of the body are to be mobilized in a particular way and the whole energy of the body is to be concentrated on this particular achievement. Consequently, the body is unable to spare any great amount of energy for other muscular endeavors. When nearly all the available energy of the body is utilized in specialized muscular development, a lack of desire usually appears that discourages the individual to make real efforts in other directions.

We know that for the attainment of a high degree of mental development, continued and intensified efforts are the sine qua non. The lack of desire associated with specialized muscular development is the natural means to protect the body from being severely damaged. This condition of existence is unfavorable for the development of a high order of mental life. The energy and concentration required for it are not sufficient in this state. This is why in many an instance we find men who have attained a high degree of physical development without a corresponding mental development. These instances certainly do not prove that physical development is antagonistic to mental development or that physical education is detrimental to mental life. Physical development and physical education are not

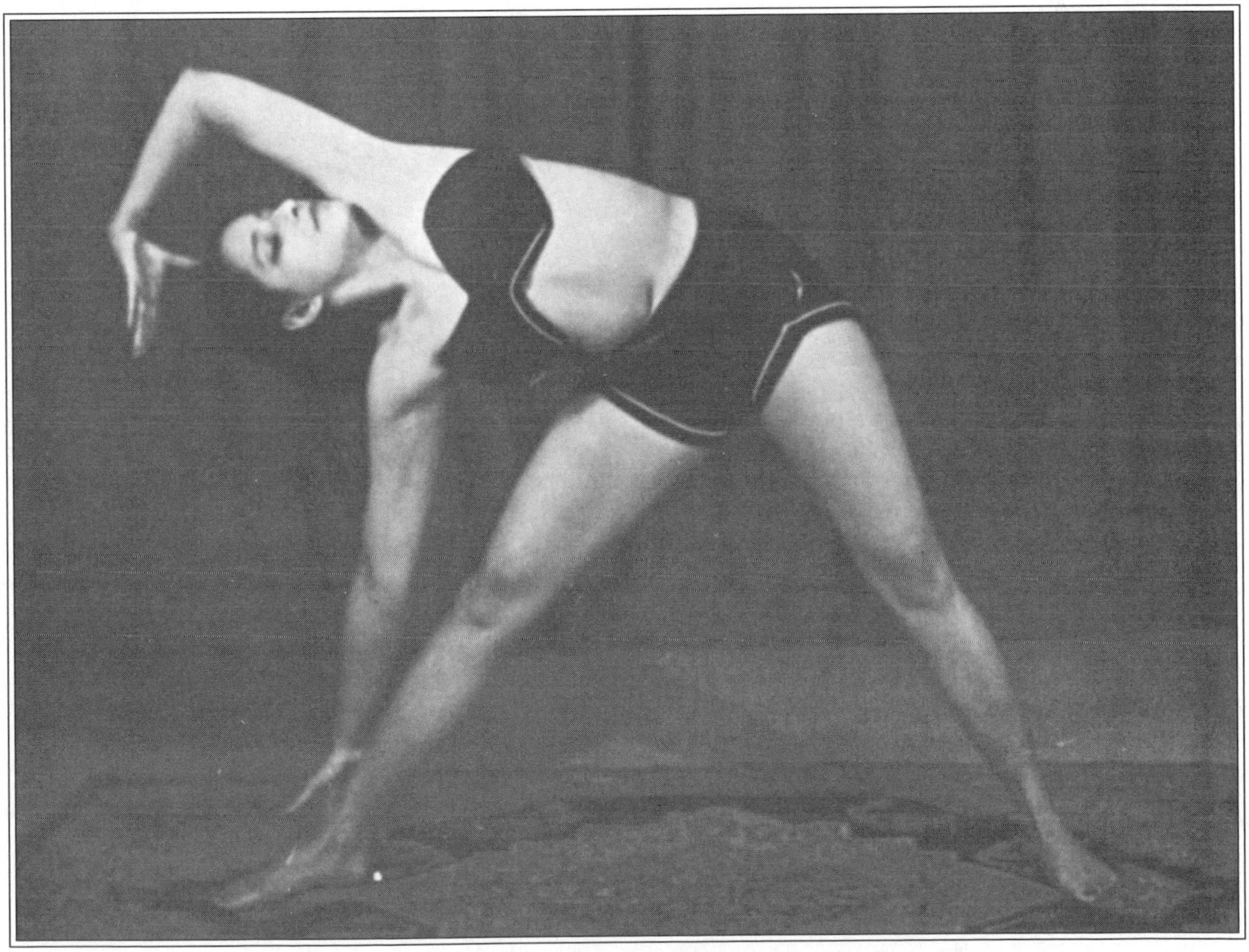

Fig. 3.6. Flexibility and grace in a symmetrically developed body. Posed by Leela Ghosh

responsible for underdeveloped mental faculties. Rather they are caused by a lack of proper understanding and an approach that is neither physiologically nor psychologically correct, resulting in an overemphasis on muscles.

It is true that our human specialty lies more in our mental life, especially in our full manifestation of higher mental powers. Human development will be hopelessly impeded if we create an artificial state of the body by wrong application of physical education in which mental life is sacrificed, to a great extent, for physical specialization. Then the body is unable to play its proper role in mental life. The body needs to take part in exhibiting mental and spiritual activities.

On the other hand, we should not forget that the body is indispensable to the mind and its activities. In a well-developed mental life, thoughts and attitudes, as well as actions and behaviors, are molded into a definite form, indicating a close relationship between the physical and mental life. The functional efficiency of the bodily organs plays a part in shaping mental activities. The vital organs, the endocrine organs, the blood, the nervous system, the muscles, all have to play definite parts in the functioning of the mind. So the state of the body cannot be overlooked in mental life.

There are, of course, cases in which a giant mind dwells in a frail body. The thought-machine is an exceptionally efficient machine, which is able to maintain its functional power even under very unfavorable conditions. But this does not prove that physical health and development are unconnected to or unnecessary for mental development. Bodily negligence should not be encouraged for the glorification of the mind by picking out exceptional cases.

A careful analysis of such cases discloses many interesting and instructive facts. First, a large number of such people are not actually physically inferior; rather they are above the average. However, their physical vigor is usually overlooked, because they do not happen to show it through appreciably increased muscular growth. There is also a slender type of person in whom great muscular development does not take place. But such people may not actually lack vitality. The slenderness of many vigorous people may also be due to their extremely abstemious habits of eating and living. There are also people who are constitutionally vigorous by birth, who utilize their congenital advantage in developing the mind alone, neglecting the body. They may do well up to a certain age, then begin to show signs of mental sluggishness, with diminution of health and vigor. These mental giants ultimately become the victims of various chronic diseases, and their minds also become dull.

Gautama the Buddha, the great spiritual teacher and founder of Buddhism, developed his body by regular exercise. His well-developed and vital body was not antagonistic to his spiritual awakening and realization of the invisible higher reality. It is erroneous to suppose that the Bible does not approve of physical education and that Jesus was a weakling. Jesus Christ kept his body healthy, vigorous, and clean by physical exercise and mental and physical disciplines, and by leading a simple and well-controlled life. He worked hard in his younger days in Joseph's carpenter shop, which helped to strengthen his body. He walked long distances, up and down hills, day after day when preaching his gospel. Says St. Paul: "Know ye not that ye are the temple of God? If any man defile the temple of God, him shall God destroy, for the temple of God is holy, which temple ye are. Therefore glorify God in your body."

The type of muscular development in which the mind is ignored is not encouraged in Haṭha Yoga, which in fact aims at developing a balanced type of body, not a specialized type. The necessity of keeping the body full of vitality, healthy, strong, and purified for higher spiritual achievements has been fully recognized in Yoga.

Health Level of Physical Development

The aim of physical education in Yoga is the level of development that is associated with a high degree of vital vigor, enabling the body to perform all activities of daily life with ease and efficiency and for a prolonged period when necessary, to accumulate plenty of reserve force, to mobilize bodily resources to the maximum degree, and to endure a heavy expenditure without unhealthful effects on the organism. The amount of muscle tissue that is actually needed or associated with this type of physical development is developed by Yoga exercise. As the body functions organically most efficiently in this state, thus maintaining perfect health, this is what we call the "health level of physical development."

In this condition of the body, strength, speed, and endurance are developed into a balanced state. There is sufficient strength to maintain all activities of daily life, plus various other activities requiring strength to a reasonable extent. There is sufficient endurance to be able to carry out activities for a prolonged period. Vital endurance is associated with it, which enables the body to endure lack of food, sleep, and other privations and inclemency of weather. Bodily movements are usually easy, graceful, and well-controlled. There is power to execute nonlocomotor and locomotor movements reasonably swiftly. The muscle mass is in proportion to the physical development, and the body is muscularly beautiful and symmetrical.

In this state of the body the healthful functioning of the vital organs is not interrupted by the factors associated with muscular development. The body is in balance with the internal organs and the muscles. The figures in this chapter show the health level of physical development, both masculine and feminine, attained through Yoga exercise, combined with right diet, internal cleansing, relaxation, and concentration.

This state of the body is the most suitable for the actualization of mental powers. Under this condition the energy of the body is wasted neither in overcoming the conditions that disturb health nor in attaining too much physical specialization, but is reserved and rightly utilized for mental development. This is a state—a balanced state—in which intellectual, contemplative, organic, and muscular powers are developed harmoniously.

After successful attainment of the health level of physical development, further physical development may be attempted if desired without sacrificing the established balanced condition. This requires specialized training. If this training does not cause any disturbance in the vital functioning of the body nor prove to be unsuitable for intellectual and contemplative life, it may be undertaken. But if the time devoted to the special training, the type and amount of exercise necessary for that purpose, the type of diet, amount of sleep, and other alterations of living associated with it create a condition in which the balance between the muscles and the rest of the body and between the body and the mind is difficult to maintain, the specialization should be sacrificed in favor of balanced development.

Health is a state of the organism in which all organs function uninterruptedly and vigorously and in full cooperation with one another to support longer survival and the best development of the body, enabling a person to express his or her best through intellectual, moral, spiritual, and physical activities. A vital body and a dynamic mind are intimately associated with vital health. When health is established, the body becomes a fitter machine, more enduring, more powerful, better developed, and better controlled; the mind becomes more vigorous, more imaginative, better balanced, and more contemplative; and the emotions become more normalized and spiritualized.

Vital Endurance

The state of health is associated with the maintenance of the organic state of the body at a certain level of constancy normal to an individual in spite of the unceasing influence of extremely diverse and intense—and often very unfavorable—changes in the environment. This organic state is the result of the adaptive functions of the body in which all the functional systems take part through their incessant, but purposeful and methodical, activities. When the activities of the functional systems reach a certain level and are most successfully balanced between themselves and in relation to the steady organic state, vital endurance of the body is fully activated, resulting in natural healthfulness, increased natural disease-resisting power, and life extension.

To maintain the desired level of organic functioning most suitable for health, all of the activities of the nervous, glandular, circulatory, respiratory, alimentary, eliminative, and muscular systems need to be efficiently integrated. Abnormal activities of the functional systems and their disharmony are mainly caused by adopting a mode of life that is not properly adjusted to the organism. Various unsuitable environmental conditions also influence the functional systems adversely.

Vital endurance is congenital as well as acquired. Inherent endurance may be very much modified by an unsuitable mode of life. On the other hand, a suitable mode of life increases vital endurance.

Patterns of Thoughts and Actions

Our mode of life is actually an expression of our thoughts and actions, which influence the activities of the functional systems. The patterns of thoughts are molded by a mixture of spiritual, intellectual, emotional, and organic factors in varying proportions characteristic of an individual. Actions are manifested thoughts.

The patterns of thoughts and actions that are associated with alimentary excesses, artificial hungers, unhealthful sexual activities and inhibitions, greed, and various debilitating habits are coarse in character, obstructive to harmony and deep thinking, and cause disturbances in the organic functions. A mode of life based on such types of thoughts and actions is unsuitable for a person's optimum development. The only way to counteract the deleterious effects of such a life is to introduce some discipline in which thoughts and actions are molded into a new pattern through regulations, privations, and activations that are most suitable for establishing the vital health level of the body. In Yoga this is done through *yama, niyama,* and various exercises.

Role of Muscular Exercise

Muscular exercise plays a most important role in controlling and bringing the activities of all the functional systems to a desired level by properly utilizing the muscular-organic relations existing from the birth of muscle and developed in succeeding stages. The most fruitful approach is made through the fundamental musculature by raising its action level to a certain height through measured movements of definite patterns in which the muscles and other functional systems are in perfect balance. This we may call the body's health-level actions. Vital endurance and natural disease-resisting power are fully developed in this state of the body.

In Yoga the fundamental movements have taken the specific form of spinal, abdominal, and thoracic-diaphragmatic movements applied both statically and dynamically to effectively nurture the organic state of the body in which the health-level is most satisfactorily established. This type of exercise is not so much for muscular specialization but for natural healthfulness and immunity. Specialization, if desired, can be carried so far as it is possible without breaking the harmony between it and the health level.

4

Practical Application of Yoga Exercise

The dynamic form of posture exercise is really the first stage of Yoga exercise, which promotes health and development of the body. It also prepares the body, through the development of the degree of strength, endurance, and flexibility required for the perfection and control of a posture pattern, for the successful practice of static posture exercise. Static posture exercise is the advanced form of Yoga exercise designed for developing vital endurance to a high level, and making the body most suitable for concentration.

Time for Exercise

The afternoon or evening (before dinner) is the best time to practice dynamic posture exercise for developmental purposes. The next best time for developmental exercise is three or four hours after breakfast. If these times are not available, developmental exercise may be done in the early morning (before breakfast). The early morning is the most suitable time for breath-control exercise and static posture exercise. Constitutional exercise may be done in the morning before or after breakfast or in the evening.

If posture exercise is done in the evening, constitutional exercises may be done either before or after breakfast. If posture exercise is done in the morning, constitutional exercise may be done in the evening. When posture exercise is done both in the morning and evening (as, for example, static exercise in the morning and dynamic exercise in the evening), constitutional exercise may be done after breakfast or at any other suitable time. You should rest for an hour or at least thirty minutes, after exercise, before eating a meal.

Occupation and Exercise

If the muscles are hardly used at all in a given occupation, all the muscles of the body should be adequately used in general posture exercise. If certain groups of muscles are especially used in a particular occupation, they should be moderately exercised by posture exercise and the unused muscles should be adequately exercised. If the occupation is light, heavier forms of exercise should be performed and vice versa.

Health Condition and Exercise

The form and amount of exercise depend to a very great extent upon the health of the person doing the exercise. If you are in poor health, you should begin with a lighter form of exercise; if you are strong, begin with a heavier form. If you are weak and your work is heavy, it is good for you to stop work and do light exercise until some improvement in your health takes place. If it is not possible to stop work, it may be advisable for you to do only some light constitutional exercise. Generally, it is better for a person of poor health to start with some suitable form of constitutional exercise till his or her overall health condition improves.

When Exercise Is Contraindicated

You should not exercise when tired, for then you need rest. You should not exercise when nervously depleted, for then all your organs have been overworked and you need rest. Exercise should be avoided when there is inflammation and any acute disease.

During an acute disease the body tries to eliminate the excess of accumulated poisons by increasing the functional activities of all the eliminative organs to a maximum degree. The body needs all available energy for this purpose alone, and nothing can be spared for exercise or even digesting food. Also the nerve energy during this period is more or less depleted. Furthermore, during this period the body does not need to be stimulated by exercise, for the functional activities have been sufficiently accelerated.

Exercise is usually contraindicated at the beginning stage of tuberculosis, gastric and intestinal ulcers, polyneuritis, high blood pressure, severe heart disease, and dropsy. Exercise should not be done when you are injured. In the case of strain and sprain, especially at their acute stage, exercise should be stopped.

Exercise and Age

Muscular exercise is necessary not only for adults, but at all ages from birth to death. Of course, certain types of exercise are more suited and beneficial at one age than at another. The following suggestion may be helpful:

1st year—spontaneous movements; some play exercise.

2nd to 5th year—walking; running; various forms of games.

6th to 9th year—walking; running; games; deep breathing exercise; light dynamic posture exercise; correct posture and easier folded-leg postures (only to be assumed for a brief period).

10th to 12th year—walking; running; jumping; throwing; swimming; dancing; light dynamic posture exercise; deep breathing; correct posture; practice of folded-leg postures.

13th to 16th year—walking; running and all other forms of speed-endurance exercise; breath-control exercise; correct posture; light developmental dynamic posture exercise; practice of folded-leg postures.

17th to 30th year—all forms of constitutional exercise; breath-control exercise; heavy developmental dynamic posture exercise; static posture exercise.

31st to 40th year—same as for 17th to 30th year, with slight modifications, if necessary, according to individual health conditions.

41st to 50th year—same as 31st to 40th year, slight modifications, if necessary; distance walking.

51st to 60th year—all constitutional exercise (modified, if necessary); light and medium developmental dynamic posture exercise; static posture exercise; breath-control exercise; distance walking.

61st year and up—the amount and form of exercise should be entirely governed by the condition of the muscles, internal organs, and general health. If the body has been maintained in perfect health by previous healthy living habits, developmental and constitutional exercise, static exercise, and breath-control exercise should be continued, perhaps with modified doses. Distance walking is especially beneficial.

Exercise for Females

Alluring feminine beauty cannot be artificially made. Beauty cannot be expressed in a pimpled face, wrinkled eyes, and an emaciated or corpulent body. Soap, cream, powder, rouge, and garments cannot hide an underdeveloped and unappealing body. Ideally, feminine beauty lies in facial beauty combined with a symmetrically developed body. The attainment of a certain size of muscles together with a certain amount of fat, giving the body a beautiful shape, contour, curves, and vigorous health, are indispensable factors of beauty. Exercise, nutritious diet, internal cleanliness, and other health-building measures are factors of health and efficiency as well as of beauty.

Dynamic posture exercise, both for health-building and developmental purposes, is equally applicable to females and males, but to some extent the forms should be modified for females. These modifications, of course, depend upon individual constitution, strength, age, requirements. Static posture exercise is quite suitable for females. Breath-control exercise should be prescribed. Even Abdominal Retraction and Straight Muscle Exercise have proven to be very beneficial. Generally all forms of constitutional exercise, slightly modified, can be prescribed. Walking, swimming, and dancing should be an important part of a female exercise program.

Exercise during Menstruation

Exercise is generally omitted during menstruation. There are, of course, many healthy women who do not find any difficulty in continuing exercise during this time. However, it is best to stop heavy developmental posture exercise, inverse body posture exercise, balance posture exercise, Abdominal Retraction, and Straight Muscle Exercise. Breath-control exercise, folded-leg postures, walking, and other milder forms of constitutional exercise can be practiced.

In cases of profuse menstruation, exercise should be stopped. Proper exercise should be taken between periods. Swimming should be avoided.

Bathing

In the morning a brief cold bath is very healthful, taken either before or after morning exercise. After heavy exercise in the evening, a cold bath should be taken. After vigorous exercise, it is better to rest for a few minutes before bathing to give the heart and lungs an opportunity to return to their normal condition. It is best to rinse off perspiration first with a warm shower, followed by a cold shower or cold bath with vigorous friction with the hands. After a bath you should be able to dress without drying yourself, if the reactive power is good. Otherwise dry the body with a dry, coarse towel, and finish with a dry friction bath, then dress. Then drink a glass or two of cold water and take rest.

A warm bath, followed by a cold bath, should be taken once a week. A sweating bath is highly beneficial if taken periodically. The sweating bath should always be followed by a cold bath. A tepid or neutral immersion bath taken once or twice a week is excellent. It helps relaxation, equalizes circulation, and removes stiffness of the muscles and joints.

Sunbathing should be done regularly. It promotes muscular growth, improves muscle tone, and makes the muscles firm. Very satisfactory results are obtained if some constitutional exercise is combined with sunbathing and getting fresh air.

Mental Factor

A proper mental attitude is absolutely necessary for maintaining perfect health and a high degree of efficiency. Negative mental states lower the vitality, interfere with the normal functions of the vital organs, lower the disease-resisting power, and decrease the nerve power.

Cultivate a hopeful, cheerful, and calm attitude of mind. Have self-reliance, determination, courage, and patience. Sweeten your emotional life by carefully managing the normal and appropriate expression of emotion. Spiritual awakening will help you the most in brightening emotion, and in attaining a greater, nobler, grander, clearer, and purer mind and a better, stronger, healthier, cleaner, and fresher body. Fear, depression, worry, sorrow, and other morbid conditions can best be controlled by spiritual strength combined with the normalization of the body.

Do not allow your mind to stagnate, for it stops the creation of mental energy. Try to develop the power of clear and deep thinking. The practice of concentration and breath-control exercise will help you most.

Relaxation

Conscious relaxation is a state in which the mind becomes free from desires, agitations, and thoughts, and the body still. It is not sleep, but a mental and physical inactive state brought about consciously. On the mental side, relaxation makes the mind clear and develops thinking power, concentration, and greater power of control over the mind. On the physical side, it prevents unnecessary and excessive energy expenditure and nervous and muscular tensions. If it is practiced during exercise, it helps to delay the onset of fatigue and oxygen debt. When it is practiced after exercise it removes the tired feeling and gives freshness to body and mind.

Though relaxation is a condition in which all efforts cease, the mind becomes fully calm, and the body motionless, certain conscious effort needs to be applied in a definite manner at the preliminary stages to make the mind and the body quite still. The so-called Corpse Posture, lying flat on the back, face upward, arms by the sides, is the best posture for relaxation. First of all, assume a most comfortable position. Now withdraw the flow of consciousness from the body as much as possible, keeping it absolutely motionless. Then try to make the mind inactive by thinking no thoughts, making it more and more void. By systematic practice success will be attained.

Relaxation should also be practiced in Prone-Lying Posture, Standing Posture, and all folded-leg postures. Brief relaxation should be practiced between exercises. Prolonged relaxation should be practiced in Corpse Posture after completion of an exercise. It is highly beneficial to practice relaxation after any prolonged physical or mental work, any time of the day, if so desired, and on retiring.

5

Dynamic Application of Posture Exercise

The development value of dynamic posture exercise depends entirely upon the principle of graduation. It operates in two ways: gradually increasing the degree of muscular contraction and gradually increasing the number of repetitions.

Graduated Contraction Method

The secret of muscular development lies in the execution of movements in a manner that requires powerful contraction of the muscles in which an increasing number of muscle cells are employed. At the first stage the strength of the muscle cells is very small. Therefore, at this stage a light form of movement is enough to adequately stimulate the muscles and to develop their size and strength. But as the muscles gradually become stronger, light exercise becomes insufficient to stimulate and employ a growing number of muscle fibers in the movement. At this stage exercise should be heavy enough to cause a greater number of fibers to be employed during contraction of the muscles.

The repetition of light exercise many times will not serve this purpose. In this circumstance, before the stimuli spread to the inactive fibers, the fibers that had been previously employed will be fatigued and yet compelled to move, causing depletion of their store of potential energy. Moreover, after a certain point, light exercise does not create a demand for greater contraction, which is associated with muscular development. The most favorable condition for proper muscular development is created when most of the fibers of the muscles are involved during contraction and a maximum blood supply to the contracted muscles is caused. This can only be done by the application of a graduated contraction method.

In Haṭha Yoga neither instrument nor the body pressure of another person (as in wrestling) are used in exercise to apply resistance to the muscles in a graduated manner. Here two methods have been adopted: voluntary-full-contraction method and posture-contraction method. In the voluntary-full-contraction method, a voluntary effort is made to contract the muscles under movement as fully as possible, the movement being executed in positions most favorable for full contraction. This type of exercise is included in contraction exercise.

The posture-contraction method consists of assuming different postures, stage by stage, in which the muscles undergo contraction in a graduated manner, from light to heavy. When voluntary full contraction and posture contraction are properly combined in exercise, the most satisfactory results are obtained.

Posture-Contraction Method

For the proper development of muscles posture exercise has been evolved and the exercises are so systematically arranged as to cause contraction of a particular group of muscles in a graduated manner. Each posture exercise is so devised as to cause a desired degree of contraction.

For the sake of convenience, we may divide contraction into three grades: light contraction, medium contraction, and great contraction. In light contraction a comparatively small number of fibers in a muscle are brought into play. In medium contraction a large number of fibers are involved, whereas in great contraction most of the fibers take part in the exercise. Certain posture exercises cause light contraction, certain others medium contraction, while the rest cause great contraction. Therefore posture exercises may be labeled as light-contraction posture exercise, medium-contraction posture exercise, and great-contraction posture exercise.

When the muscles are not rightly exercised and their strength is at a low level, light-contraction posture exercise will successfully train and strengthen the inefficient and inactive muscle cells and a certain stage of development will be reached. In fact, at this stage, the medium- and great-contraction posture exercises are unsuitable. After the initial development is attained, light-contraction posture exercise becomes inadequate to stimulate the muscle properly and cause a sufficient number of muscle cells to be employed. At this stage medium-contraction posture exercise is indicated. Again a stage of development will be reached when the great-contraction posture exercise is to be applied for still further development. The main point in dynamic posture exercise is the arrangement of the posture exercises in a graduated manner in order to cause, stage by stage, light, medium, and finally great contraction in the muscles.

Repetition Factor

The gradually increasing number of repetitions of movements is also an essential part of the principle of graduation. No grade of contraction posture exercise will be fruitful unless it is repeated in a definite and graduated manner. For the sake of convenience, the repetition factor maybe divided into low repetition, medium repetition, high repetition, and very high repetition. The usual range of low repetition is from 5 to 12 times, of medium repetition from 6 to 18 times, of high repetition from 10 to 30, and of very high repetition from 24 to 50 times.

The number of repetitions also depends upon the grades of exercise. Light-contraction posture exercise requires high repetition, medium-contraction posture exercise requires medium repetition, and great-contraction posture exercise requires low repetition. On the other hand, if it is necessary to make the exercise heavy enough to bring about the desired results, high repetition may be applied for medium-contraction posture exercise and medium-repetition for great-contraction posture exercise. Great-contraction posture exercise becomes very heavy when high repetition is applied. In certain exercises and in exceptional cases very high repetition is necessary.

The number of movements, from the beginning to the maximum number, should be increased in a definite order. The following order is usually adopted.

INCREASING LOW REPETITIONS

Interval	Number of Repetitions
1st week	5
2nd to 7th week	add 1 every week
8th week	12

Points of Note: Sometimes it may be necessary to continue with the same number of movements for two weeks instead of one. It depends upon individual constitution, strength, endurance, age, sex. It may also be necessary to modify the number in certain cases.

INCREASING MEDIUM REPETITIONS

Interval	Number of Repetitions
Order A	
1st week	6
2nd to 6th week	add 2 every week
7th week	18
Order B	
1st week	6
2nd to 12th week	add 1 every week
13th week	18

Points of Note: Order A is for stronger students. However, a certain number of repetitions can be maintained longer than indicated by the table, if required. Everything depends upon the constitution, strength, endurance, age, gender, and so on, of the students. It may also be necessary to alter the number in each order in certain cases.

INCREASING HIGH REPETITIONS

Interval	Number of Repetitions
Order A	
1st week	10
2nd to 10th week	add 2 every week
11th week	30
Order B	
1st week	10
2nd to 20th week	add 1 every week
21st week	30

Points of Note: Same as for medium repetitions.

INCREASING VERY HIGH REPETITIONS

Interval	Number of Repetitions
Order A	
1st week	24
2nd to 13th week	add 2 every week
14th week	50
Order B	
1st week	24
2nd to 26th week	add 1 every week
27th week	50

Points of Note: Same as for medium repetitions.

Classification of Specific Posture Exercises

In this section, each type of dynamic posture exercise is categorized. Later chapters in the book provide detailed instruction on the performance of the exercises. Please refer to the index to locate the instructions. Here, the specific postures are listed according to light, medium, and great contraction. Even the exercises of the same contraction type may be different and graded. Within each category, the exercises are listed in an ascending order, with each exercise in the list requiring greater contraction or flexibility than the previous one. In certain cases, however, the same amount of contraction is required. In that case, the posture exercises are listed with a "+" sign between them.

Dynamic Posterior Trunk-Bend Posture Exercise

▶ **Light-Contraction Posterior Trunk-Bend Posture Exercise:**

Cobra Posture (fig. 12.1)
Modified Locust Posture (see page 111)
Cuckoo Posture (fig. 12.9)

▶ **Medium-Contraction Posterior Trunk-Bend Posture Exercise:**

Snake Posture (fig. 12.2)
Locust Posture (fig. 12.4)
Back-Raise Posture with Hands Clasped behind Head (see page 110)
Bow Posture (fig. 12.5)
Boat Posture (fig. 12.6)
Swing Posture (fig. 12.7)
Raised Bow Posture (fig. 12.10)
Modified Wheel Posture (fig. 12.12)

▶ **Great-Contraction Posterior Trunk-Bend Posture Exercise:**

Back-Raise Posture with Forearms Locked behind Head (fig. 12.3)
Bent-Head Adamantine Posture (fig. 12.11)
King-Cobra Posture (fig. 12.8)
Back Posture (fig. 12.13)
Wheel Posture (fig. 12.14)

▶ **Gradation of Exercise**

Exercise may be graded stage by stage according to the following plan:

Stage 1 (in ascending order)

Cobra Posture
Cuckoo Posture
Snake Posture
Back-Raise Posture with Hands Clasped behind Head
Back-Raise Posture with Forearms Locked behind Head
King-Cobra Posture

Stage 2 (in ascending order)

Modified Locust Posture
Locust Posture
Bow Posture
Raised Bow Posture
Boat Posture
Swing Posture
King-Cobra Posture

Stage 3 (in ascending order)

Raised Bow Posture
Modified Wheel Posture
Bent-Head Adamantine Posture
Back Posture
Wheel Posture

Dynamic Anterior Trunk-Bend Posture Exercise

▶ **Light-Contraction Anterior Trunk-Bend Posture Exercise:**

Spinal-Stretch Posture (fig. 12.15)
Head-Knee Posture (fig. 12.16)
Foot-Hand Posture (fig. 12.21)

▶ **Medium-Contraction Anterior Trunk-Bend Posture Exercise:**

Head-Bend Lotus Posture (fig. 12.19)
Forward Head-Bend Posture (fig. 12.17)

▶ **Great-Contraction Anterior Trunk-Bend Posture Exercise:**

Head-Bend Posture (fig. 12.18)
Forward Body-Bend Posture (fig. 12.20)

▶ **Gradation of Exercise:**

Spinal-Stretch Posture
Foot-Hand Posture
Head-Knee Posture
Head-Bend Lotus Posture
Forward Head-Bend Posture
Head-Bend Posture
Forward Body-Bend Posture

Dynamic Lateral Trunk-Bend Posture Exercise

▶ **Light-Contraction Lateral Trunk-Bend Posture Exercise:**

Half-Moon Posture (fig. 12.22)

▶ **Medium-Contraction Lateral Trunk-Bend Posture Exercise:**

Hip-Bend Posture (fig. 12.23)

▶ **Great-Contraction Lateral Trunk-Bend Posture Exercise:**

Moon Posture (fig. 12.24)

▶ **Gradation of Exercise:**

Half-Moon Posture
Hip-Bend Posture
Moon Posture

Dynamic Trunk-Twist Posture Exercise

▶ **Light-Contraction Trunk-Twist Posture Exercise:**

Twist Posture (fig. 12.25)

▶ **Medium-Contraction Trunk-Twist Posture Exercise:**

Modified Spinal-Twist Posture (fig. 12.26)
Ankle-Hold Modified Spinal-Twist Posture (figs. 12.27 and 12.28)

▶ **Great-Contraction Trunk-Twist Posture Exercise:**

Spinal-Twist Posture (fig. 12.29)
Sideward Head-Bend Posture (fig. 12.31)

▶ **Gradation of Exercise:**

Twist Posture
Modified Spinal-Twist Posture
Ankle-Hold Modified Spinal-Twist Posture
Sideward Head-Bend Posture
Spinal-Twist Posture

Dynamic Neck Posture Exercise

▶ **Light-Contraction Neck Posture Exercise:**

Neck Flexion-Extension
Neck Rotation (see page 137)
Lateral Neck Flexion (see page 137)

▶ **Medium-Contraction Neck Posture Exercise:**

Neck Posture (fig. 13.1)

▶ **Great-Contraction Neck Posture Exercise:**

Neck-Bridge Posture (fig. 13.2)

▶ **Gradation of Exercise:**

Neck Flexion-Extension + Neck Rotation + Lateral Neck Flexion
Neck Posture
Neck-Bridge Posture

Reminder: The "+" mark indicates that the three exercises are of the same contraction type but each of them is intended either to exercise the neck muscles in different manners or to exercise different muscles brought into play.

Dynamic Anterior Trunk-Raise Posture Exercise

▶ **Light-Contraction Anterior Trunk-Raise Posture Exercise:**

Spine Posture (fig. 14.1)

▶ **Medium-Contraction Anterior Trunk-Raise Posture Exercise:**

Spine Posture with Hands Clasped behind Head (fig. 14.2)

▶ **Great-Contraction Anterior Trunk-Raise Posture Exercise:**

Spine Posture with Forearms Locked behind Head (fig. 14.3)
Risen Balance Posture (fig. 14.4)

▶ **Gradation of Exercise:**

Spine Posture
Spine Posture with Hands Clasped behind Head
Spine Posture with Forearms Locked behind Head
Risen Balance Posture

Dynamic Oblique Trunk-Raise Posture Exercise

▶ **Light-Contraction Oblique Trunk-Raise Posture Exercise:**

Oblique Spine Posture (fig. 14.5)

▶ **Medium-Contraction Oblique Trunk-Raise Posture Exercise:**

Oblique Spine Posture with Hands Clasped behind Head (fig. 14.6)

▶ **Great-Contraction Oblique Trunk-Raise Posture Exercise:**

Oblique Spine Posture with Forearms Locked behind Head (fig. 14.7)

▶ **Gradation of Exercise:**

Oblique Spine Posture
Oblique Spine Posture with Hands Clasped behind Head
Oblique Spine Posture with Forearms Locked behind Head

Dynamic Lateral Trunk-Raise Posture Exercise

▶ **Light-Contraction Lateral Trunk-Raise Posture Exercise:**

Lateral Spine Posture (when performed with legs supported and raised only partially) (see page 147)

▶ **Medium-Contraction Lateral Trunk-Raise Posture Exercise:**

Lateral Spine Posture (when performed with legs supported) (see page 147)

▶ **Great-Contraction Lateral Trunk-Raise Posture Exercise:**

Lateral Spine Posture (fig. 14.8)

▶ **Gradation of Exercise:**

Lateral Spine Posture (with legs supported and raised partially)
Lateral Spine Posture (with legs supported)
Lateral Spine Posture

Dynamic Pelvis-Raise Posture Exercise

▶ **Light-Contraction Pelvis-Raise Posture Exercise:**

Plow Posture (fig. 14.9)
Ear-Pressing Posture (fig. 14.11)

▶ **Medium-Contraction Pelvis-Raise Posture Exercise:**

Plow Posture with Forearms Locked behind Head (fig. 14.10)

▶ **Great-Contraction Pelvis-Raise Posture Exercise:**

Risen Back Posture (fig. 14.12)
Lotus-Plow Posture (fig. 14.13)

▶ **Gradation of Exercise:**

Plow Posture + Ear-Pressing Posture
Plow Posture with Forearms Locked behind Head
Risen Back Posture
Lotus-Plow Posture

Dynamic Leg-Raise Posture Exercise

▶ **Light-Contraction Leg-Raise Posture Exercise:**

Single Risen Leg Posture (see page 153)

▶ **Medium-Contraction Leg-Raise Posture Exercise:**

Sideward Leg-Motion Posture (fig. 14.15)
Right-Angle Leg Posture (fig. 14.16)

▶ **Great-Contraction Leg-Raise Posture Exercise:**

Risen Leg Posture (fig. 14.14)

▶ **Gradation of Exercise:**

Single Risen Leg Posture
Sideward Leg-Motion Posture
Right-Angle Leg Posture
Risen Leg Posture

Dynamic Anterior Trunk Leg-Raise Posture Exercise

▶ **Light-Contraction Anterior Trunk Leg-Raise Posture Exercise:**

Head-Knee Spine Posture (fig. 14.17)

▶ **Medium-Contraction Anterior Trunk Leg-Raise Posture Exercise:**

Knee-Touching Spine Posture (fig. 14.18)

▶ **Great-Contraction Anterior Trunk Leg-Raise Posture Exercise:**

Pillow Posture (fig. 14.19)

▶ **Gradation of Exercise:**

Head-Knee Spine Posture
Knee-Touching Spine Posture
Pillow Posture

Dynamic Lateral Trunk Leg-Raise Posture Exercise

▶ **Light-Contraction Lateral Trunk Leg-Raise Posture Exercise:**

Toe-Hold Lateral Spine Posture (performed with the support of the disengaged arm and raised only partially) (see page 159)

▶ **Medium-Contraction Lateral Trunk Leg-Raise Posture Exercise:**

Toe-Hold Lateral Spine Posture (performed with the partial support of the disengaged arm and raised fully) (see page 159)

▶ **Great-Contraction Lateral Trunk Leg-Raise Posture Exercise:**

Toe-Hold Lateral Spine Posture (fig. 14.20)

▸ **Gradation of Exercise:**

Toe-Hold Lateral Spine Posture (with full arm support and raised partially)

Toe-Hold Lateral Spine Posture (with partial arm support and raised fully)

Toe-Hold Lateral Spine Posture

Dynamic Pelvic Posture Exercise

▸ **Light-Contraction Pelvic Posture Exercise:**

Pelvis-Raise Posture (fig. 15.1)

Arm-Head Posture (fig. 15.2)

▸ **Medium-Contraction Pelvic Posture Exercise:**

Single Foot-Head Posture (fig. 15.3)

Single Foot-Head Head-Knee Posture (fig. 15.5)

▸ **Great-Contraction Pelvic Posture Exercise:**

One-Leg Pillar Posture (fig. 15.6)

Pillar Posture (fig. 15.7)

Double Foot-Head Posture (fig. 15.4)

Noose Posture (fig. 15.8)

▸ **Gradation of Exercise:**

Pelvis-Raise Posture

Arm-Head Posture

Single Foot-Head Posture

Single Foot-Head Head-Knee Posture

Double Foot-Head Posture

Noose Posture supplemented by One-Leg Pillar Posture

Pillar Posture

Dynamic Pectoral Limb Posture Exercise

▸ **Light-Contraction Pectoral Limb Posture Exercise:**

Risen Lotus Posture (fig. 16.1)

Four-Point Posture (fig. 16.4)

Arm Motion (fig. 16.9)

▸ **Medium-Contraction Pectoral Limb Posture Exercise:**

Cock Posture (fig. 16.2)

Three-Footed Posture (fig. 16.5)

▸ **Great-Contraction Pectoral Limb Posture Exercise:**

One-Arm Cock Posture (fig. 16.3)

Arm-Leg Posture (fig. 16.6)

Opposite Arm-Leg Posture (fig. 16.7)

Arm Posture (fig. 16.8)

▸ **Gradation of Exercise:**

Stage 1 (in ascending order)

Risen Lotus Posture

Cock Posture

One-Arm Cock Posture

Stage 2 (in ascending order)

Four-Point Posture + Arm Motion

Three-Footed Posture

Arm-Leg Posture

Opposite Arm-Leg Posture

Arm Posture

Dynamic Pelvic Limb Posture Exercise

▸ **Light-Contraction Pelvic Limb Posture Exercise:**

Toe Posture (fig. 17.7)

Thigh Posture (fig. 17.1)

Knee-Touching Thigh Posture (fig. 17.2)

▸ **Medium-Contraction Pelvic Limb Posture Exercise:**

Feet-Extending Thigh Posture (fig. 17.3)

Sideward Feet-Extending Thigh Posture (fig. 17.4)

- **Great-Contraction Pelvic Limb Posture Exercise:**

  One-Legged Toe Posture (fig. 17.8)
  Leg-Raise Thigh Posture (fig. 17.5)
  One-Legged Squat Posture (fig. 17.6)

- **Gradation of Exercise:**

  Stage 1 (in ascending order)
  Toe Posture—One-Legged Toe Posture

  Stage 2 (in ascending order)
  Thigh Posture
  Knee-Touching Thigh Posture
  Feet-Extending Thigh Posture
  Sideward Feet-Extending Thigh Posture
  Leg-Raise Thigh Posture
  One-Legged Squat Posture

Abdominal Retraction (Uḍḍīyāna)

There are two repetition methods for Abdominal Retraction. One is to maintain the retraction as long as the breath is suspended. Then the abdomen should be relaxed along with inhalation. Then the whole process should be repeated.

The second method consists of performing the retraction movement from 5 to 10 times (or more) in one suspension of breath. This is one round. Each retraction should be executed quickly, but should be complete. In this work the second method has been adopted.

REPETITION METHOD

Week		Repetitions
1st week:	2 rounds (10 in each round)	= 20
2nd week	4 rounds (10 in each round)	= 40
3rd week	6 rounds (10 in each round)	= 60
4th week	8 rounds (10 in each round)	= 80
5th week	10 rounds (10 in each round)	= 100

Points of Note: Maintain 100 times until it becomes quite easy. Then gradually increase—one round a week or in two weeks or more, depending upon the condition—until 500 times are reached.

Straight Muscle Exercise (Naulī)

The following is the repetition method:

SECTION 1 REPETITIONS

Week	Central Isolation
1st week	10
2nd week	20
3rd week	30
4th week	40
5th week	50
6th week	60
7th week	70
8th week	80
9th week	90
10th week	100

SECTION 2 REPETITIONS

Week	Central	Right	Left
1st week	100	10	10
2nd week	110	15	15
3rd week	120	20	20
4th week	130	25	25
5th week	140	30	30
6th week	150	35	35
7th week	160	40	40
8th week	170	45	45
9th week	180	50	50
10th week	190	50	50
11th week	200	50	50

Points of Note: The number of repetitions may be modified according to the condition of the student.

SECTION 3 REPETITIONS

Week	Central	Right	Left	Right-Left Turn
1st week	200	50	50	5
2nd week	210	55	55	5
3rd week	210	55	55	10
4th week	220	60	60	10
5th week	220	60	60	15
6th week	230	65	65	15
7th week	230	65	65	20
8th week	240	70	70	20
9th week	240	70	70	25
10th week	250	75	75	25

Points of Note: The number of repetitions may be modified according to the condition of the student.

SECTION 4 REPETITIONS

	Central	Right	Left	Right-Left Turn	Rolling
1st week	250	75	75	25	5
2nd week				30	5
3rd week				30	10
4th week				35	10
5th week				35	15
6th week				40	15
7th week				40	20
8th week				45	20
9th week				45	25
10th week				50	25

Points of Note: The number of repetitions may be modified according to the condition of the student. If it is desired and suitable, the number of repetitions of the central, right, and left isolations may be increased.

Anal Exercise (Aśvinī Mudrā)

The following is the repetition method:

Commence with 25 times. Then increase 25 times each week until you reach 500 times.

6
Static Application of Posture Exercise

The main feature of posture exercise when utilized statically is to maintain the final attitude for a certain time limit. This time limit is not constant. The maintenance of a posture should be gradually increased in a definite manner from the lowest to the highest time limit. The effectiveness of the static posture exercise depends upon the time factor.

Suitable postures should be selected for static exercise. Each posture should be first perfected and controlled by its regular dynamic use. Only a perfected and well-controlled posture is utilizable as a static exercise.

In the static form of exercise the whole body that is in a particular attitude should remain absolutely motionless. This physical motionlessness, apart from its great health value, has far-reaching effects. It is essentially connected with the development of the concentration of the mind. As different posture exercises are intended to exercise the body and all its parts in different manners, so the physical motionlessness attained in different postures influences the mind in different ways favoring deep concentration. One who is able to concentrate in different postures gains sufficient power of control over the mind. But whatever posture is adopted for the purpose, physical motionlessness should be attained in that posture, otherwise the body will not be at all suitable for concentration.

The ease stage of a posture is inseparably connected with the physical motionlessness. As soon as the final attitude is assumed, the body will be perfectly motionless, if the posture is perfected and controlled, and the ease stage will immediately follow. This is the stage most suitable for mental relaxation and concentration. The duration of the ease stage should be gradually increased by regular practice.

Usually the posture is discontinued at the onset of discomfort. The discomfort stage may be subdivided into four phases: discomfort phase, endurance phase, willpower phase, and intolerance phase. When discomfort turns into pain, it is called pain or endurance phase. If the posture is continued up to this point, the power of toleration of pain is increased and along with it vital endurance is increased. As a result natural health and natural immunity are established in the body. The endurance phase should be very carefully and gradually lengthened. However, when pain becomes intense, the willpower phase is reached. In bearing the intense pain calmly with the body maintained motionless, willpower is called into play and developed to a high level. The willpower phase also should be increased in a systematic manner. At a certain point the intense pain becomes intolerable. At this phase the posture must be discontinued.

Time Period for Holding Static Posture Exercises

The time period is the length of time a static posture is held. As mentioned earlier, a static posture exercise has three stages: preliminary stage (in which there is movement), comfort stage, and discomfort stage. The time period of a static posture exercise includes the comfort stage, as well as the endurance and willpower phases within the discomfort stage. The duration of time is regulated according to the type of exercise. The increase of the length of the overall time period should be done in a graduated manner and should be adjusted according to the practitioner's general physical condition, strength, endurance, age, gender, and so on.

Time Periods for the Comfort Stage

The period of time during which the posture can be maintained with ease, that is, without the feeling of discomfort, varies according to the type of posture as well as the perfection and control achieved by training in the posture. As a rule, when the posture is perfected and controlled by dynamic exercise, the comfort stage becomes longer. The scale of increasing the time period of the comfort stage may be divided into four categories: low, medium, high, and very high.

In the low scale, the time is increased by half a minute at a time until the maximum of six minutes is reached. In the medium scale, the time is increased by half a minute or a minute at a time until the maximum of fifteen minutes is reached. The ability to maintain a posture for fifteen minutes qualifies the practitioner for the high scale, in which the time is increased by one or two minutes at a time until the maximum of thirty minutes is reached. In the very high scale, the time is increased by three, four, or five minutes at a time until the maximum of an hour, or even more, is reached. It is not necessary to give any timetable for very high time period. Only an advanced practioner can adopt this measure.

The scale of increase and the intervals may be modified according to the general physical condition, strength, endurance, age, sex, and individual requirements of the practitioner. According to the capacity of the practitioner, order A or B (or C or D if given) can be adopted, keeping in mind that order D is for those endowed with greatest strength and endurance. It may also be necessary to modify the scale of increase in certain cases.

Timetables follow.

LOW-SCALE TIME PERIOD TABLE (COMFORT STAGE)

Interval	Increment
Order A	
1st week	1 minute
2nd to 10th week	increase ½ minute every week
11th week	6 minutes
Order B	
1st week	1 minute
2nd to 20th week	increase ½ minute every second week
21st week	6 minutes

MEDIUM-SCALE TIME PERIOD TABLE (COMFORT STAGE)

Interval	Increment
Order A	
1st week	6 minutes
2nd to 9th week	increase 1 minute every week
10th week	15 minutes
Order B	
1st week	6 minutes
2nd to 18th week	increase ½ minute every week
19th week	15 minutes
Order C	
1st week	6 minutes
2nd to 18th week	increase 1 minute every second week
19th week	15 minutes
Order D	
1st week	6 minutes
2nd to 36th week	increase ½ minute every second week
37th week	15 minutes

HIGH-SCALE TIME PERIOD TABLE (COMFORT STAGE)

Interval	Increment
Order A	
1st week	15 minutes
2nd to 8th week	increase 2 minutes every week
9th week	30 minutes
Order B	
1st week	15 minutes
2nd to 16th week	increase 2 minutes every second week
17th week	30 minutes
Order C	
1st week	15 minutes
2nd to 15th week	increase 1 minute every week
16th week	30 minutes
Order D	
1st week	15 minutes
2nd to 30th week	increase 1 minute every second week
31st week	30 minutes

Time Periods for the Endurance and Willpower Phases

The duration of time of the endurance phase should be very slowly increased. The usual scale of increase at a time is from ten to twenty seconds at intervals of one to four weeks. The usual maximum time period is ten minutes. In exceptional cases, it may go beyond ten minutes.

The willpower phase starts when the endurance phase is carried to a point where intense pain is experienced. The duration of time of the willpower phase should also be very slowly and carefully increased. The usual scale of increase at a time is from five to ten seconds at intervals of one to four weeks. The maximum time period is five minutes. In exceptional cases, it may go beyond that.

Practical Application of Time Periods

The name of each exercise together with the suitable time period is given in the following tables, organized according to light, medium, and heavy contraction.

STATIC POSTERIOR TRUNK-BEND POSTURE EXERCISE

Exercise Name	Time Period Scale
Light-Contraction Exercise	
Cobra Posture	Low
Cuckoo Posture	Low

Exercise Name	Time Period Scale
Medium-Contraction Exercise	
Snake Posture	Low
Locust Posture	Low
Back-Raise Posture with Hands Clasped behind Head	Low
Bow Posture	Low
Boat Posture	Low
Swing Posture	Low
Raised Bow Posture	Low
Great-Contraction Exercise	
Back-Raise Posture with Forearms Locked behind Head	Low
King-Cobra Posture	Low
Wheel Posture	Low

STATIC ANTERIOR TRUNK-BEND POSTURE EXERCISE

Exercise Name	Time Period Scale
Light-Contraction Exercise	
Spinal-Stretch Posture	Low
Head-Knee Posture	Low
Foot-Head Posture	Low
Medium-Contraction Exercise	
Head-Bend Lotus Posture	Low
Forward Head-Bend Posture	Low
Great-Contraction Exercise	
Head-Bend Posture	Low
Forward Body-Bend Posture	Low

STATIC LATERAL TRUNK-BEND POSTURE EXERCISE

Exercise Name	Time Period Scale
Light-Contraction Exercise	
Half-Moon Posture	Low
Medium-Contraction Exercise	
Hip-Bend Posture	Low
Great-Contraction Exercise	
Moon Posture	Low

STATIC TRUNK-TWIST POSTURE EXERCISE

Exercise Name	Time Period Scale
Light-Contraction Exercise	
Twist Posture	Low
Medium-Contraction Exercise	
Modified Spinal-Twist Posture	Low
Ankle-Hold Modified Spinal Twist Posture	Low
Great-Contraction Exercise	
Spinal-Twist Posture	Low
Sideward Head-Bend Posture	Low

SUPPLEMENTARY STATIC ABDOMINAL POSTURE EXERCISE

Exercise Name	Time Period Scale
Fish Posture	Low and Medium

STATIC NECK POSTURE EXERCISE

Exercise Name	Time Period Scale
Neck-Bridge Posture	Low

SUPPLEMENTARY STATIC NECK POSTURE EXERCISE

Exercise Name	Time Period Scale
Chin Lock	Low and Medium

Points of Note: Chin Lock is the most important static neck exercise and is also utilized in breath control exercise. After Chin Lock, static Fish

Posture should be practiced to stretch the neck muscles. Static neck rotation is effected by Modified Spinal-Twist Posture, Ankle-Hold Modified Spinal-Twist Posture, and Spinal-Twist Posture. Therefore, the right combination of all these exercises is necessary for the static exercise of the neck.

STATIC ANTERIOR TRUNK-RAISE POSTURE EXERCISE

Exercise Name	Time Period Scale
Light-Contraction Exercise	
Spine Posture	Low
Medium-Contraction Exercise	
Spine Posture with Hands Clasped behind Head	Low
Great-Contraction Exercise	
Spine Posture with Forearms Locked behind Head	Low

STATIC PELVIS-RAISE POSTURE

Exercise Name	Time Period Scale
Light-Contraction Exercise	
Plow Posture	Low and Medium
Ear-Pressing Posture	Low
Medium-Contraction Exercise	
Plow Posture with Forearms Locked behind Head	Low
Great-Contraction Exercise	
Risen Back Posture	Low
Lotus-Plow Posture	Low

STATIC ANTERIOR TRUNK-LEG-RAISE POSTURE EXERCISE

Exercise Name	Time Period Scale
Light-Contraction Exercise	
Head-Knee Spine Posture	Low
Medium-Contraction Exercise	
Knee-Touching Spine Posture	Low
Great-Contraction Exercise	
Pillow Posture	Low

STATIC LATERAL TRUNK-LEG-RAISE POSTURE EXERCISE

Exercise Name	Time Period Scale
Great-Contraction Exercise	
Toe-Hold Lateral Spine Posture	Low

SUPPLEMENTAL STATIC ABDOMINAL POSTURE EXERCISE

Exercise Name	Time Period Scale
Bent-Knee Inverse Lotus Posture	Low

STATIC PELVIC POSTURE EXERCISE

Exercise Name	Time Period Scale
Light-Contraction Exercise	
Pelvis-Raise Posture	Low
Arm-Head Posture	Low
Medium-Contraction Exercise	
Single Foot-Head Posture	Low
Single Foot-Head Head-Knee Posture	Low
Great-Contraction Exercise	
One-Leg Pillar Posture	Low
Pillar Posture	Low
Double Foot-Head Posture	Low
Noose Posture	Low

SUPPLEMENTARY STATIC PELVIC POSTURE EXERCISE

Exercise Name	Time Period Scale
Happy Posture	Low

Sideward Leg-Stretch Posture	Low
Backward-Forward Leg-Stretch Posture	Low

STATIC PELVIC CONTROL EXERCISE

Exercise Name	Time Period Scale
Anal Lock	Low

Points of Note: Anal Lock may be repeated from 3 to 12 times in one sitting.

STATIC PECTORAL LIMB POSTURE EXERCISE

Exercise Name	Time Period Scale
Light-Contraction Exercise	
Risen Lotus Posture	Low
Four-Point Posture	Low
Medium-Contraction Exercise	
Cock Posture	Low
Great-Contraction Exercise	
One-Arm Cock Posture	Low

STATIC PELVIC LIMB POSTURE EXERCISE

Exercise Name	Time Period Scale
Light-Contraction Exercise	
Toe Posture	Low
Knee-Touching Thigh Posture	Low
Medium-Contraction Exercise	
Feet-Extending Thigh Posture	Low
Sideward Feet-Extending Thigh Posture	Low
Great-Contraction Exercise	
One-Legged Toe Posture	Low
Leg-Raise Thigh Posture	Low

STATIC BALANCE POSTURE EXERCISE

Exercise Name	Time Period Scale
Eagle Posture	Low
Standing Head-Knee Posture	Low
Wing Posture	Low
Bent-Head Wing Posture	Low
Knee-Heel Posture	Low
Standing Single Foot-Head Posture	Low
Standing Leg-Stretch Posture	Low
Mountain Posture	Low
Peacock Posture	Low
Crab Posture	Low
Rolling Posture	Low
Arm-Stand Posture	Low
Modified Scorpion Posture	Low
Scorpion Posture	Low

STATIC INVERSE BODY POSTURE EXERCISE

Exercise Name	Time Period Scale
Inversion Posture	Low, Medium, and High
Shoulder-Stand Posture	Low
Head Posture	Low, Medium, High, and Very High
Inverse Lotus Posture	Low and Medium

FOLDED-LEG POSTURES

Exercise Name	Time Period Scale
Accomplished Posture	Low, Medium, High, and Very High
Lotus Posture	Low, Medium, High, and Very High
Pleasant Posture	Low, Medium, High, and Very High
Toe-Hold Lotus Posture	Low and Medium

7
Diet

Diet plays a most important role through the supply of certain elements that must come to the system from outside. These are needed to maintain the structure and functions upon which a person's state of physical and mental life depends to a very great extent. These elements are contained in what we call food. Diet exercises its influence in a general as well as specific manner. In a general way, it maintains the forms and structure of the tissues and their functional efficiency by supplying substances that are utilized for construction and repair, and for the production of heat and energy. When there is a lack of one or more such substances, a disturbance takes place in the system.

The character of the tissues is mostly determined by the character of the food that is eaten habitually. Many factors are involved in the selection of food, such as: established dietetic habits, environmental conditions, country, muscular activities, individual preferences, education, and ideals. The physical and mental standards of a person depend so much on the selection of food. The selective power of the organism operating in relation to the digestion and absorption of food is a check against allowing certain substances to pass into the blood. It contributes to the building of a specific constitution of the body, which is related to the individual specificity of the mind. When the selection of food is done in conformity with this inner selective principle, a most suitable condition for physical and mental health and growth is created.

The state of health depends on the supply of various elements from the outer world in the correct proportion and combination. When there is a deficiency or complete absence of one or more of these elements, or an oversupply of one or more elements or all elements, the balance between alimentation and elimination is disturbed, health is impaired, vital vigor is decreased, the functional efficiency of the body is lowered, and normal growth is affected. Two factors are most important in this connection: selection of right food in the right amount and the digestive power.

In selecting food, long-standing dietetic habits should be carefully considered. The effects of a certain mode of alimentation are both immediate and far-reaching. The dietetic influence on bodily growth and strength is observable within a short period of time. But its influence in giving the body and the mind a characteristic shape—a speciality—cannot be noticeable within a few years. It may not even be well marked during the lifetime of an individual. But it will be fully manifested in the person's descendants. Each of us is the product of our ancestors' dietetic habits. Real improvement lies more in this specific molding of the body and mind through diet than in increased size and strength of the body. It is, therefore, not wise to make a radical change away from the ancestral mode of diet without considering many factors.

The earliest human diet seems to have been mainly based on plants, including leaves, shoots, roots, flowers, and fruits. At the next stage meat and fish were added. Human beings lived on this mixed diet for hundreds of thousands of years. With the domestication of animals, milk and eggs were added to this diet of vegetables, fruits, and meat. Finally, with the introduction of agriculture, cereals and pulses were added.

While this is considered to be the general order, it is not to be supposed that the whole human race followed this order of diet uniformly and at the same time. The relative proportion of meat, milk, fruits, vegetables, and grains depended on the flora and fauna of a particular region, the fertility of the land, stage of culture, type of life, opportunity, racial, class, and individual characteristics, religious beliefs, and so forth. On the whole, human dietetic habits took three main forms: mixed diet, lacto-vegetarian diet, and meat diet. In the meat diet meat is the main item. In the lacto-vegetarian diet meat has been discarded. The greater part of the human race has adopted the mixed diet consisting of fruits, vegetables, grains, milk, and meat.

Yogic Diet

In Yoga the lacto-vegetarian diet has been mainly adopted. The yogic diet is based on the principle of maintaining a perfect balance between alimentation and elimination, upon which the natural health of the body depends so much. The power of concentration also depends on their balance. The lacto-vegetarian diet is most suitable for maintaining the normal nutritional level of the body, gastro-intestinal efficiency, normal colonic activity and cleanliness, and general increased elimination. The yogins found that a diet consisting of fruits, vegetables, and milk is well suited to this purpose.

It is not that meat is an unsuitable food for human beings. In fact it is a most ancient food, much older than milk. A normal human alimentary canal is equally efficient in handling meat and milk. Moreover, it has been observed that a diet with meat or one with milk but without meat are equally nourishing. Meat eating has proved more satisfactory in those conditions of life in which physical exercise plays a predominant part. But to one leading a life that is characterized by decreased physical activities and increased mental activities meat does not seem to be as satisfactory. Many people have experienced that meat increases the sluggishness and poor bacterial health of the colon, along with general impurification. Furthermore, meat has been found to be unsuitable for concentration. This is one of the reasons why meat has been replaced by milk in the yogic diet.

It may also be noted in this connection that not everyone experiences meat as an adverse influence on concentration. At a higher stage of Yoga, diet, of course, does not play a prominent part. Both milk and meat prove to be equally good for health and concentration. More restriction is necessary at the elementary stages. Furthermore, persons with a strong propensity for meat may find it difficult to give it up altogether all at once. When meat eating has been an established habit, individual as well as ancestral, it is not easy and perhaps not wise to discard it completely without carefully considering other important factors. On the other hand, if meat is foreign to an ancestral and individual diet, it would be equally unwise to adopt a meat diet because of the unfounded belief that meat has a special strength-giving value or that muscle and strength cannot be built without it.

A lacto-vegetarian diet is quite as satisfactory in promoting the health, growth, and strength of the body as mixed or meat diets. And in many respects it seems to be superior to both. Milk can meet all the protein needs of the body even for persons doing heavy muscular exercise. It has also been observed that milk is much more suitable for maintaining increased colonic activity and the bacterial health of the colon. Milk, fruits, and vegetables are the best laxative foods and most useful in relieving constipation.

Classification of Foods

The yogic lacto-vegetarian diet consists of fruits, vegetables, cereals, pulses, nuts, sugars, milk, and milk products. From a practical point of view these foods can be classified as follows:

1. Acid Fruits
2. Sweet Fruits
3. Nonstarchy Vegetables
4. Starchy Vegetables
5. Cereals
6. Pulses
7. Nuts
8. Milk
9. Sugars

To determine correctly the nutritional value of each food, each type of food is to be considered from the point of view of the following ten categories:

I. Carbohydrates
II. Fats
III. Proteins
IV. Mineral salts
V. Acid-alkaline balance
VI. Vitamins
VII. Laxative foods
VIII. Foods to be used raw
IX. Weight-reduction foods
X. Weight-gain foods

I. Carbohydrates

From a chemical point of view foods are classified into carbohydrates, fats, proteins, minerals, and vitamins. Carbohydrates are the chief source of heat and energy for activity. They consist of simple sugars (monosaccharides), double sugars (disaccharides), and starch and cellulose (polysaccharides). The sugars and starch supply energy. The simple sugars are glucose, fructose, and galactose. Disaccharides consist of cane sugar, malt sugar, and milk sugar or lactose. Cellulose is not digested in the human alimentary canal. Its main function is to add to the bulk of the contents of the alimentary canal, which helps the onward march of the food toward the rectum.

II. Fats

Fats also supply heat and energy. They are more concentrated fuel foods than carbohydrates and give about two and a quarter times more calories of heat for a given amount. However, carbohydrates are the main fuel food for muscular activities. The muscle will utilize them first, if available. But muscle is also able to utilize fat if it is in available form, especially when the carbohydrates stored in the liver and muscles have been depleted by prolonged muscular exercise. Fat has a special value as food. It seems to supply certain essentials, not well understood at present, which enable a person to make prolonged respiratory effort in connection with breath control. The fat within the body is formed from fatty foods as well as carbohydrates, and also possibly from proteins.

III. Proteins

Proteins build and repair tissues. Their value as a fuel is of minor importance. Heavy muscular exercise does not require a larger protein intake. The power of the body to utilize proteins is limited. By consuming more protein we cannot attain greater muscular growth. Excess protein is neither utilized nor stored in the body, but in fact is the source of the impurification of the body and disease. Not all protein foods are equal in value. Foods containing those amino acids that are good for both growth and maintenance are of superior type. The others are of inferior type.

The nutritional value of an inferior protein is increased when combined with a superior protein. The proteins of milk, nuts, meats, and eggs are of superior type. Among all the superior proteins, milk is considered the best. When vegetable proteins are combined with milk or other superior proteins, they become nutritionally more satisfactory.

IV. Mineral Salts and V. Acid-Alkaline Balance

The mineral salts have no fuel value but are essential to the growth, functional efficiency, health, and vitality of the body. They include calcium, phosphorus, potassium, sulfur, sodium, chlorine, magnesium, iron, manganese, iodine, silicon, fluorine, copper, zinc, aluminum, and others. Calcium, in conjunction with phosphorus and vitamin D, is the most important element concerned with the development of bone and teeth. It plays an important role in maintaining cardiac efficiency and the capacity for physical and mental work, blood coagulation, and increasing disease-resisting power.

Sodium chloride is necessary for growth and vitality. Sodium affects the rhythmic action of the heart. Potassium is involved in maintaining the normal action of the heart and the normal osmotic pressure in the tissues. Sulfur plays a role in oxidation. Silicon is connected with the enamel of the teeth, nails, and hair. Fluorine also affects the enamel of the teeth. Iron is concerned with the carrying of oxygen and carbon dioxide. Copper and perhaps manganese are concerned with the formation of hemoglobin. Iodine plays an important role in the normal functioning of the thyroid gland.

Minerals also play a role in maintaining the acid-alkaline balance. The normal alkalinity of the blood should be maintained by the right selection of foods. Lowered alkalinity of the blood lowers the vitality and causes disease. Calcium, potassium, sodium, magnesium, and iron are alkaline elements. Foods rich in these elements are alkaline foods. Phosphorus, sulfur, chlorine, and iodine are acid elements.

VI. Vitamins

Vitamins are essential for health, vitality, growth, and efficiency, and for the prevention of specific diseases caused by their deficiency. The better-known vitamins are: A, B_1, B_2 complex, C, D, E, and K. Vitamin B_2 complex consists of nicotinamide (nicotinic acid), riboflavin, pyridoxin, pantothenic acid, and others.

Vitamin A deficiency causes the failure of growth, night blindness, xerosis, xerophthalmia, and multiple infections. Vitamin B_1 affects carbohydrate metabolism and its deficiency causes beri-beri. A deficiency of nicotinamide causes pellagra. A deficiency of riboflavin causes cheilosis. The deficiency of pyridoxin is probably also associated with cheilosis. Not much is known these days about pantothenic acid. Its deficiency may be associated with "burning-feet" syndrome and some other troubles. Vitamin C is needed for a person doing heavy muscular exercise and also during pregnancy and lactation. Its deficiency causes scurvy and increased susceptibility to infection. Vitamin D is especially connected with bone growth. Its lack causes rickets. Vitamin E is associated with sexual health and efficiency, and its deficiency causes sterility in women and degeneration of the germ cells in men. The deficiency of vitamin K lowers the prothrombin content of the blood.

VII. Laxative Foods; VIII. Foods To Be Used Raw; IX. Weight-Reduction Foods; X. Weight-Gain Foods

Laxative foods are those that promote normal bowel evacuation and prevent constipation. Foods rich in cellulose are generally laxative. But there are certain other foods that are also laxative due to their specific properties.

For better health and increased vitality certain foods, especially fruits and certain vegetables, should be eaten raw. Certain foods are more suitable and useful when taken raw. So laxative and raw foods should be added to a well-balanced diet.

Foods that support weight-gain are generally those that have a high caloric value. They should be discarded or reduced in a reducing diet. Foods having low caloric value are suitable for weight reduction.

Examples of Food

In the following lists, examples are given for each of the types of food in the lacto-vegetarian diet listed above, such as acid fruits and starchy vegetables. In addition, particular examples of the ten categories (such as carbohydrates, fats, and so on) are noted.

▶ Acid Fruits

Foods listed as acid fruits promote vitality and health. They contain glucose and fructose and in general are rich in mineral salts and vitamins, antitoxic and laxative, and suitable for the purification of the body.

1. Āmalakas (fruit of the Emblic myrobalan)
2. Apples
3. Apricots
4. Blackberries
5. Blueberries
6. Cantaloupes
7. Cherries
8. Currants
9. Figs (fresh)
10. Gooseberries
11. Grapes
12. Grapefruits
13. Honeydew melons
14. Lemons
15. Lichis
16. Limes
17. Mangoes
18. Musk melons
19. Oranges
20. Peaches
21. Pears

22. Persimmons
23. Pineapples
24. Plums
25. Pomegranates
26. Prunes
27. Shaddocks
28. Strawberries
29. Tangerines

▸ Ten Category References

I. Carbohydrates—glucose and fructose: especially in 8, 9, 11, 13, 17, 18, 19, 20, 21, 23, 25, 28, 29
II. Fats
III. Proteins
IV. Mineral salts—calcium, magnesium, phosphorus, iron, and copper: 11
V. Acid-alkaline balance—acid-forming: 10, 24, 26; alkaline: all except 10, 24, and 26
VI. Vitamins—Vitamin C: 2, 8, 12, 14, 16, 19, 20, 23, 28
VII. Laxative foods—8, 9, 11, 17, 20, 26, 28
VIII. Foods to be used raw—all
IX. Weight-reduction foods—1, 2, 7, 9, 12, 14, 15, 16, 19, 23, 24, 25, 27, 29
X. Weight-gain foods—11, 17

▸ Sweet Fruit Group

1. Bananas (ripe)
2. Bilva (wood apple)
3. Dates
4. Figs (dry)
5. Panasa (ripe Indian jackfruit)
6. Papayas
7. Raisins
8. Watermelons

▸ Ten Category References

I. Carbohydrates—glucose and fructose: all
II. Fats
III. Proteins
IV. Mineral salts—calcium and magnesium: 3, 7; phosphorus: 1, 7; iron: 1, 3, 7; copper: 1, 3
V. Acid-alkaline balance—alkaline: all
VI. Vitamins—vitamin C: 6
VII. Laxative foods—2, 4, 5, 6, 7
VIII. Foods to be used raw—all
IX. Weight-reduction foods—2, 6, 8
X. Weight-gain foods—1, 3, 5

▸ Nonstarchy Vegetables

Foods listed in this group are, in general, rich in mineral salts and vitamins, antitoxic, and laxative, more suitable for weight reduction and conducive to health, vitality, and bodily purification.

1. Asparagus
2. Beans (green)
3. Beet tops
4. Broccoli
5. Brussels sprouts
6. Cabbage
7. Cauliflower
8. Celery
9. Chard
10. Chives
11. Collards
12. Corn (green)
13. Cress
14. Cucumbers
15. Dandelion greens
16. Dumbari
17. Eggplants
18. Endives
19. Leaves (green)

20. Lettuce
21. Melons (green)
22. Paprika
23. Parsley
24. Patola
25. Peas (green)
26. Plantain stems
27. Radishes
28. Spinach
29. Squash
30. Tomatoes
31. Turnip tops
32. Watercress

▸ Ten Category References

I. Carbohydrates
II. Fats
III. Proteins
IV. Mineral salts—calcium and magnesium: 1, 6, 8, 19, 20, 28, 30; phosphorus: 1, 6, 8, 20, 25, 28, 30; iron: 1, 6, 8, 15, 17, 20, 27, 28, 30; copper: 17, 27; manganese: 19; iodine: 19, 27
V. Acid-alkaline balance—alkaline: all
VI. Vitamins—vitamin A: 19, 28, 30; vitamin B_1: 25; vitamin C: 6, 7, 19, 22, 25, 28, 30; vitamin E: 19, 20; vitamin K: 6, 7, 19, 28
VII. Laxative foods—1, 2, 19 and raw vegetable group
VIII. Foods to be used raw—6, 7, 8, 12, 13, 14, 18, 19, 20, 21, 22, 25, 27, 28, 30
IX. Weight-reduction foods—all
X. Weight-gain foods

▸ Starchy Vegetables

1. Beets
2. Jackfruit (Indian)
3. Bulb of *Arum Indicum*
4. Carrots
5. Parsnips
6. Plantains (green)
7. Potatoes (sweet)
8. Potatoes (white)
9. Pumpkins (sweet)
10. Roots
11. Turnips

▸ Ten Category References

I. Carbohydrates—starch: all
II. Fats
III. Proteins
IV. Mineral salts—calcium and magnesium: 4, 10, 11; phosphorus: 4, 11
V. Acid-alkaline balance—alkaline: all
VI. Vitamins—vitamin A: 4; vitamin C: new potatoes; vitamin K: 4, 8
VII. Laxative foods—1, 2, 4, 5, 9, 10, 11
VIII. Foods to be used raw—1, 4, 7, 8, 11
IX. Weight-reduction foods—1, 2, 4, 5, 6, 11, if taken moderately
X. Weight-gain foods—especially 7, 8

▸ Cereals

1. Barley
2. Barley meal (ground)
3. Corn (whole)
4. Oat (whole)
5. Rice (brown)
6. Rice flour (whole)
7. Wheat (whole grain)
8. Wheat flour (whole)

▸ Ten Category References

I. Carbohydrates—starch: all
II. Fats
III. Proteins
IV. Mineral salts—phosphorus: 4, 5, 6, 7, 8;

potassium: 7, 8; sulfur: 4, 7, 8; iron: 1, 2, 4, 5, 6, 7, 8; copper: 1, 2, 4, 5, 6, 7, 8; manganese: all; iodine: 4, 7, 8

V. Acid-alkaline balance—acid-forming: all

VI. Vitamins—vitamin B_1: all, wheat germ; nicotinamide: 7, 8, bran, yeast (dried); pyridoxin: all (in general); wheat germ, yeast (dried); riboflavin: yeast (dried); vitamin E: all (in general), wheat germ, wheat germ oil, rice germ oil

VII. Laxative foods—7, 8, wheat bran

VIII. Foods to be used raw—all (in moderate quantities)

IX. Weight-reduction foods

X. Weight-gain foods—all

▶ Pulses

1. Beans (dry)
2. Canaka (dry)
3. Masa (dry)
4. Mudga (dry)
5. Peas (dry)

▶ Ten Category References

I. Carbohydrates—starch: all

II. Fats

III. Proteins—all

IV. Mineral salts—sulfur, iron, copper, and manganese: all

V. Acid-alkaline balance—alkaline: all

VI. Vitamins—vitamin B_1:. all (in general); vitamin D: perhaps in sun-dried pulses

VII. Laxative foods

VIII. Foods to be used raw: 2, 3, 4

IX. Weight-reduction foods

X. Weight-gain foods

▶ Nuts

1. Almonds
2. Cashew
3. Coconut
4. Pistachios
5. Walnuts

▶ Ten Category References

I. Carbohydrates—all, especially 2

II. Fats—all

III. Proteins—especially 1, 4, 5

IV. Mineral salts

V. Acid-alkaline balance—acid-forming: 2, 4, 5; alkaline: 1, 3

VI. Vitamins

VII. Laxative foods—3, 5

VIII. Foods to be used raw—all

IX. Weight-reduction foods

X. Weight-gain foods—all

▶ Milk

1. Buttermilk
2. Chānā (Indian fresh cheese)
3. Milk (whole)
4. Skimmed milk
5. Sour milk
6. Butter
7. Cream
8. Ghee (clarified butter)

▶ Ten Category References

I. Carbohydrates—lactose: 3

II. Fats—6, 7, 8

III. Proteins—2, 3, 4, 5

IV. Mineral salts—calcium: all; phosphorus: all; potassium: 3; sulfur: 3; iron: 3 (less in quantity but superior in value; it should be supplemented with iron-rich foods); copper and iodine: 3

V. Acid-alkaline balance—alkaline: 1, 3, 4, 5 (2 is neutral)
VI. Vitamins—vitamin A: 3, 6, 8; vitamin B_1, nicotinamide, and riboflavin: 3; vitamin D: 3, especially summer milk, 6, 8
VII. Laxative foods—3
VIII. Foods to be used raw—1, 2, 3, 4, 5
IX. Weight-reduction foods—1, 4
X. Weight-gain foods—2, 3, 6, 7, 8

▶ Sugars

1. Honey
2. Milk sugar (lactose)
3. Molasses
4. Sugar (brown)
5. Sugar candy
6. Syrup

▶ Ten Category References

I. Carbohydrates—glucose and fructose: 1; cane sugar: 1, 3, 4, 5, 6; lactose: 2
II. Fats
III. Proteins
IV. Mineral salts—iron: 3; pyridoxin: 3
V. Acid-alkaline balance
VI. Vitamins
VII. Laxative foods—2
VIII. Foods to be used raw
IX. Weight-reduction foods
X. Weight-gain foods—all

Balanced Diet

In a well-balanced diet, acid fruits, nonstarchy vegetables, and milk should form the important parts. Sweet fruits, starchy vegetables, and cereals should be used as fuel foods to supply energy. For additional energy sugars and fats may be used. Nuts may also be added. For protein requirements one should depend mainly on milk, which can be supplemented by cereals, pulses, and nuts. A certain quantity of raw foods should be eaten daily. Most suitable for the purpose are acid and sweet fruits, nonstarchy vegetables, and certain starchy vegetables. The quantities of the laxative foods should be determined according to the condition of the bowels. If there is constipation, more laxative foods should be added. The best laxative food is raw milk. To it may be added acid fruits such as figs, grapes, mangoes, and prunes; sweet fruits such as wood apple, dry figs, and ripe Indian jackfruit; and coconuts. Milk sugar may be used in exceptional cases. For reducing purposes more acid fruits (except grapes and mangoes) and nonstarchy vegetables should be taken. More sweet fruits, fats, sugars, nuts, and plenty of milk should be added to a generally nourishing diet for weight gain.

The protein requirement depends on various factors, such as body weight. As a general guideline, from sixty to seventy-five grams of protein per day will meet all the needs of the body, even if you are getting plenty of physical exercise. In many cases less than sixty grams may be enough. Milk, whole-wheat flour, almonds, spinach, cabbage, and tomatoes may meet the daily requirements of protein, taken in right quantities.

Either twenty-four ounces of milk or sixteen ounces of milk along with one large orange and two ounces of carrots will meet the daily requirements of calcium for an adult. Milk, fruits, vegetables, and cereals will supply the necessary phosphorus. For the iron requirements a more careful selection of food is necessary. Milk, whole-wheat flour, potatoes, carrots, green peas, tomatoes, cabbage, spinach, bananas, raisins, dates, figs, oranges, and almonds in the right amounts will meet the daily requirements of iron for an adult. But there are exceptional cases. If it is not possible to maintain the right number of red cells and right percentage of hemoglobin on the lacto-vegetarian diet, egg yolks, whole eggs, or lean meat may be added.

The daily vitamin A requirements may be met by a daily intake of one ounce of butter, one ounce of carrots, and half an ounce of spinach. For vitamin B_1 it is desirable to add edible food yeast to a diet consisting of whole wheat, peas, and milk. Barley germ, wheat germ, or rice bran may also be added. A diet consisting of whole wheat, milk, and dried yeast in the correct quantities will meet the requirements of nicotinamide. Cereals, pulses, molasses, and dried yeast will supply pyridoxin. For riboflavin, milk and dried yeast should be added to the daily diet. Two ounces of orange juice and one ounce of lemon juice will supply all the necessary vitamin C. In a lacto-vegetarian diet the only reliable source of vitamin D is summer milk and butter. Egg yolks are richer in this vitamin than milk or butter. A liberal quantity of milk and butter combined with sunbathing may supply the needed amount of vitamin D. However, if this does not prove satisfactory, a few drops of tunny-liver oil or halibut-liver oil should be taken. Regular use of green leaves is necessary for vitamin E. Half an ounce of dry lettuce or half a teaspoonful of wheat germ oil will meet the daily requirements of this vitamin. The use of green leaves will supply vitamin K.

Right Eating Habits

Eating habits should be strictly regulated for better health, greater efficiency, and longer life. Any error in diet is injurious in some way or other and should be avoided. Overeating—which is a very common error—must be abandoned. You should not eat unless you feel hungry and can enjoy the food. Three meals a day are sufficient even for a person getting very vigorous muscular exercise. Two meals may be sufficient for many persons taking light exercise or leading practically sedentary lives. Three light meals may be eaten by those doing light exercise. More than three meals a day should be allowed only in exceptional cases, such as some cases of emaciation, gastric ulcer, or hyperacidity. In many cases it is more useful to have only two meals, such as in obesity, reduced gastric efficiency, high blood pressure, gastritis, and so on. Eating once a day is not wise; such a habit should be abandoned.

Do not eat many kinds of foods at one meal. Avoid all sorts of wrong food combinations, namely, combining different kinds of fats, different kinds of proteins, and different kinds of starches at one meal. Do not make foods complicated by adding too many spices, salts, flavorings, fat, sugar, and so on. Adulterated foods should be taboo. An adequate quantity of raw vegetables, especially greens, and fresh fruits should be a part of the daily diet. Natural foods are always good. All refined foods should be avoided as much as possible.

A cooking method by which all the food values are retained should be adopted, especially in cooking vegetables. Fried foods should be avoided. The best method of cooking is to prepare natural foods in a simple way. Overcooking and complicated cooking should be given up. Avoid excessive tea or coffee drinking, excessive salt, refined flour, refined sugar, rhubarb, and hot spices. Do not use food preserved with sodium benzoate or sulphur dioxide.

Suggested Menus

We are presenting here for your convenience a number of healthy and nutritious food combinations for specific meals.

Breakfasts:

A. Acid fruits
B. Acid fruits, sweet fruits
C. Acid fruits, milk
D. Acid fruits, sweet fruits, milk
E. Acid fruits, sweet fruits, nuts, milk
F. Acid fruits, sweet fruits, nuts, milk, honey

Lunches:

A. Raw nonstarchy vegetables, sour milk
B. Raw nonstarchy and starchy vegetables, sour milk
C. Raw nonstarchy vegetables, cooked starchy vegetables, butter, sour milk
D. Raw nonstarchy vegetables, cooked starchy vegetables, cereals, butter, sour milk
E. Raw nonstarchy vegetables, cooked starchy vegetables, cereals, pulses, butter, sour milk
F. Nonstarchy and starchy vegetables, cereals, butter, nuts

Dinners:

A. Raw vegetables, cooked vegetables, cereals, butter, milk, honey
B. Acid and sweet fruits, cereals, pulses, butter, chānā, molasses
C. Acid fruits, sweet fruits, nuts, milk, honey
D. Raw nonstarchy and starchy vegetables, acid and sweet fruits, nuts, milk, honey
E. Cooked vegetables, cereals, pulses, butter, milk, acid fruits
F. Acid fruits, sweet fruits, chānā, nuts, honey

8

Fasting and Special Diets

Fasting is a natural means of rejuvenating the whole body and eliminating various wastes and other surplus materials accumulated in the body. When the body is forced to nourish itself from its accumulated materials, a higher form of efficiency is developed. The alimentary organs are rested by fasting; as a result the power of digestion and absorption is remarkably improved. In addition the bacterial decomposition in the alimentary canal is checked.

The functional efficiency of the heart is improved by fasting. The blood is cleansed of all impurities and its efficiency increased. Elimination through all the eliminative organs is greatly increased during fasting. The mucus membrane of the gastrointestinal tract acts as an organ of elimination when a fast is undertaken. Even the liver eliminates some wastes in the bile.

Mental and sensory powers are improved by a fast. The memory is strengthened and the power of clear thinking is developed. The vital activities of the cells are increased. The ability of the cells to reconstruct themselves is improved to an extraordinary degree. The increased power of digestion and absorption and the increased ability of the cells to utilize building materials promote growth.

Fasting Defined

Fasting is the abstaining from all kinds of foods, solid and liquid, with the exception of water. In certain cases even drinking water is not permitted. In many cases lemon juice is allowed with water. In some cases even orange juice, about a cup, may be allowed once or twice a day.

The types of fasts may be divided into short, medium, and long. A short fast is from one to three days. A medium fast is from five to twelve days. Beyond a twelve-day period, it is considered a long fast.

Short (and occasionally medium) fasts are employed when there is no specific disease in the system. Usually a short fast is enough to give the body a physiological rest, improve digestion and absorption, cleanse the system, build vitality, increase disease-resisting power, and stimulate growth. When undertaking a fast for these purposes, water should be drunk freely. This helps elimination.

A particular kind of long fast is known as a "finish fast." The effects of the "finish fast" are the following:

The return of hunger
The clearing of the tongue
The clean condition of breath
Disappearance of bad taste from the mouth

Conducting a Fast

The following plan may be adopted when undertaking a short or medium fast (one to twelve days):

1. Drink a cup of warm water with fresh lemon juice, which should be taken at intervals of 30 to 45 minutes for 3 hours in the morning. Thereafter drink a cup of cold water now and then.
2. Cleanse the stomach and colon with water daily during the fast. Colonic Auto-Lavage may be done after drinking the warm water. After the Colonic Auto-Lavage, Gastric Auto-Lavage may be done.
3. A mild type of exercise, especially walking and light breathing exercise, may be done.
4. During a fast, you should also spend time outdoors in the sun and fresh air, take general water baths, and get plenty of rest, relaxation, and sleep. A cheerful attitude of mind is to be developed for best results.
5. The duration of a fast is thoroughly dependent on the health, age, sex, and requirements of the person.

Fast-Breaking

After a short fast adopt the following plan:

1st day: Drink 8 oz. of orange juice three times. Pineapple juice may also be used if orange juice is not available.

2nd day: Eat three meals of acid fruits. Drink water freely. Take Colonic Auto-Lavage if required.

3rd day and thereafter: either a milk diet or milk and fruit diet may be adopted.

The following fast-breaking routine may be adopted after the medium fast:

1st day: Drink 8 oz. of orange juice three times.

2nd day: Eat three meals of acid fruits, drink water freely between meals, and do Colonic Auto-Lavage if required.

3rd day: Same as 2nd day.

4th day and thereafter: either a milk diet or milk and fruit diet may be adopted.

Milk Diet

The milk diet presents three great advantages: it promotes growth; it encourages the growth of lactic-acid-forming bacteria in the colon and stimulates peristalsis; it is rich in endocrine gland secretions. The milk to be used in a milk diet should not be boiled or pasteurized. However, it should be clean and handled with care. Milking should be very carefully done. For the most satisfactory results milk should be drunk while it is naturally warm—that is, not long after it is drawn from the udder. Such milk is rich in endocrine secretions and very beneficial.

Cow milk should be used. Goat milk can also be used. The animals should be perfectly healthy, well developed, and young. They should be well fed and given plenty of fresh grass and greens and sprouted grains. They should get fresh air, sunshine, and exercise. If it is not possible to get milk as mentioned above, the best possible available milk can be used.

During a milk diet, get moderate exercise, sun, and fresh air. A warm or rather neutral immersion bath should be taken daily. Colonic Auto-Lavage may be done, if necessary.

Following a Milk Diet

Before commencing with milk, 8 oz. of orange juice should be taken daily. A cup or two of milk may be replaced by the same quantity of orange juice in the afternoon.

The dose and the number of feedings often need to be modified to suit individual conditions. In certain cases skimmed milk or buttermilk may be taken instead of milk. This diet may be followed with great advantage once or twice a year for two weeks or more.

1st day: 8 oz. of milk every second hour for 12 hours.
2nd day: 8 oz. of milk every hour for 12 hours.
3rd day: 8 oz. of milk every 45 minutes for 12 hours.
4th day and thereafter: 8 oz. of milk every 30 minutes for 12 hours.

Milk-Fruit Diet

A milk-fruit diet consists of acid and sweet fruits and milk. Skimmed milk and buttermilk may also be taken instead of milk. If necessary, Colonic Auto-Lavage may be done.

Milk-Fruit Diet Plan 1

1st meal: Acid fruits
2nd meal: Acid fruits, milk
3rd meal: Same as 2nd meal

Milk-Fruit Diet Plan 2

1st meal: Acid and sweet fruits
2nd meal: Acid fruits and milk
3rd meal: Acid and sweet fruits, milk

Milk-Fruit Diet Plan 3

1st meal: Acid fruits and milk
2nd meal: Acid and sweet fruits, milk
3rd meal: Same as 2nd meal

Fruit Diet

In certain cases a fruit diet is very beneficial. Eating only fruit for a day or two now and then produces excellent results in the purification and vitalization of the body. Colonic Auto-Lavage may be done, if necessary. Water should be drunk freely. The following plans may be adopted.

Fruit Diet Plan 1

1st meal: Acid fruits
2nd meal: Acid and sweet fruits
3rd meal: Same as 2nd meal

Fruit Diet Plan 2

1st meal: Acid fruits
2nd and 3rd meals: Same as 1st meal

Fruit Diet Plan 3

1st meal: Acid and sweet fruits
2nd and 3rd meals: Same as 1st meal

Raw Food Diet

A raw food diet is very useful under certain health conditions. It purifies and alkalinizes the blood. In this diet only raw foods are used. Foods used in this diet consist of raw vegetables, fruits, nuts, and some cereals or pulses in raw form. Included are all acid and sweet fruits, cabbage, cauliflower, celery, green corn, cress, cucumber, endive, green leaves, lettuce, green melon, paprika, green peas, radish, spinach, tomato, beet, carrot, sweet potato, white potato, turnip, cereals, canaka, masa, mudga, and nuts. Sometimes milk, buttermilk, skimmed milk, or sour milk may be added. Cereals and pulses should be soaked in cold water sufficiently long to be softened. Sprouted pulses may be used.

This diet may be followed for a day or two or even for a week with great advantage. Sometimes it may be necessary to continue it longer. Water should be drunk regularly. Colonic Auto-Lavage may be done, if necessary. The following plans may be adopted.

Raw Food Diet Plan 1

1st meal: Acid fruits
2nd meal: Nonstarchy vegetables
3rd meal: Nonstarchy and starchy vegetables

Raw Food Diet Plan 2

1st meal: Acid and sweet fruits
2nd meal: Non-starchy and starchy vegetables
3rd meal: Acid and sweet fruits, nuts

Raw Food Diet Plan 3

1st meal: Acid and sweet fruits
2nd meal: Nonstarchy and starchy vegetables
3rd meal: Sweet fruits, pulses

Raw Food Diet Plan 4

1st meal: Acid and sweet fruits
2nd meal: Nonstarchy and starchy vegetables, cereals
3rd meal: Acid and sweet fruits, nuts

Raw Food Diet Plan 5

1st meal: Acid and sweet fruits
2nd meal: Nonstarchy and starchy vegetables, sour milk
3rd meal: Acid and sweet fruits, milk

Orange Juice Diet

An orange juice diet is very useful in general toxemia. It increases elimination and alkalinizes the blood. In many cases it may be adopted in place of fasting. When the vitality is low, the bowels sluggish, and the appetite dull, it is highly beneficial to adopt an orange juice diet.

The orange juice diet consists of drinking eight ounces of orange juice every hour, twelve or fifteen times a day. At least six to ten glasses of water should be drunk. Colonic Auto-Lavage should be done daily during this period. The usual duration of the diet is from three to seven days. It can be done once or twice a year.

9

The Yoga Method of Internal Cleansing

The internal cleansing method of Yoga, termed *śodhana,* consists of six principal techniques, which can be divided into two main groups: alimentary and nasopharyngeal. The cleansing of the alimentary canal consists of oral, esophageal, gastric, colonic, and alimentary canal cleansing processes. The nasal cavities and upper part of the throat are cleansed by water baths and nasal thread cleansing.

Oral Cleansing (Danta Dhautī)

Oral cleansing is necessary to clean the teeth, tongue, and palate and to keep the mouth sweet. It consists of teeth cleansing, tongue cleansing, and palatine cleansing.

A good tooth powder or a fresh semi-hard twig of some suitable tree, called a tooth-stick, is used to clean the teeth. A tooth-stick cleans better than a toothbrush. During the teeth cleansing plenty of water should be used. The teeth should be cleaned twice a day, morning and evening.

The cleansing of the tongue should be done in connection with the teeth cleansing. It is very important, as it removes deposited matter from the tongue. It is done with an instrument called a tongue scraper, a smooth-edged, thin implement about a quarter of an inch wide and preferably made of silver, copper, brass, or celluloid. The tongue scraper should be pulled with both hands with moderate pressure several times from the back of the tongue to the tip, never in a reverse way. Then the tongue should be cleaned with the index, middle, and ring fingers and plenty of water. Lastly, the tongue should be rubbed with the inner surface of a piece of lemon from which the juice has been squeezed. This cleanses the tongue and sweetens the mouth.

The palate should also be cleansed with water and with the help of the right thumb. It should be done after the cleansing of the tongue. Other important aspects of oral prophylaxis are chewing of apples and some raw foods, exposing the open mouth to the sun, deep breathing through the mouth, and rinsing the mouth with warm or cold water mixed with salt.

Esophageal Cleansing (Daṇḍa Dhautī)

The cleansing of the esophagus removes the minute particles regurgitated into it. It also helps gastric emptying through the mouth by exciting vomiting. The circulation in the mucus membrane is also stimulated by the rubbing action of the process.

Esophageal Cleansing consists of inserting a straight flexible rod-like implement, such as a flexible fresh twig of *Jhāu* (*Tamarix* spp.) or *Vetra* (*Calamus rotang*), wrapped with cloth, or a rubber catheter of suitable size, into the mouth and pushing it down to the stomach. This should not be attempted without proper instruction from an expert. It is not necessary for ordinary students of physical education to practice it.

Gastric Cleansing

There are two methods of gastric cleansing: Gastric Auto-Lavage (Vamana Dhautī) and Gastric Cloth-Cleansing (Vāsa Dhautī).

Gastric Auto-Lavage is an excellent means to remove any filthy accumulation from the stomach and to keep it clean and sweet. If there is any morbid coating on the gastric mucus membrane, either due to incomplete gastric emptying or regurgitation of intestinal contents, it will be removed. The gastric muscles and nerves will also be stimulated.

According to Yoga, Gastric Auto-Lavage is absolutely necessary for maintaining a high degree of gastric efficiency. It gives a feeling of well-being and a sense of cleanliness and aids in concentration. It is also very helpful in conditions of failing appetite, coated tongue, diminished energy, and hyperacidity.

The process consists of drinking four to six glasses of water and then vomiting it completely. The distention of the stomach may help to induce vomiting. The application of pressure on the stomach by Abdominal Retraction is very helpful. However, at the beginning stage, vomiting may be induced by inserting the fingers into the throat. Either a squatting or a standing posture may be assumed.

Ordinarily cold water is used. Sometimes lukewarm water may be necessary. Gastric Auto-Lavage should be done in the morning after oral cleansing. It may be done five or six days a week for the first four weeks. Thereafter it may be done once or twice a week or every ten days. Whenever there is a lack of appetite and a dull feeling it should be done in conjunction with a fast. One should not eat any food immediately after the lavage.

Gastric Cloth-Cleansing is a special method of gastric cleansing. If there is an accumulation of excess mucus, unused juices, and debris, they are completely eliminated by this process. It is also an excellent process of internal massage of the esophagus and stomach. Various kinds of automatic movements of the gastric musculature cause the gastric mucosa to come into direct contact with the cloth swallowed, causing them to be properly massaged. This massage stimulates circulation and the vital activities of the mucus membrane.

In Gastric Cloth-Cleansing a long, clean, and narrow piece of fine cloth is necessary. The usual length is about twenty feet and width three inches. The cloth should first be boiled for a while and soaked in clean, cool water and then gradually swallowed. Of course, the whole piece of cloth should not be swallowed. About ten inches of the cloth should always be kept outside the mouth. After the desired length of the cloth is swallowed, it should be very slowly and gently withdrawn by using both hands. When the process is mastered, the swallowing only takes a few minutes.

Gastric Cloth-Cleansing should be performed when the stomach is quite empty. The best time for its practice is in the morning after the usual oral cleansing. Neither Esophageal Cleansing nor Gastric Auto-Lavage should be done on the days when cloth-cleansing is practiced. At the initial stages it is better to practice it more frequently, say two or three times a week. Thereafter it may be done once a week.

Gastric Cloth-Cleansing is a very healthful practice if done in the right way. Many of the author's students, both in India and Sweden, have practiced it for a long time with very satisfactory results. But this technique should be learned from an expert. An ordinary student of physical education may omit it. It is contraindicated in gastritis, enteritis, colitis, gastric ulcer, duodenal ulcer, and in certain other pathological conditions of the body.

Colonic Cleansing

The necessity of maintaining a clean condition of the colon for the attainment of perfect health and a high degree of vital vigor is often overlooked. Colonic cleanliness is also absolutely necessary for the attainment of success in breath control and concentration.

Colonic cleanliness is closely associated with three factors: the bacterial state of the colon, the character of the colon contents, and the colonic motility. These three factors are interrelated and interdependent. Colonic bacteria may be divided into two groups: poison-forming and poison-destroying. There is a biological antagonism between the two groups. When one group predominates, the other succumbs. The growth of poison-forming bacteria is mainly encouraged by protein foods, especially meat, fish, and eggs, which readily undergo putrefaction in the colon. If this type of contents remains in the colon for a long period of time, the putrefactive bacteria will be given a greater opportunity to develop there, and consequently there will be more toxic products.

On the other hand, if the colon contents contain more starch and lactose, the growth of the poison-destroying micro-organisms will be promoted and the putrefactive bacteria will be reduced in number and strength. Two important changes take place when benign intestinal bacteria predominate in the colon: increased colonic activity and the disappearance of bad odor from the feces. Thus, a diet rich in vegetables, fruit, and milk is conducive to the growth of antipoison bacteria in the colon. It may be noted here that milk protein does not putrefy in the colon because of the presence of lactose. A milk diet makes the sluggish colon active by building up its muscles and nerves and changing the character of the intestinal flora.

Colonic sluggishness is often due to nervous and muscular weakness and the excessive growth of poison-forming bacteria in the colon. When the contents of the colon do not remain longer than is necessary, the putrefactive bacteria get less chance to thrive. The power of the colon to pass its contents at a normal rate depends upon the building up of a high degree of nervous and muscular efficiency of the colon by right diet and exercise as well as the encouragement of the acid-forming bacteria in the colon by appropriate diet.

In addition to exercise and diet, colon cleansing plays a very important role in maintaining the health and cleanliness of the colon. It is a very useful hygienic measure to eliminate fecal accumulation, excess gases, and products of bacterial decomposition, to remove the morbid coating of the colonic mucus membrane, and cleanse the haustra, the most inactive parts of the colon. It also stimulates the colon to increased activity. Our experience teaches us that even when the bowels move regularly, the extra elimination obtained by colon lavage is of much help. Colon washing is especially important for those who cannot keep themselves internally clean by sufficient exercise and a good diet.

Colonic Auto-Lavage (Jala Vasti)

In Haṭha Yoga, a process known as Jala Vasti (also called Vasti) has been developed for cleansing the colon thoroughly with water without any instrument. The technique of Colonic Auto-Lavage begins with assuming a squatting posture in a bathtub filled navel-deep with water. Even a basin that allows the anus to be immersed an inch or two below the surface of the water will serve the purpose. From one and a half to two pints of water will be sufficient to reach the cecum.

The process consists of two parts. First, water is sucked up through the rectum and then it is brought into the entire colon. The suction of water entirely depends upon the changing of the intracolonic pressure by abdominal control and the voluntary opening of the anal sphincters by anal control. The passage of water through the colon up to the cecum is effected by specialized controlled abdominal muscular movements. Special training is necessary to gain full control over the abdominal and pelvic muscles for the Colonic Auto-Lavage.

First, any fecal accumulation in the anal canal should be removed by a process called Mūlā Śodhana (Anal Cleansing). This process also helps to bring about relaxation of the anal region, which is useful in the suction of water. The process consists of the insertion of the middle finger into the anal canal and the execution of circular movements with the finger. Before insertion, the nail of the finger should be cut and the finger cleansed and lubricated.

The bowels should be evacuated before the practice of Colonic Auto-Lavage. The best time for beginners is in the morning. When the process is mastered, three to five suctions are advised for a thorough cleansing of the entire colon. After each suction the water should be discharged. After the final ejection of water and washing the area, a few minutes rest should be taken, preferably lying on the left side of the body. Then Straight Muscle Exercise (fig. 14.24) should be practiced a few times, followed by remaining in Peacock Posture (fig. 18.9) for a minute or two. These practices will help the elimination of the remaining water, if there is any. The intra-abdominal pressure is increased in Peacock Posture, which helps the expulsion of fluid from the colon. It is a suitable position for attaining control over the anal sphincters.

Colonic Auto-Lavage should be done twice a week in the evening. The evening practice should consist of only one suction. Once a month from three to five suctions may be done in the morning for a thorough cleansing of the colon. It is necessary to learn the technique of Colonic Auto-Lavage directly from an expert.

X-Ray Documentation of Colonic Auto-Lavage

By a special invitation, the author's pupil Dinabandhu Pramanick gave a demonstration of Colonic Auto-Lavage before a number of distinguished medical men on August 8, 1949, at the Karolinska Sjukhuset, Stockholm, one of the greatest X-ray centers in the world. Pramanick was first stripped naked and then asked to expose his body to X-rays. His colon was examined via X-rays and an X-ray picture was taken. The observations and the picture showed that the colon was empty. He was then asked to take a liquid contrast medium of barium sulfate into his rectum from a sitz basin, which he did without any instrumental aid. He then again exposed his naked body to X-rays, which showed that he had been able to suck the contrast medium into the rectum. Then, by his power of muscular control, he brought the contrast medium to a point on the right side beyond the middle of the transverse colon. The whole process was observed through X-rays and at every stage X-ray pictures were taken. Two of the many X-ray pictures taken at the Karolinska Sjukhuset are reproduced here. Fig. 9.1 shows the stage after suction and fig. 9.2 shows the passing of the contrast medium beyond the middle of the transverse colon. The medical statement follows:

> We have seen Dr. Pramanick demonstrate his ability to take a liquid contrast medium of barium sulphate into his rectum without mechanical aid from a sitz basin. The accompanying X-ray pictures were taken to prove the absence of such medium before and then to show the height to which the medium was taken. Within 30 minutes, under observation

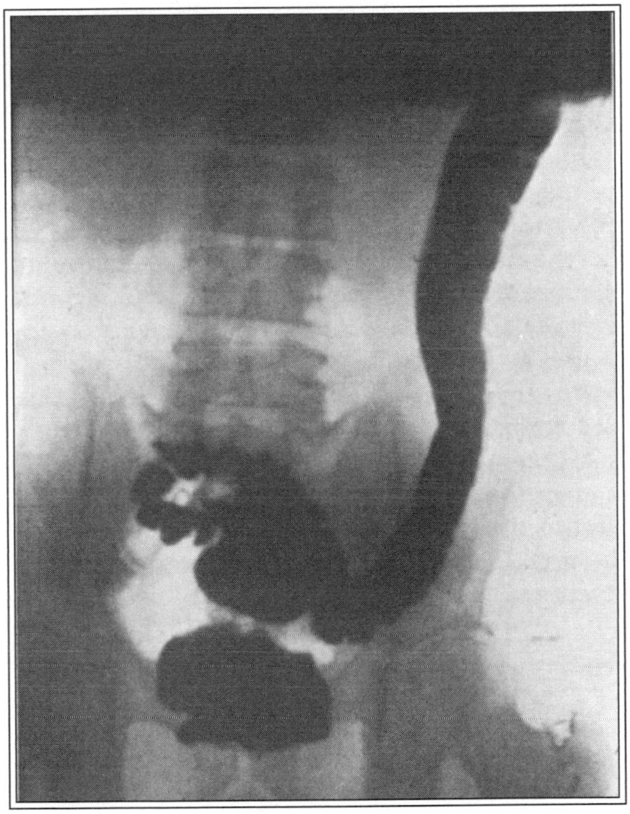

Fig. 9.1. Radiograph I was taken after the suction of fluid into the colon through the process of Colonic Auto-Lavage (Vasti) without instrumental aid. Auto-Lavage was performed by Dinabandhu Pramanick at the Karolinska Sjukhuset, Stockholm, on August 8, 1949.

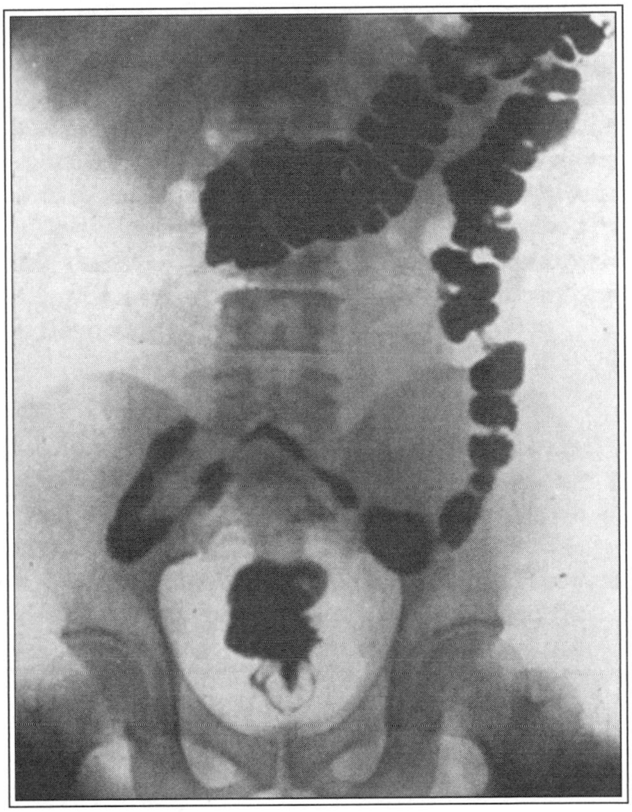

Fig. 9.2. Radiograph II shows the contrast medium brought up into the right half of the transverse colon by muscular control as performed by Dinabandhu Pramanick at the Karolinska Sjukhuset, Stockholm, on August 8, 1949.

all the time, and in standing position, he was able to bring the contrast medium up into the right half of the transverse colon.

(Signed) Sven-Roland Kjellberg, M.D., X-ray Diagnosis Department

(Signed) Ulf Rudhc, Certified X-ray Technician, X-ray Diagnosis Department

(Signed) Robert P. Marshall, M.D., X-ray Diagnosis Department

Dinabandhu Pramanick also demonstrated Colonic Auto-Lavage at: the British Medical Association, South Indian and Hyderabad branches; St. Luke's Hospital, Chicago; American Naturopathic Association, Pittsburgh; Imperial University, Physiology Department, Tokyo; St. Luke's International Medical Center, Tokyo; Madras Medical Association; Hyderabad Medical Association; Physical Therapy Institute of the University of Zurich; Human Morpho-Physiological Society, Paris; Salpêtrière Hospital, Paris; and elsewhere.

Enema

Those who are not able to perform Colonic Auto-Lavage are advised to take enemas. Only clean water should be used. You should not eat for at least half an hour after an enema. The knee-chest position is the best. For cleansing purposes, lukewarm water enemas are most suitable. They are also relaxing. The quantity of water should not exceed two quarts. Three or four warm water enemas may be taken for a thorough cleansing of the colon. After each enema the bowels should be evacuated. The last lukewarm enema should be followed by a small cold one for its tonic effect. This thorough cleansing should be done once a month, in the morning after normal evacuation of the bowels. A small (about one or one and a half pints) cold water enema may be taken twice a week in the evening before dinner.

Colonic Auto-Air Bath (Śuṣka Vasti)

A process of introducing air into the colon for its purification and stimulation is advised for advanced students. It is performed without any instrumental aid. The air is sucked in the same way as the water is in Colonic Auto-Lavage. It is to be practiced in the morning and after the Colonic Auto-Lavage.

Colonic Auto-Air Bath is an advanced colonic exercise suitable for advanced students. It should be learned directly from an experienced teacher. Ordinary students may omit it and depend more upon Colonic Auto-Lavage and diet for maintaining colonic cleanliness and health.

Alimentary Canal Auto-Lavage (Vāri Sāra)

Alimentary Canal Auto-Lavage is an excellent means for cleansing the whole alimentary canal with water without any instrumentation. It consists of drinking water at certain intervals and passing it from the stomach into the small intestine and thence into the colon, from which it is ejected from the body with the contents of the alimentary canal. However, an advanced control over the abdominal muscles is required to be able to do this. Once the process is mastered, and the required amount of water drunk, it usually takes from ten to fifteen minutes.

Morning is the best time for this practice. The student should first evacuate the bowels and then cleanse the colon with water before commencing. This method should be learned from a competent teacher.

There is another natural alternative for cleansing the whole alimentary canal that is as efficient as Vāri Sāra, though much easier to perform, and yet preferably instructed by an experienced teacher This auto-lavage method is called Śankprakṣalana. It is recommended before starting a short or long fast, or when adopting a fruit diet. Śankprakṣalana may also be used under normal health conditions whenever there is need to cleanse the entire digestive tract.

Śankprakṣalana

The method consists of repetitive rounds of drinking one glass of warm, salty water—use one full teaspoon salt per liter of water used—in alternation with four movements repeated six times, respectively:

1. Standing with your feet slightly apart, flex the body to the right and the left in Half-Moon posture.
2. Standing upright with your feet slightly apart and arms stretched forward, rotate the trunk and arms swiftly from side to side.
3. Assume Plank Pose (supporting the body in a strictly straight position on hands and toes as though you were about to do a pushup) but set your feet a little further apart than you would for a pushup. Your head should be in line with your body, bending neither upward nor downward. Gently twist your head to the left and look over your left shoulder until you can see the heel of your right foot on the opposite side of your body. Then twist your head to the right until you can see your left foot.
4. Squatting with your hands on your knees, twist the body to the right and left so as to have the abdomen squeezed by the thighs.

Each round in this cleansing exercise consists of drinking one glass of warm, salty water in alternation with the series of four movements, repeated six times each. These rounds should be carried out until bowel movements appear and until the alimentary canal is actually emptied of its contents, that is, when the liquid contents of the last bowel movement are nearly as clear as drinking water. The whole process may be completed within one hour for experienced practitioners, while it may take a little more time for beginners. It is advisable then to rest a while, preferably lying on your left side, and to take a relaxing bath.

This thorough cleansing should be done once a fortnight or once a month, in the morning after normal evacuation of the bowels.

Easy Method of Alimentary Canal Cleansing

We are presenting here two simplified processes of the cleansing of the alimentary canal for ordinary students: one based on drinking water and the other on drinking water with exercise.

In the water-drinking process six or eight glasses of warm water are drunk at intervals of thirty or forty minutes. It should be done in the morning when the stomach is empty and after normal evacuation of the bowels. After drinking the water, rest should be taken for an hour, followed by an enema. No breakfast should be eaten. At noon only orange juice or some fruits should be eaten, followed by a light dinner in the evening. This may be done once a week or twice a month.

The other alternative is to first drink a cup of warm water and then commence exercise. Then six to eight cups of water should be drunk in between doing various exercises. The abdominal and spinal exercises are more suitable for this purpose. This should be done in the morning when the stomach is quite empty and after the normal evacuation of the bowels.

It can be performed once or twice a week. Breakfast should be omitted on those days, followed later by a very light lunch of fruits and milk and a light dinner in the evening.

Alimentary Canal Auto-Air Bath (Vāta Sāra)

The Alimentary Canal Auto-Air Bath is a very difficult process, a yogic technique that can only be mastered by an advanced practitioner having extraordinary control over the abdominal muscles and certain inner control. This process is very helpful in prolonged breath suspension. By this process atmospheric air is first swallowed, then made to pass into the stomach and thence into the small intestine and large intestine and finally expelled from the body. No instrumental aid is necessary for its performance.

The knee-elbow position is the best for air swallowing and passing. Air should be taken through crow-beak shaped lips. It should be practiced in the morning when the stomach is quite empty. Before commencing the practice, the bowels should be evacuated and the stomach and colon should be cleansed with water. It does not take more than twenty minutes to perform the Alimentary Canal Auto-Air Bath when it is fully mastered.

Natural Nasopharyngeal Water Baths

There are two processes of cleansing the nasal and pharyngeal passages. The first one is the drawing of salty, lukewarm water through the nostrils and its expulsion through the mouth. This is called Vyutkrama Kapālabhātī (Nasopharyngeal Water Bath). The second one, called Śītkrama Kapālabhātī (Inverted Nasopharyngeal Water Bath), consists of taking a mouthful of water and expelling it through the nostrils. A glass or cup may be used for the purpose. A beginner may use lukewarm water for some time, but cold water should be used in general. These nasal baths may be taken in the morning after oral cleansing.

The nasal baths are useful in removing any waste materials accumulated in the nasopharyngeal passages. The circulation in the mucus membrane of the passages is accelerated, its functional efficiency is improved and the local nerves and the brain are invigorated. It has a soothing effect on the brain and the nervous system. After prolonged mental work these baths are a great restorative when followed by breathing exercise.

Nasal Thread-Cleansing (Sūtra Neti)

Nasal Thread-Cleansing consists of passing a fine soft thread, moistened with water, through one nostril, and then ejecting it through the mouth. Another supplementary act is to pass the thread through one nostril and eject it through the other nostril. Both methods can be used together. These acts are best performed in the morning after oral cleansing.

Thread-cleansing cleanses the passages, absorbs morbid secretions, and massages the mucus membrane. The regular use of cold nasal baths and thread-cleansing, according to our experience, prevents colds and catarrh, especially when combined with right diet and exercise. The Nasopharyngeal Water Baths should be taken before and after Nasal Thread-Cleansing. They may be practiced three or four times a week or even more. They may also be taken alternately.

10
The Yoga Method of Endocrine Development

The endocrine glands play an important role in maintaining the health and efficiency of the body. When the functional efficiency of these glands begins to decline, the general decline of the bodily and mental powers starts. It becomes, therefore, evident that the building up of the health and functional efficiency of the endocrine system is absolutely necessary.

Gland Transplantation and Vasoligature

Various attempts have been made to reenergize devitalized endocrine glands by gland transplantation, vasoligature, and organo-therapy. A popular form of gland transplantation was hetero-transplantation in which the glands of a monkey, a goat, or a ram were generally used. Various devices were tried in order to keep the implanted glands alive and functioning in the human body. But in the majority of cases it was found that the implanted gland did not survive. In some cases, it worked only temporarily.

The claim leading to the practice of vasoligature was that the interstitial cells are stimulated and developed by the ligature of the vas deferens, while the generative tissue undergoes degeneration by the constant pressure caused by the accumulated external gonadal fluid. It was further claimed that while the generative part of the glands fails to function, the interstitial part tries to compensate with increased functioning. Unfortunately, this practice did not produce the desired effects. Moreover, the generative part, which is voluntarily made inactive by vasoligature, may play an important role in the chemical balance of the blood, the exact nature of which is not quite known at present. The destruction of the external function of the gonads by vasoligature is not a sane procedure. We also cannot depend upon glandular preparations for permanent results.

Yoga Method

It should be borne in mind that endocrine degeneration is not an isolated phenomenon, but is indicative of the failure of all the tissues of the body to play their parts in maintaining that chemical and physiological state in which the body as a whole functions efficiently. Are we provided with a mechanism through which we can maintain the harmony of organic functions? According to Yoga, two factors form the essential parts of the mechanism: muscular exercise and the state of the blood.

An inseparable functional relationship between the muscles and the various organs has existed for millions of years. In fact, the development of specialized cells, leading to the development of the organs, was intimately related to the demands of the muscles. The cells of the organs as well as of the muscles know how to act in the interest of each other and of the whole body. According to this principle, all the tissues of the body prepare themselves by suitable morphological and physiological changes, and in these changes muscles play a prominent part.

Muscles in action stimulate the activities of the organic system as a whole to maintain the constancy of the inner medium, the blood. Changes in the blood caused by muscular activity demand greater and coordinated activities of all the vital organs including the nervous and endocrine systems. So, in endocrine development, muscular exercise plays a prominent part that is often overlooked.

Blood Purification

Blood purification is a very important factor in making the endocrine glands function efficiently for a prolonged period. Fasting, internal cleansing, fruit and milk diets, and other factors are involved in blood purification. Exercise will prove most fruitful in energizing these glands when rightly combined with the blood purification method.

Blood Purification

1st Stage

Fast for 3 to 5 days, drinking warm water.

Perform Gastric Auto-Lavage and Colonic Auto-Lavage.

Add sunbathing, exposure to fresh air, general bathing, and restricted exercise, if required.

2nd Stage: Special Diet

Break the fast with orange juice.

Take acid fruits for a day or two.

Then take exclusive milk diet or milk-fruit diet for 10 or 12 days.

3rd Stage: Normal Diet

A lacto-vegetarian diet is generally most suitable, as it is eliminative as well as nourishing.

Exercise should be a regular part of the daily program.

Proper application of Gastric Auto-Lavage and Colonic Auto-Lavage should be made.

Sunbathing, fresh air, cold baths, and occasional warm baths should be taken.

Periodical fruit diet, raw diet, or milk-fruit diet are very helpful.

The milk for a milk diet should be raw milk from a healthy and young cow. Such milk is rich in endocrine substances and very suitable for the purpose. The most satisfactory results are obtained when the milk is drunk immediately after it is drawn from the udder.

When following an ordinary diet, care should be taken to maintain the blood in a normal and pure condition. That means the diet should consist of sufficient minerals and vitamins. Adequate quantities of antitoxic and laxative foods should be added. A liberal quantity of fresh, clean, naturally warm milk should be added to the daily diet. This will supply an adequate amount of the most suitable protein, calcium, and vitamins, which are are necessary to prolong the youth of and give life and efficiency to the tissues, the glandular tissues included. All dietetic errors, especially overeating, should be strictly abandoned. The yogic lacto-vegetarian diet is an ideal form of diet to maintain a normal blood condition. Increased elimination should be maintained by cleansing processes. Bacterial healthfulness of the alimentary canal and increased colon activity should be specially maintained by yogic diet, exercise, internal cleansing, and so on.

Exercise for Endocrine Development

Endocrine exercise is that type of exercise that, when rightly applied, causes an accelerated circulation in the endocrine organs. Endocrine exercise may be divided into two groups: dynamic and static. The dynamic form consists of local muscular movements in which the circulation is increased both in the glands and the muscles involved in the exercise. For better results in endocrine development a condition should be created in which there will be a maximum active glandular hyperemia with a minimum muscular hyperemia; this glandular state should be maintained for a prolonged period. This can best be achieved by static posture exercise. However, the most satisfactory results are obtained when both types are combined.

▶ Exercise for the Pineal and Pituitary Glands

Dynamic Form:

General posture exercise
Neck posture exercise
Spinal posture exercise
Breath-control exercise, especially Abdominal Short-Quick Breathing

Static Form:

Head Posture
Head Posture exercises
Inversion Posture
Inverse Lotus Posture
Breath suspension with Chin Lock

▶ Exercise for the Thyroid and Parathyroid Glands

Dynamic Form:

Same as for pineal and pituitary glands. Also speed-endurance exercise.

Static Form:

Shoulder-Stand Posture
Inversion Posture
Breath suspension with Chin Lock

▶ Exercise for the Adrenal Glands

Dynamic Form:

General posture exercise
Spinal posture exercise
Abdominal posture exercise
Abdominal Retraction
Straight Muscle Exercise
Breath-control exercise, especially Abdominal Short-Quick Breathing

Static Form:

Inversion Posture
Head Posture
Head Posture exercises

11
Sexual Efficiency and Control

The gonads play an extraordinary role in extracting and concentrating vital elements from the whole body and producing a replica of the person, and in converging the sexual urge through which the human creative hunger is satisfied. The seminiferous tubules of the male gonads produce the creative substance, the sperm, which unites with the ovum to give rise to a new individual. The testicular hormone plays an important part in influencing muscular development and strength. It helps in maintaining the development and strength of the heart. It regulates the accumulation and distribution of fat characteristic of the male body. It stimulates the blood-making organs and serves to increase the formation of hemoglobin.

Interstitial Cells and Seminiferous Tubules

Today, it is generally accepted, though by no means conclusively proved, that groups of interstitial cells contained in loose connective tissue in the spaces between the seminiferous tubules manufacture the hormone. An attempt was made to develop the interstitial tissue by the ligature of the vas deferens. It was believed that vasoligature would create a more suitable condition for the development of the interstitial cells and their increased functioning by destroying the seminiferous tubules. It is now known that vasectomy does not stop spermatogenesis. Moreover, it has not been demonstrated that there is an actual increase in the interstitial cells as a result of vasoligature.

In cases of undescended testes or engrafted male gonads in the abdominal cavity, degeneration of the generative tissue occurs, and finally almost all its parts may disappear. The impairment of the generative part of the gonads is mainly due to greater temperature in the abdomen than in the scrotum. The interstitial tissue is not much affected by cryptorchidism. The degeneration of the generative tissue does not cause any improvement in hormonic function. Rather there is much less hormone production than normal. Such observations and experiments do not prove that degeneration of the generative part of the gonads causes greater development of the interstitial part, rather they show that the latter is also affected but not to the same degree. Moreover, these experiments do not conclusively prove that the generative tissue is not involved in the production of the sex hormone. They simply demonstrate that the interstitial tissue can influence the accessory sex organs even in the absence of the generative tissue.

Under normal conditions, spermatogenesis and hormone production run more or less parallel. It appears that both functions are normally interrelated and interdependent. In the developmental period, spermatogenesis, hormone production, and bodily development go hand in hand. So far as our experiences go we find that gonadal wastage in the early developmental period is unsuitable. Moreover, our observations suggest that external gonadal secretion also influences the body when wastage is prevented. It is also likely that at least at a certain stage of development, the spermatogenic cells of the tubules may manufacture a hormone that strengthens the hormone produced by the interstitial cells and that they may both work in a harmonious manner and most efficiently. Perhaps this joint action is more suitable for the better development of the body and mind, though the hormone of the interstitial cells alone is capable of maintaining the development of the accessory organs of sex.

Most probably, normally both the tissues influence the organism, one acting in cooperation with the other, in such a way that the most satisfactory manly type of body and mind, strength, and character will be developed. We also consider, and this is backed by our experience, that the conservation of the gonadal energy is a highly important factor in maintaining the joint action of the two parts of the gonads and their influence on health, vitality, and vigor.

Control of Ejaculation

We do not know much about the influence of the gonadal external secretion on the body except its reproductive function. A certain period of time is necessary for the maturation of the sperm cells in the epididymis. Just how much time is necessary for their full growth, no one knows—here we can only guess. Nor is it known how long they remain young. On the other hand, frequent ejaculations give less or almost no opportunity for them to attain their physiological maturity in the epididymis. Even from the point of view of fertilization, excessive gonadal wastage is contraindicated.

If ejaculations are postponed for a reasonably long time, the matured sperm cells will be forced out from the epididymis into the vas deferens by the pressure of the incoming new sperm cells from the seminiferous tubules, as the production of spermatozoa is constant after puberty. The various external secretions, especially of the seminal vesicles and the prostate gland, will be added to the released well-developed sperm cells. The prostatic secretion seems to prolong their life. If ejaculation is checked for a sufficiently prolonged period, the entire system of ducts, especially the epididymis, vas deferens, the ampulla of the vas deferens, and the seminal vesicle will be filled with the vital fluid. Normally, seminal vesicles do not serve as reservoirs for sperm cells. But under these conditions the sperm cells are forced to enter into these hollow bags. The life of the released sperm cells from the epididymis seems to be prolonged here because of their having a comparatively free motility and a more favorable environment.

Two factors may be associated with the control of ejaculation. One of the two relates to whether the retained sperm cells in a living state produce any substance having some specific influence on the revitalization of the body and mind. And after their death, do the sperm cells become a source of supplying precious materials to the body, when reabsorbed? Do they aid in maintaining a healthy and efficient condition of both the generative and interstitial parts of the gonads? It seems to us that the external secretion (śukra) with its high concentration of *ojas,* is a highly precious substance, which may be utilized in the construction and reconstruction of the body. The yogins found in it the secret of the prolongation of youth, efficiency, and life.

The second factor in connection with the control of ejaculation is the transformation of the sex energy by its repression into a suprasexual form, which is utilized in developing higher physical, mental, and spiritual powers. That sexual control is conducive to the maintenance of individual vigor has been demonstrated. The spirit of continued struggle, the power of concentrating emotional, mental, and physical energy, and the arousing of the dormant powers are really associated with sexual control. Excessive indulgence has the opposite effects.

Yogic Method for Sexual Control

It is not an easy matter to prevent the waste of seminal fluid. The fluid, especially the internal secretion, supplies some chemicals to the blood, which is one of the chief factors responsible for the psychosexual phenomena in man. The emotion and the urge are governed to a very great extent by the chemicals elaborated by the gonads. This is beyond the field of mere psychical adventure. Desire is stirred by imagination, association, and various local and general disturbances; when it is strengthened by experience it becomes extremely difficult to harness this powerful creative force.

In Yoga, a highly scientific method of gonadal control has been evolved. It has been termed Vajrolī Mudrā.

Sexual Control Exercise (Vajrolī Mudrā)

The sexual control process consists of three main stages. At the first stage, students aim at building up sexual health and efficiency to a high level. Gonadal efficiency is intimately associated with the following factors: vigorous health of the body, a high degree of nerve power and control, and a very powerful contractile power of the orifices of the ejaculatory ducts. All these are attained through the practice of exercise combined with blood purification and other health-building measures.

The exercises to be practiced include general posture exercises and special exercises, such as abdominal posture exercise, spinal posture exercise, pelvic posture exercise, abdominal control exercise, and pelvic control exercise. In addition to these exercises, a special measure is to be taken to relieve pelvic congestion. This is most fruitfully effected by inverse body posture exercise, especially when the inverse postures are maintained for a prolonged period. Inversion Posture (fig. 19.1) and Head Posture (fig. 19.3) are the best for the purpose.

A high degree of retentive power and gonadal vigor with well-controlled urge and decongested organs will be attained if the exercises are practiced according to the direction of a competent teacher. At this stage, a student will be able to use sexual vigor reasonably, avoiding all sexual excesses. He will experience that intercourse is health-giving and has a vitalizing effect on the body.

At the second stage, the pelvic control exercises are carried to a point where it is not only possible to prolong intercourse to a very great extent, but to control orgasm, too. In a prolonged intercourse, the system is given full opportunity to produce the internal and external secretions of the gonads in large quantities, to cause an increased absorption of the internal secretion into the blood, and to distribute the vital chemicals from the gonadal secretions to all the cells of the body. In other words, the whole system is reenergized by this process.

The second stage may be subdivided into two parts. At first, special abdominal-pelvic exercises are practiced in conjunction with indirect contact and direct passive contact. When this phase is mastered, students are advised to practice the exercises with dynamic contact. Three important factors are involved in the gonadal exercises: internal muscular control, special breathing technique, and special concentration.

It is extremely difficult to reach the final stage of the control process, but when it is acquired, maximum sexual control and efficiency are attained. To attain success in the final stage, the practitioner should master the following two practices: penile contraction and urethral suction. In the penile contraction the male organ can be completely drawn inside the body by voluntary effort. The writer has demonstrated this in India and abroad. The attainment of urethral control culminates in the development of urethral suction power demonstrated by fluid being sucked into the bladder through the urethra without any instrumental aid. The purpose of such a demonstration is not cystic lavage. Rather, it demonstrates the mastery of sexual control.

At the last stage atmospheric air can be sucked through the urethra without instrumentation. The suction of milk and air through the urethra without any mechanical help was demonstrated worldwide by Dinabandhu Pramanick at: the Physicians' Square Club of Greater New York; St. Luke's Hospital, Chicago; the 43rd Congress of the American Naturopathic Association; Macfadden's Physical Culture Institute, New York; the Physiology Department of the Imperial University, Tokyo; St. Luke's International Medical Center, Tokyo; 1949 World Physical Education Congress, Stockholm; Human Morpho-Physiological Society, Paris; Salptriére Hospital, Paris; Kinesitherapy Society, Paris; and before many eminent medical men in India, America, and Europe.

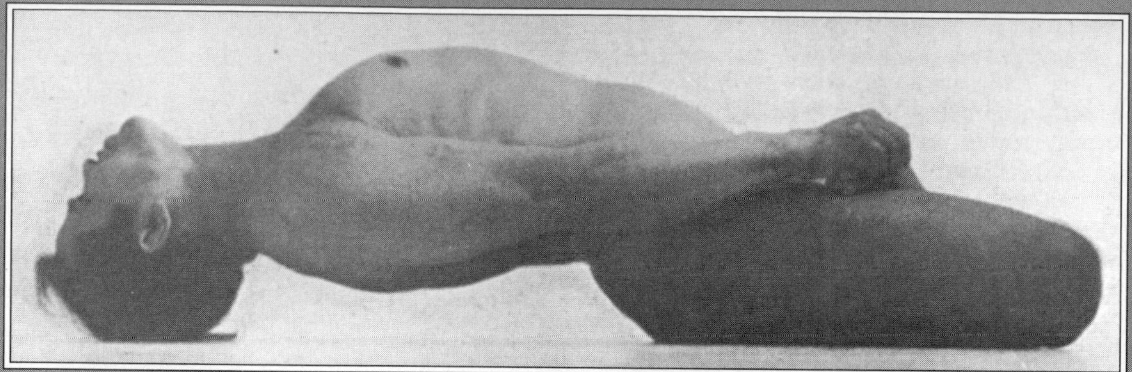

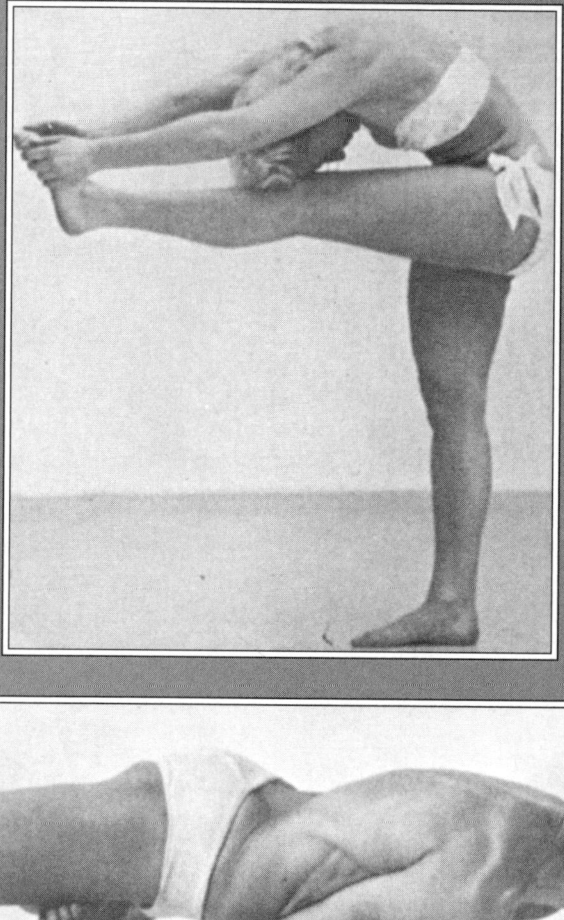

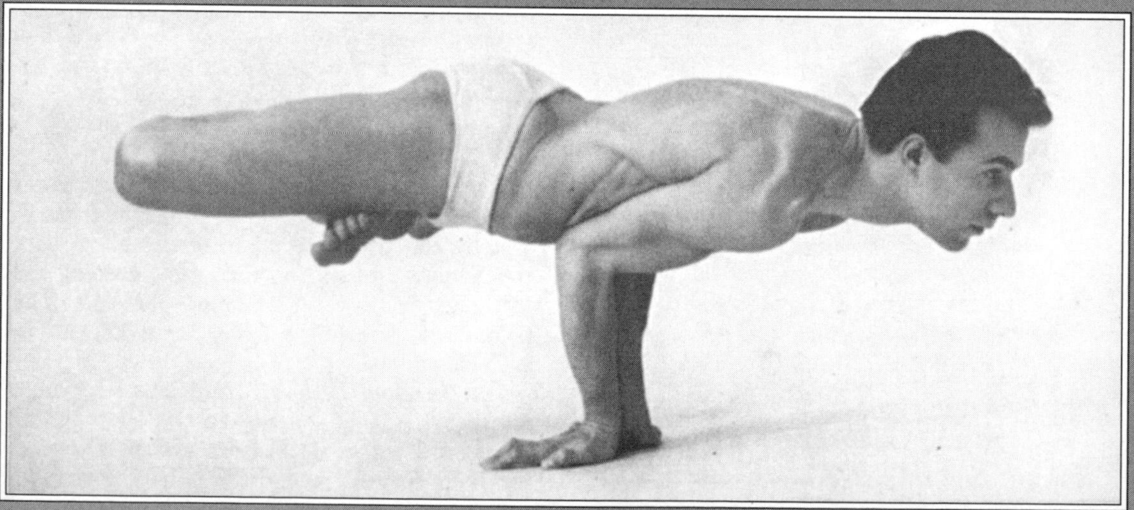

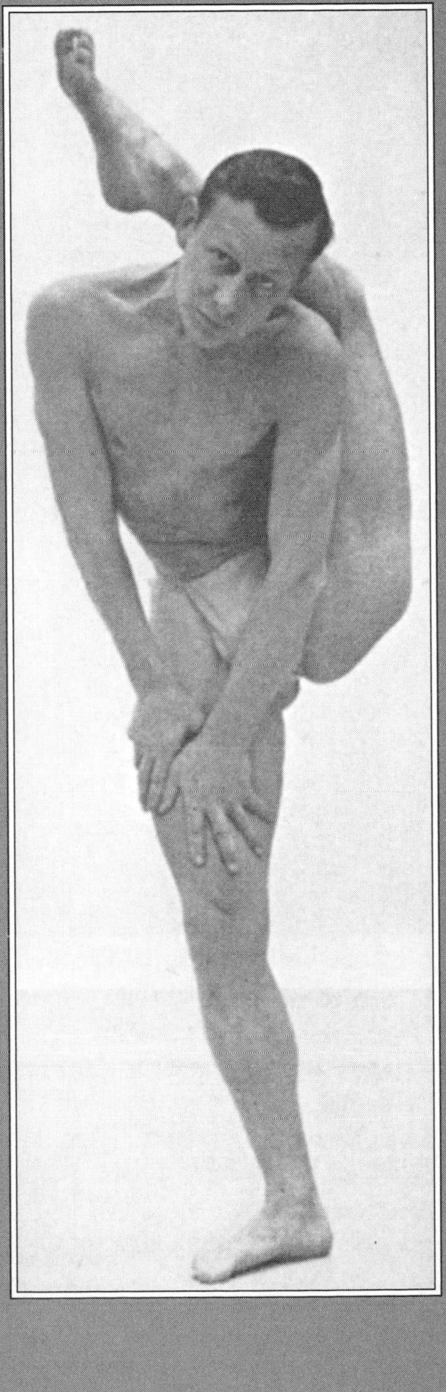

PART TWO

TECHNICAL ASPECTS OF YOGA EXERCISE

12

Spinal Posture Exercise

Posture exercise is of two types: dynamic and static. It is not necessary to consider each type of exercise separately except for a few folded-leg postures. It is more convenient to consider each exercise from both standpoints.

Starting Positions

Certain positions are assumed when starting posture exercise. These may be called starting positions. They may be classified into two: horizontal positions and vertical positions. Still there is another type of position in which the body is inverted.

The horizontal starting positions consist of three main positions: Corpse Posture or Supine Posture, Prone Posture, and Side-Lying Posture.

In Corpse Posture the body is lying on the floor with the face upward, arms by the sides.

In Prone Posture the body lies on the floor with face downward, arms by the sides.

In Side-Lying Posture the body lies on the right or left side with the upper trunk, pelvis and legs in straight line, the top arm by the side and the lower arm as advised.

The principal vertical starting positions are Standing Posture, Kneeling Posture, Adamantine Posture, Squat Posture, and Right-Angle Posture.

In Standing Posture the individual stands with the body erect, the arms hanging by the sides, either with the feet slightly separated and parallel or with the heels together and the toes pointing slightly outward.

In Kneeling Posture the individual stands on the knees, the body erect, hands resting on the thighs.

In Adamantine Posture the individual sits on the heels with the legs bent at the knees and folded back under the thighs, the feet placed under the buttocks by the sides of the anus, with soles upward, and the palms on the knees.

In Squat Posture the squatting position is assumed.

In Right-Angle Posture the body is erect, with the legs extended in front and the arms by the sides.

Spinal Posture Exercise Defined and Classified

Spinal posture exercise is based on the normal movements of the spinal column. These movements are flexion, extension, lateral flexion, and rotation. When the body is bent forward and downward from the erect position, the movement is called flexion. Where the body goes back to the erect position or bent backward and downward, it is called extension. Lateral flexion is the sideward bending of the body, and rotation is the twisting of the body. Flexion occurs most freely in the cervical, upper thoracic, and lumbar regions of the spine, extension in the cervical and lumbar regions, lateral flexion in the cervical and lumbar regions, and rotation in the cervical and thoracic regions.

Spinal posture exercise is a form of exercise designed to bring the muscles concerned in the spinal movements into play in a graduated manner, thus creating a most suitable condition for their development and control and, through them, to benefit the whole body. It develops nervous, glandular, circulatory, digestive, respiratory, and eliminative efficiency, increases vital vigor and endurance, promotes health, and invigorates the general system. It is an indispensable part of any form of exercise program.

Spinal posture exercise consists of four forms of exercise: posterior trunk-bend posture exercise, anterior trunk-bend posture exercise, lateral trunk-bend posture exercise, and trunk-twist posture exercise. The thoracic and the lumbar regions of the spine are principally involved in these exercises. The cervical spine needs special exercise, which is termed neck posture exercise, considered separately for convenience. In fact, spinal exercise is incomplete without neck exercise.

In posterior trunk-bend posture exercise the spinal muscles are contracted and the abdominal muscles are stretched. On the other hand, in anterior trunk-bend posture exercise the abdominal muscles are contracted and the spinal muscles are stretched. For full muscular development full contraction and stretching are the sine qua non. The abdominal muscles are spinal muscles and abdominal exercise is in reality spinal exercise. Spinal development is intrinsically related to nerve vigor, organic efficiency, and the natural healthfulness of the body. Abdominal development is a most important part of the alimentary purificatory processes and breath control. It is so important in Yoga that a special form of posture exercise termed abdominal posture exercise has been developed for its attainment (see chapter 14).

Posterior Trunk-Bend Posture Exercise

The exercises listed under this heading cause contraction of the spinal muscles and stretching of the abdominal muscles. The spinal muscles that are directly involved in this form of exercise are the sacrospinalis group (thoracic and lumbar portions), which includes the iliocostalis lumborum, iliocostalis dorsi, longissimus dorsi, and spinalis dorsi, and the semispinalis dorsi. These muscles are assisted by the multifidus (thoracic, lumbar, and sacral portions), rotatores, interspinales (thoracic and lumbar portions), intertransversarii (thoracic and lumbar portions), and levatores costarum. The spinal muscles are assisted by the trapezius, latissimus dorsi, and quadratus lumborum.

As with all posture exercises these exercises should be applied in a graduated manner for the most satisfactory results. At the preliminary stage attention should be focused on perfecting the exercise. After the exercise is mastered, the mind should be fully concentrated on the muscles principally involved in the exercise. In all posterior trunk-bend posture exercises the mind should be concentrated on the spinal and back muscles.

Cobra Posture

1. Assume a prone position with feet together, palms flat on the floor by the shoulders.
2. Raise the head and the trunk from the lower part of the abdomen upward and backward as much as possible by straightening the arms almost fully or fully. Maintain the final attitude for a few seconds (fig. 12.1).
3. Return to step 1.

Breathing: Inhale in step 2, exhale in step 3, when the movements are executed rhythmically after the exercise is mastered. In mastering the movements it may be necessary to take more time in executing the raising movement. In that case breathing should be normal. This applies to all exercises. Moreover, breath should not be held in any exercise unless specially mentioned.

Dynamic Application: Steps 2 and 3 should be alternately executed without any break.

Static Application: Maintain the final attitude (step 2) as instructed by a qualified Yoga teacher. Breathing is usually normal. This applies to all exercises.

Relaxation: After completion of the exercise, either dynamic or static, relax in Prone Posture.

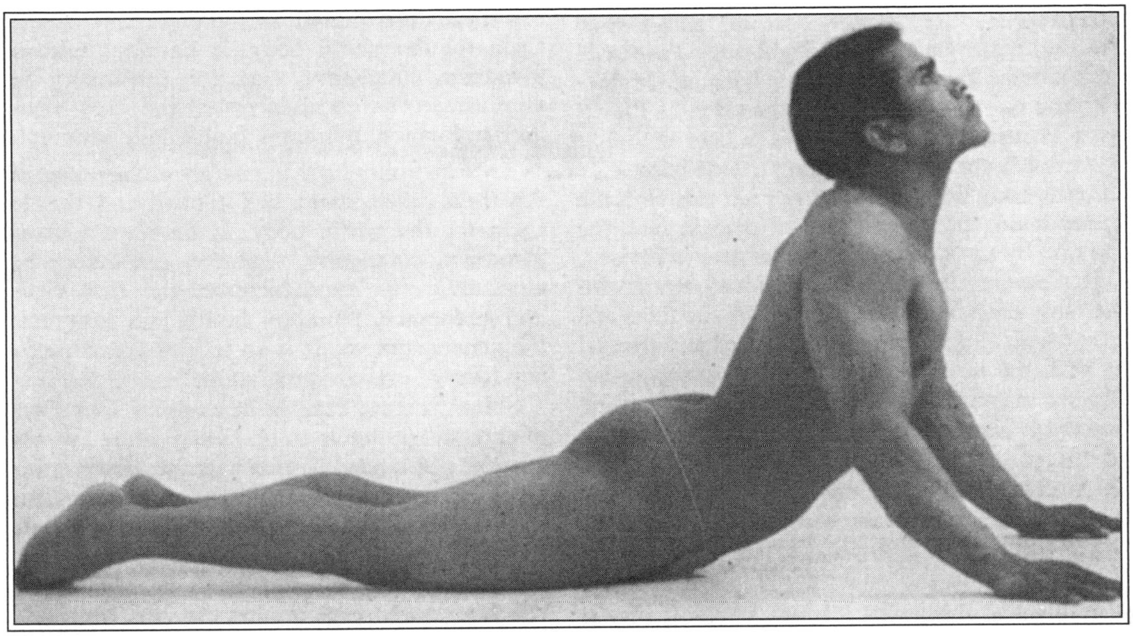

Fig. 12.1. Cobra Posture (Bhujangāsana)

Snake Posture

1. Assume a prone position with the hands clasped behind the back.
2. Raise the head and the trunk from the lower part of the abdomen upward and backward as much as possible without any jerk. Maintain the final attitude for a few seconds (fig. 12.2).
3. Return to step 1.

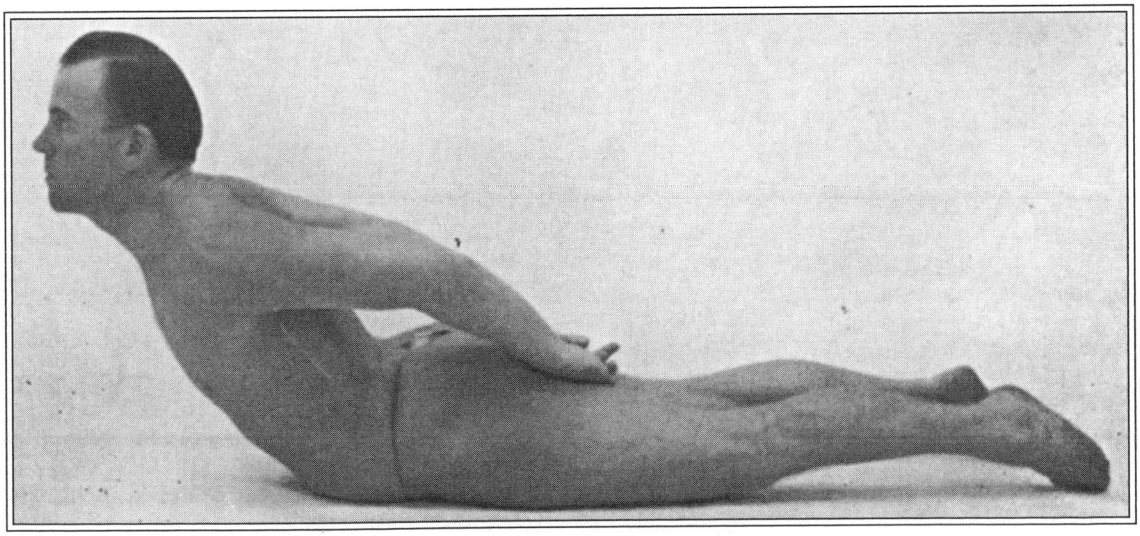

Fig. 12.2. Snake Posture (Sarpāsana)

Breathing: Inhale in step 2 and exhale in step 3.

Dynamic Application: Steps 2 and 3 should be alternately executed.

Static Application: Maintain the final attitude (step 2) as instructed by a qualified Yoga teacher.

Relaxation: After completion of the exercise, either dynamic or static, relax in Prone Posture.

Back-Raise Posture with Forearms Locked behind Head

1. Assume a prone position with the forearms locked behind the head (i.e. arms bent at elbows, folded elbows placed one upon the other, resting on the head, hands on the scapular region, right on the left side and left on the right side).
2. Raise the head and the trunk from the lower part of the abdomen upward and backward as much as possible without any jerk. Maintain the final attitude for a few seconds (fig. 12.3).
3. Return to step 1.

Breathing: Inhale in step 2 and exhale in step 3.

Dynamic Application: Steps 2 and 3 should be alternately executed.

Static Application: Maintain the final attitude (step 2) as instructed by a qualified Yoga teacher.

Relaxation: After completion of the exercise, dynamic or static, relax in Prone Posture.

Points of Note: It is desirable in many cases for the development of strength and flexibility to first practice Back-Raise Posture with the hands clasped behind the neck instead of the forearms being locked behind the head.

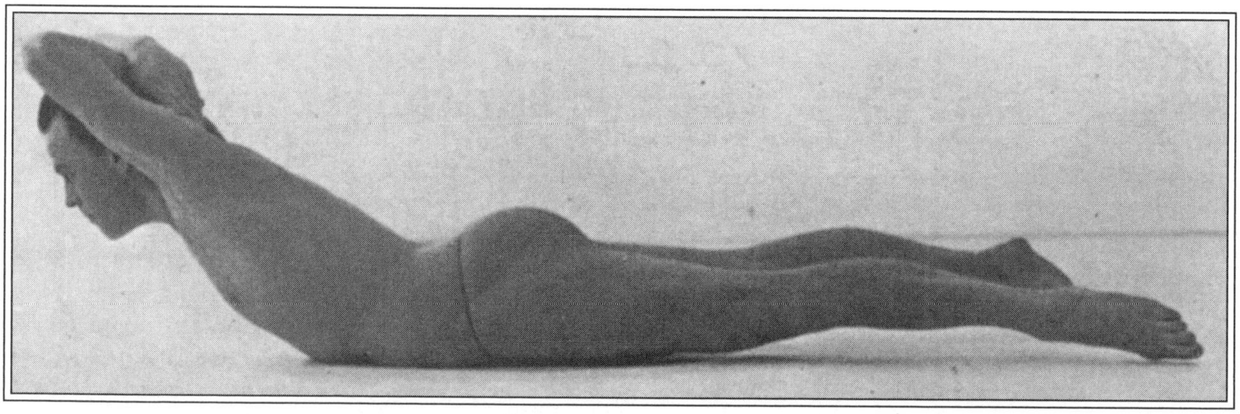

Fig. 12.3. Back-Raise Posture with Forearms Locked behind Head (Makarāsana)

Locust Posture

1. Assume a prone position with arms by the sides and palms either upward or downward.
2. Raise the legs as high as possible, with the body supported by the hands and the upper part of the body. Maintain the final attitude for a few seconds (fig. 12.4).
3. Return to step 1.

Breathing: Inhale in step 2 and exhale in step 3.

Dynamic Application: Steps 2 and 3 should be alternately executed.

Static Application: Raise the legs while inhaling, or first inhale and hold the breath and then raise the legs to the maximum point. Maintain the final attitude while holding the breath as instructed by a qualified Yoga teacher. Then lower the legs while exhaling.

Relaxation: After completion of the exercise, dynamic or static, relax in Prone Posture.

Points of Note: As with all posterior trunk-bend posture exercise, concentration is on the spinal and back muscles, especially the lumbar region and latissimus dorsi. It is desirable in many cases to increase the strength of the muscles involved in Locust Posture by first practicing Modified Locust Posture, in which one leg is raised at a time instead of both legs. Both legs, of course, should be exercised in this way.

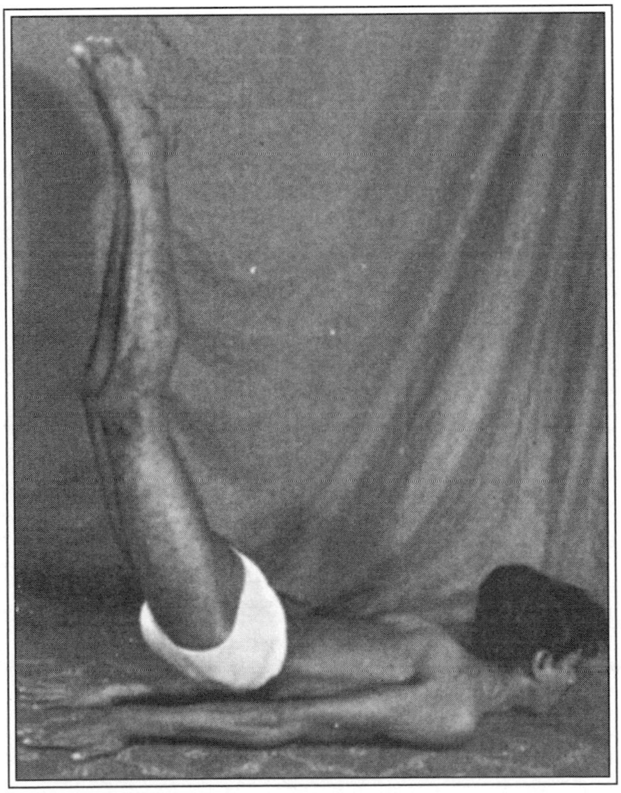

Fig. 12.4. Locust Posture (Śalabhāsana)

Bow Posture

1. Assume a prone position with arms by the sides.
2. Bend the legs back over the thighs, extend the arms, and grasp the ankles with the hands. The knees may either be kept close to each other or a few inches apart.
3. Raise the head, trunk, and thighs as high as possible without any jerk. Maintain the final attitude for a few seconds (fig. 12.5).
4. Return to step 2.
5. After completion of the exercise, return to step 1.

Breathing: Inhale in step 3 and exhale in step 4.

Dynamic Application: Steps 3 and 4 should be alternately executed.

Static Application: Maintain the final attitude (step 3) as instructed by a qualified Yoga teacher.

Relaxation: After completion of the exercise, dynamic or static, relax in Prone Posture.

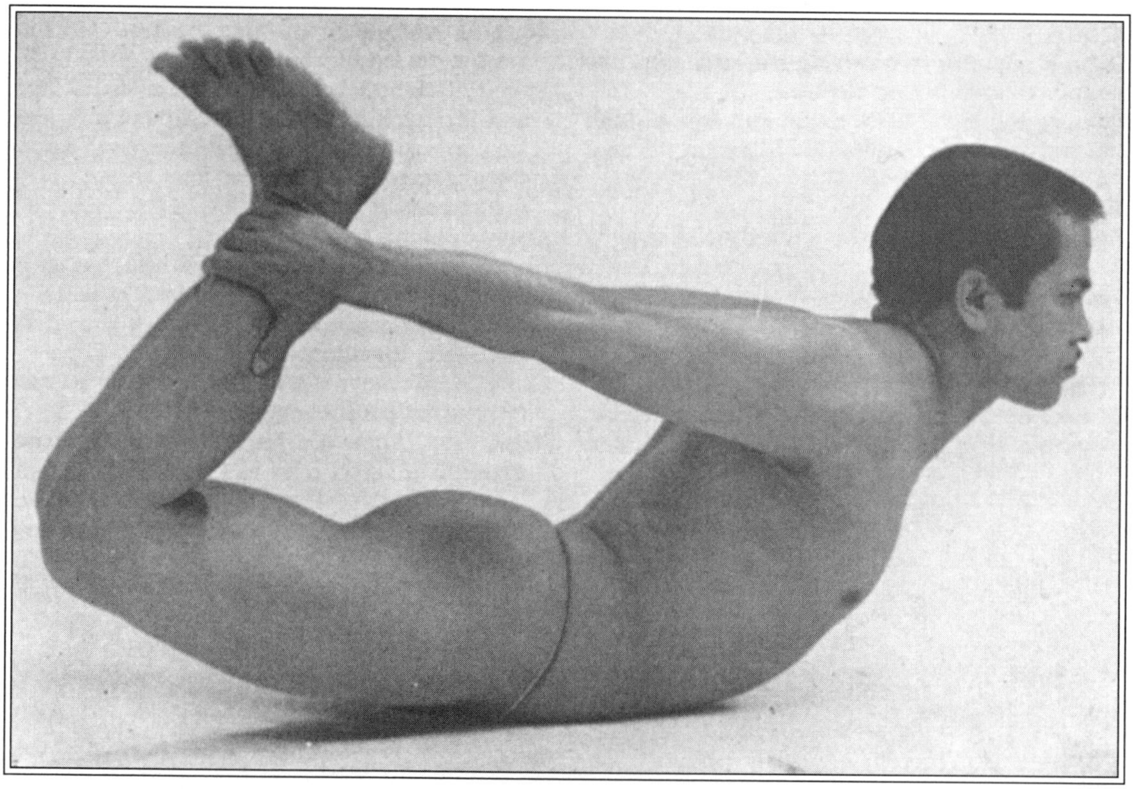

Fig. 12.5. Bow Posture (Dhanurāsana)

Boat Posture

1. Assume a prone position with the hands clasped behind the back.
2. Raise the head, trunk, and legs as high as possible without any jerk. Maintain the final attitude for a few seconds (fig. 12.6).
3. Return to step 1.

Breathing: Inhale in step 2 and exhale in step 3.

Dynamic Application: Steps 2 and 3 should be alternately executed.

Static Application: Maintain the final attitude (step 2) as instructed by a qualified Yoga teacher.

Relaxation: After completion of the exercise, dynamic or static, relax in Prone Posture.

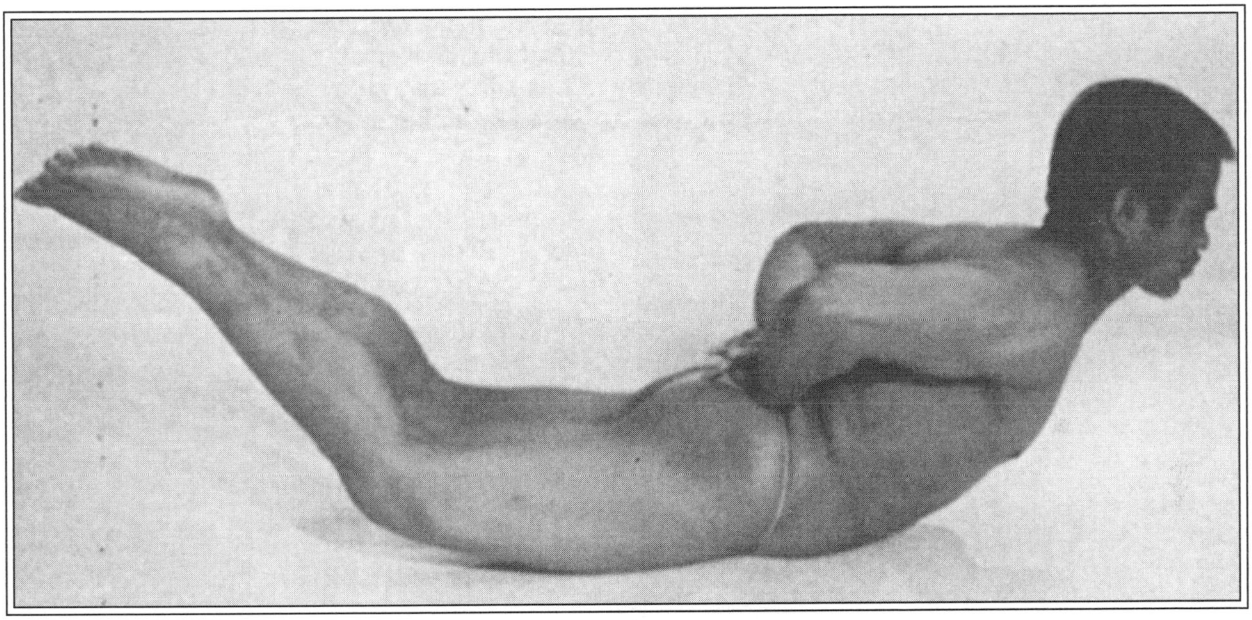

Fig. 12.6. Boat Posture (Naukāsana)

Swing Posture

1. Assume a prone position with the arms extended forward.
2. Raise the head, trunk, and the extended arms and legs as high as you can without any jerk, supporting the body mainly on the lower part of the abdomen. Maintain the final attitude for a few seconds (fig. 12.7 on page 114).
3. Return to step 1.

Breathing: Inhale in step 2 and exhale in step 3.

Dynamic Application: Steps 2 and 3 should be alternately executed.

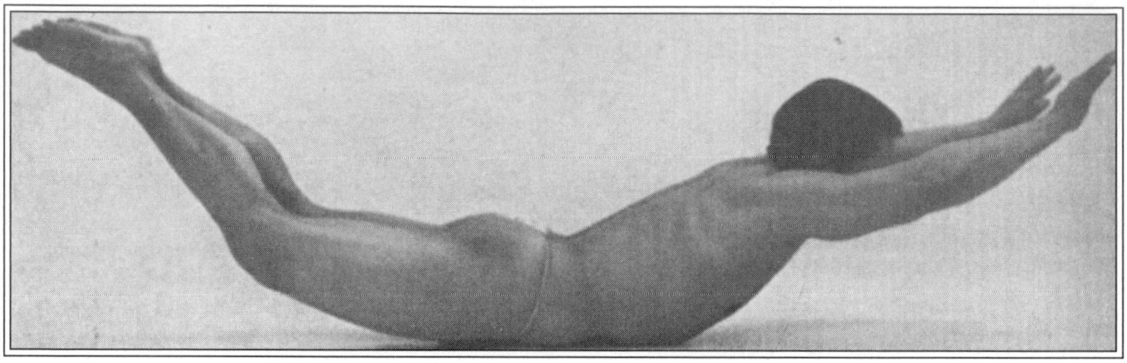

Fig. 12.7. Swing Posture (Dolāsana)

Static Application: Maintain the final attitude (step 2) as instructed by a qualified Yoga teacher.

Relaxation: After completion of the exercise, dynamic or static, relax in Prone Posture.

King-Cobra Posture

1. Assume a prone position with feet together and palms flat by the shoulders.
2. First raise the head and the trunk upward and backward to the fullest extent by straightening the arms fully. Then carry the movement further by bending the head and the trunk and especially the dorso-lumbar region of the spine backward. At the same time, raise up the hips and thighs and elevate the legs, bending them at the knees, until the toes meet the back of the head. The movement should be continuous and not jerky. The final attitude should be maintained for a few seconds (fig. 12.8).
3. Return to step 1.

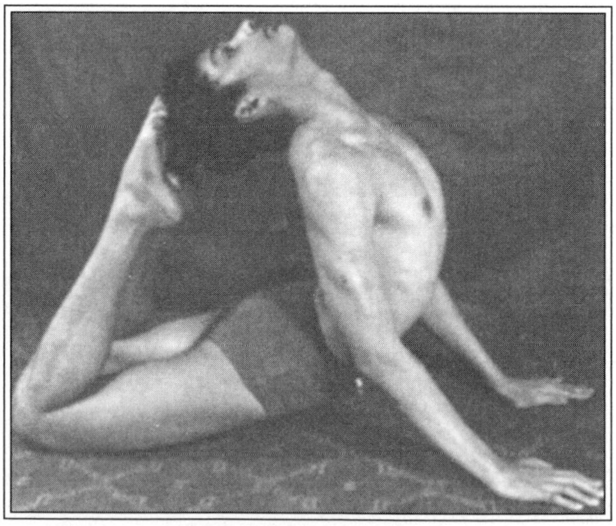

Fig. 12.8. King-Cobra Posture (Bhujangendrāsana)

Breathing: (a) Before the movement is mastered, breathing should be normal throughout step 2; (b) after the movement is well controlled, inhale in step 2, exhale in step 3.

Dynamic Application: Steps 2 and 3 should be alternately executed.

Static Application: Maintain the final attitude (step 2) as instructed by a qualified Yoga teacher.

Relaxation: After completion of the exercise, dynamic or static, relax in Corpse Posture or Prone Posture.

Cuckoo Posture

1. Assume a prone position with feet together or a few inches apart and palms flat by the shoulders.
2. Raise the whole body a few inches off the floor, supporting it on the hands and toes.
3. Raise the head and the trunk upward and backward from the hips as much as possible by straightening the arms without allowing the legs to touch the floor. Now try to bend the trunk still further backward. Finally, make the whole range of movement into a continuous one. Maintain the final attitude for a few seconds (fig. 12.9).
4. From the final attitude (step 3) raise the hips as high as you can. From this position return to step 3.
5. On completion of the exercise return to step 1.

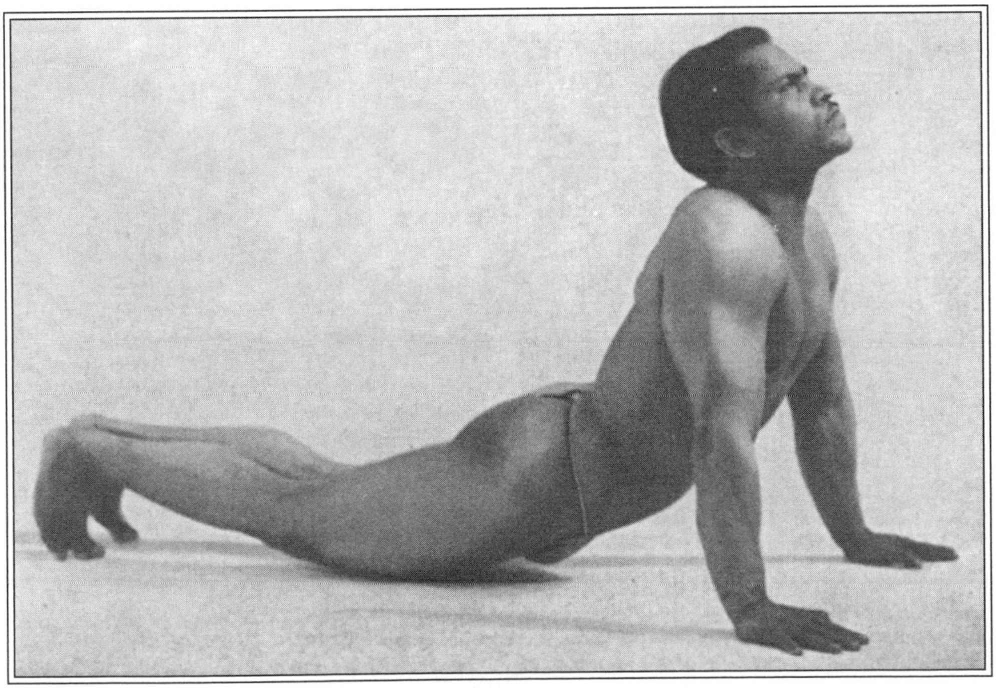

Fig. 12.9. Cuckoo Posture (Cātakāsana)

Breathing: Breathing should be normal until the whole range of movement becomes continuous. Thereafter inhale in step 3 and exhale in step 4.

Dynamic Application: Steps 3 and 4 should be alternately executed.

Static Application: Maintain the final attitude (step 3) as instructed by a qualified Yoga teacher.

Relaxation: After completion of the exercise, dynamic or static, relax in Prone Posture.

Raised Bow Posture

1. Assume a supine position with the legs bent at the knees and drawn to the buttocks and the palms placed on the floor by the shoulders, bending at the elbows.
2. Raise the body upward into a bridge position by straightening the arms and legs and supporting the body on the palms and feet. Maintain the final attitude for a few seconds (fig. 12.10).
3. Lower the body to step 1.

Breathing: Inhale in step 2 and exhale in step 3.

Dynamic Application: Steps 2 and 3 should be alternately executed.

Static Application: Maintain the final attitude (step 2) as instructed by a qualified Yoga teacher.

Relaxation: After completion of the exercise, dynamic or static, relax in Corpse Posture.

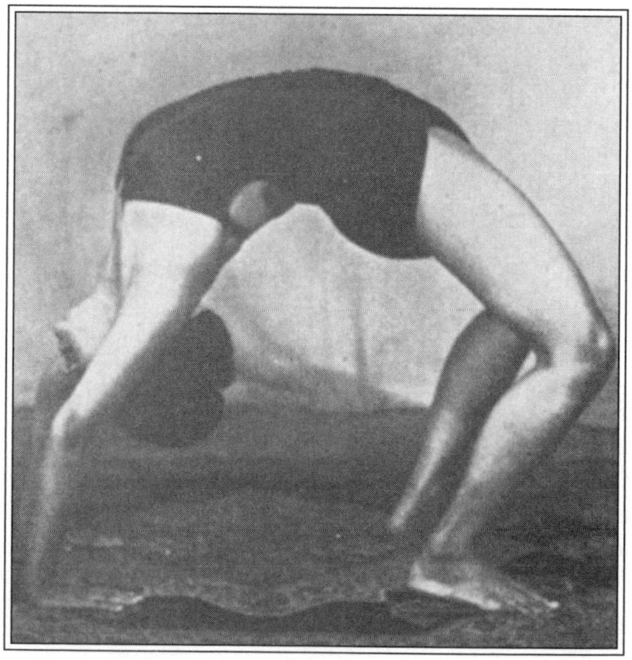

Fig. 12.10. Raised Bow Posture (Ūrdhva Dhanurāsana)

Bent-Head Adamantine Posture

1. Assume kneeling position with the forearms locked behind the head.
2. Slowly bend the head and the body backward and downward until the head touches the floor (fig. 12.11).
3. Return to step 1 slowly.

Breathing: Normal.

Dynamic Application: Steps 2 and 3 should be alternately executed.

Static Application: Not suitable.

Relaxation: After completion of the exercise, relax in Adamantine Posture.

Points of Note: This is an advanced exercise for both back and abdomen. To gradually attain sufficient strength and flexibility of the back, it is advantageous to practice this exercise first with the hands on the thighs and then with the hands clasped behind the neck.

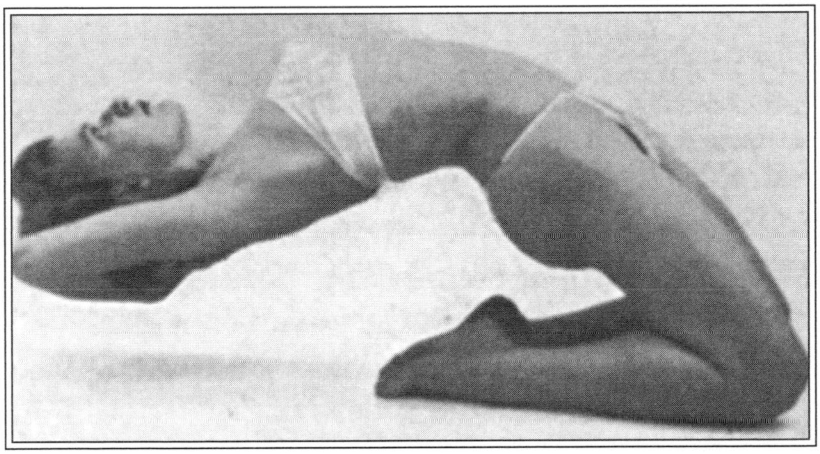

Fig. 12.11. Bent-Head Adamantine Posture (Natašira Vajrāsana)

Modified Wheel Posture

1. Assume standing position with the feet together or a few inches apart and the arms overhead.
2. Bend the trunk slowly from the waist backward and downward until it is horizontal. Maintain the final attitude for a few seconds (fig. 12.12 on page 118).
3. Return to step 1.

Breathing: Normal.

Dynamic Application: Steps 2 and 3 should be alternately executed.

Static Application: Not suitable.

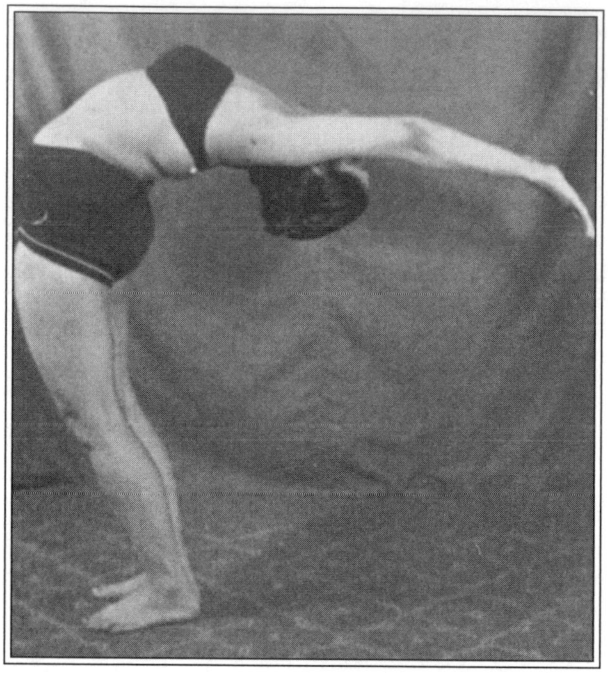

Fig. 12.12. Modified Wheel Posture
(Ardha Cakrāsana)

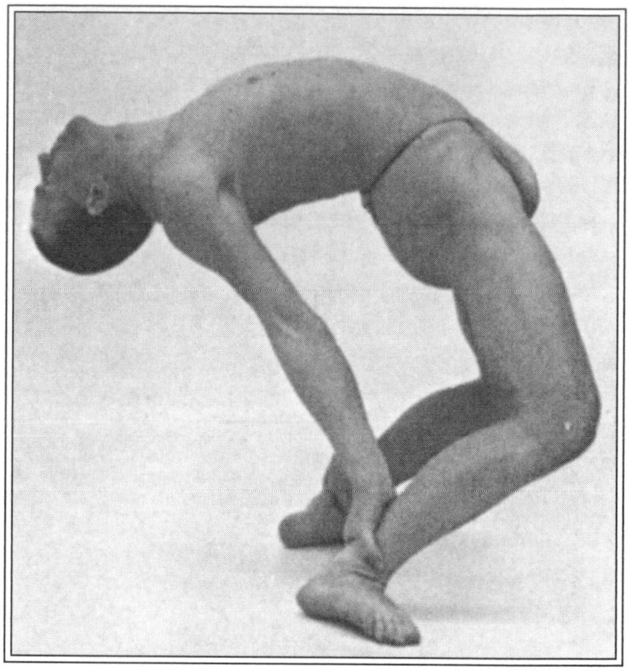

Fig. 12.13. Back Posture
(Pṛiṣṭhāsana)

Relaxation: After completion of the exercise, relax in Standing Posture.

Points of Note: The movement should be executed slowly and without any jerk. The legs should not be allowed to bend at the knees.

Back Posture

1. Assume standing position with the feet apart and the arms by the sides.
2. Slowly bend the trunk from the waist backward and downward until you are able to hold the ankles with the hands of the extended arms. Maintain the final attitude for a few seconds (fig. 12.13).
3. Return to step 1. Ordinarily the movement is discontinued after the final attitude is assumed. Then the movement is started again from the standing position.

Breathing: Normal.

Dynamic Application: Steps 2 and 3 can be alternately executed after sufficient strength is developed.

Static Application: Not suitable.

Relaxation: After completion of the exercise, relax in Standing Posture.

Points of Note: This is an advanced spinal exercise.

Wheel Posture

1. Assume standing position with the feet a few inches apart and the arms overhead.
2. Slowly bend the trunk and the arms along with the head from the waist backward and downward until the palms are placed on the floor. Then bring the hands into contact with the heels. Maintain the final attitude for a few seconds (fig. 12.14).
3. Unusual abdominal strength is required to return to step 2 slowly. Ordinarily the movement is discontinued after the final attitude is assumed (step 2). Then the movement is started again from the standing position.

Breathing: Normal.

Dynamic Application: Steps 2 and 3 can be alternately executed after sufficient strength is developed.

Static Application: Maintain the final attitude (step 2) as instructed by a qualified Yoga teacher.

Relaxation: After completion of the exercise, relax in Standing Posture.

Points of Note: This is an advanced spinal exercise.

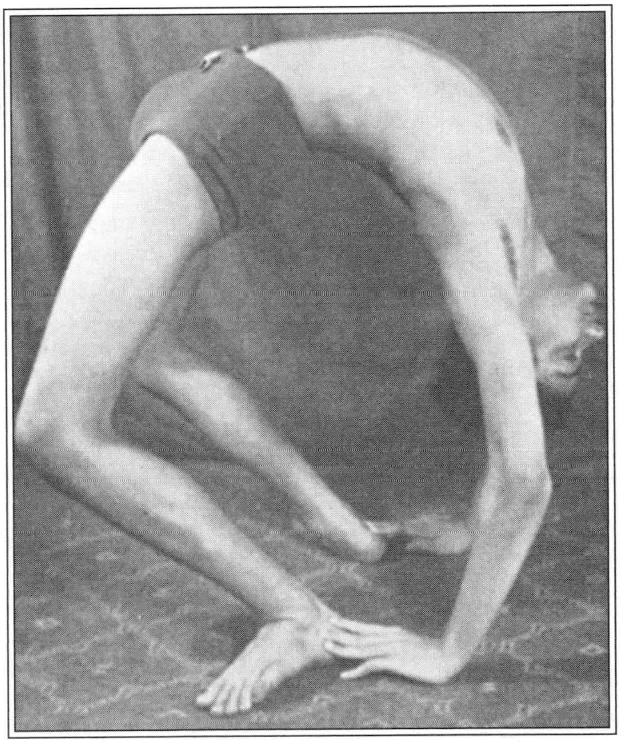

Fig. 12.14. Wheel Posture (Cakrāsana)

Anterior Trunk-Bend Posture Exercise

The exercises listed under this heading cause contraction of the abdominal muscles and stretching of the spinal muscles. The principal muscles involved are the rectus abdominis, obliquus externus abdominis, and obliquus internus abdominis. These muscles are assisted by the abdominal muscles, the psoas major and psoas minor. This type of spinal exercise is, in fact, abdominal exercise. The mind should be concentrated upon the abdominal muscles during these exercises.

Spinal-Stretch Posture

1. Sit with the legs extended in front, feet together, arms bent at the elbows and at the level of the shoulders, forearms and fingers extended forward, body erect.
2. Bend the body forward and downward and simultaneously extend the arms forward and grasp the big toes or all the toes with the hands. Then bend the head until the forehead touches the knees. The legs should be kept perfectly straight throughout the exercise. The arms may either be bent at the elbows or kept straight while holding the toes. Maintain the final attitude for a few seconds (fig. 12.15).
3. Return to step 1.

Breathing: Exhale in step 2, inhale in step 3.

Dynamic Application: Steps 2 and 3 should be alternately executed.

Static Application: Maintain the final attitude (step 2) as instructed by a qualified Yoga teacher.

Relaxation: After completion of the exercise, dynamic or static, relax in the sitting position with the legs extended forward and the arms hanging by the sides.

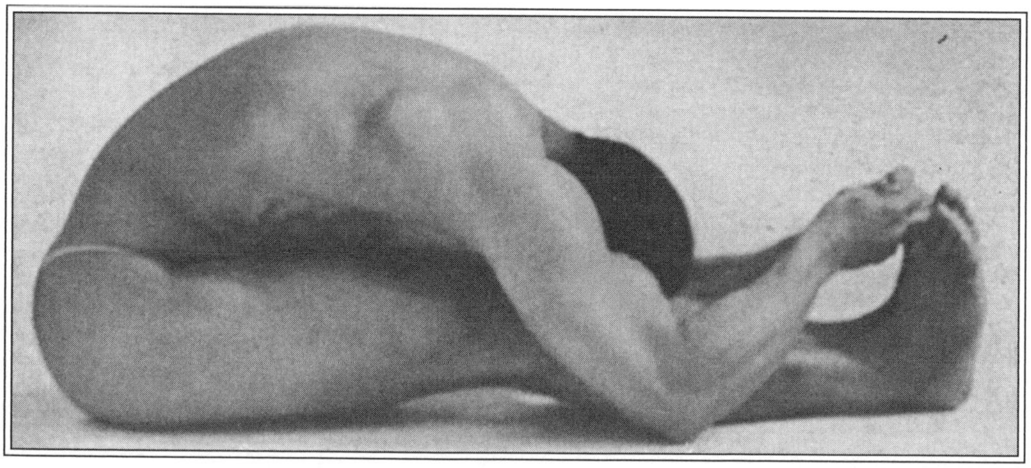

Fig. 12.15. Spinal-Stretch Posture (Paścimatānāsana)

Points of Note: This exercise relaxes and stretches the hamstring muscles and helps in securing full flexion at the hip joints.

Head-Knee Posture

1. Sit with the right heel pressed against the perineum, the left leg fully extended forward, the arms bent at the elbows and held at the level of the shoulders, the forearms and fingers extended forward, and the body erect.
2. Bend the body forward and downward and simultaneously extend the arms forward and with both hands grasp the big toe or all the toes of the left foot. Finally, bend the head until the forehead touches the left knee. The extended leg should be kept perfectly straight throughout the exercise. Maintain the final attitude for a few seconds (fig. 12.16).
3. Return to step 1.

Breathing: Exhale in step 2 and inhale in step 3.

Dynamic Application: Steps 2 and 3 should be alternately executed.

Static Application: Maintain the final attitude (step 2) as instructed by a qualified Yoga teacher.

Relaxation: After completion of the exercise, dynamic or static, relax in the sitting position with the legs extended forward and the arms by the sides.

Points of Note: The exercise should also be performed with the right leg extended. This exercise relaxes and stretches the hamstring muscles and helps in securing full flexion at the hip joints.

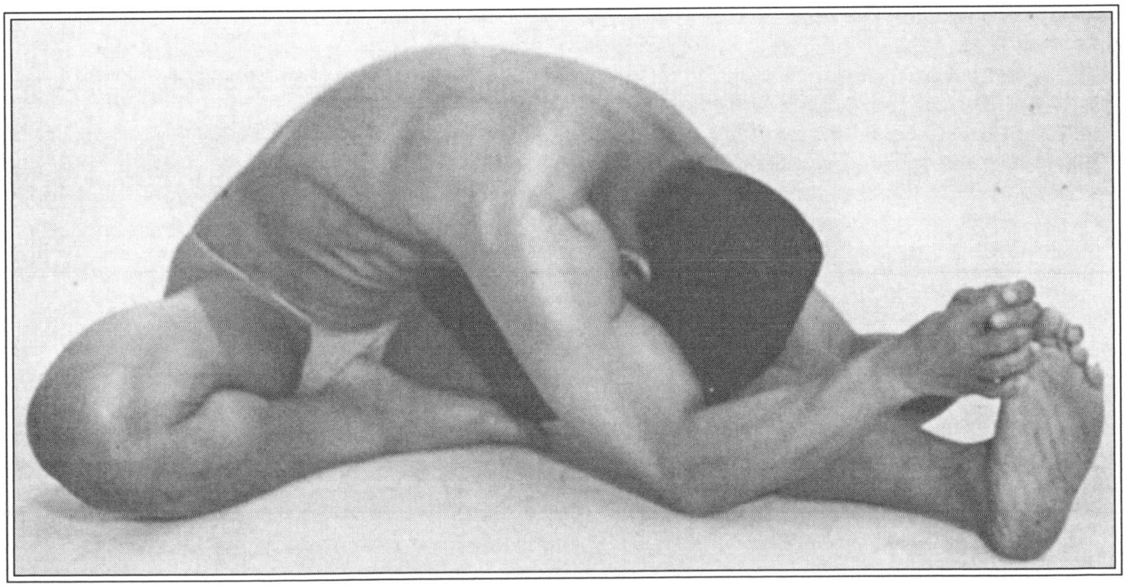

Fig. 12.16. Head-Knee Posture (Jānuśirāsana)

Forward Head-Bend Posture

1. Sit with the legs extended but kept far apart, the arms bent at the elbows and held at the level of the shoulders, the forearms and the fingers extended forward, the body erect.
2. Bend the body forward and downward and at the same time extend the arms forward and grasp the big toe or all the toes of both feet with the hands. Finally, bend the head until the forehead touches the ground. The legs should be kept perfectly straight throughout the exercise. Maintain the final attitude for a few seconds (fig. 12.17).
3. Return to step 1.

Breathing: Normal until the posture is perfected and mastered. Thereafter, exhale in step 2 and inhale in step 3.

Dynamic Application: Steps 2 and 3 should be alternately executed.

Static Application: Maintain the final attitude (step 2) as instructed by a qualified Yoga teacher.

Relaxation: After completion of the exercise, dynamic or static, relax in the sitting position with the legs extended forward and the arms by the sides.

Points of Note: This exercise causes the relaxation and stretching of the hamstring muscles to an extraordinary degree.

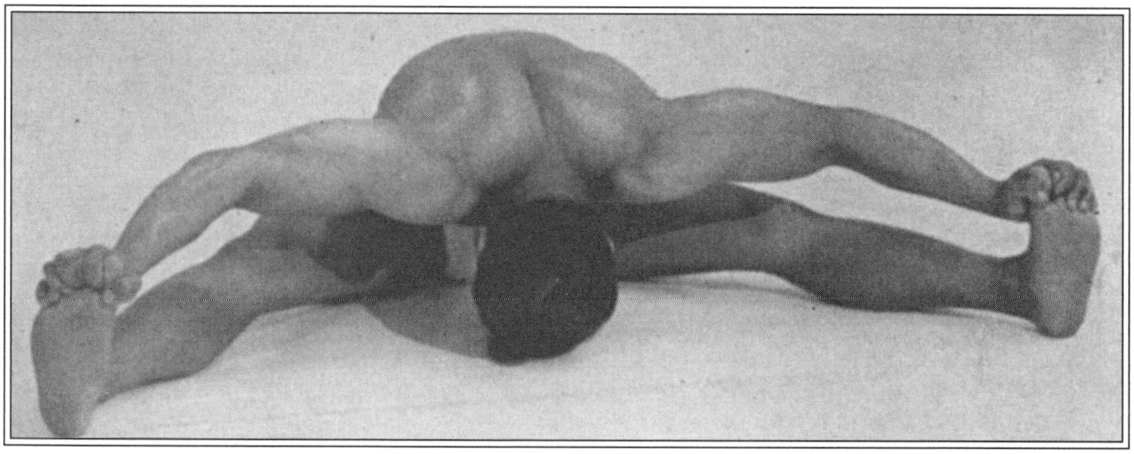

Fig. 12.17. Forward Head-Bend Posture (Bhūnamanāsana)

Head-Bend Posture

1. Sit with the legs extended but kept far apart, the hands clasped behind the back, the body erect.
2. Bend the body forward and downward until the head touches the ground. The legs should be kept perfectly straight throughout the exercise. Maintain the final attitude for a few seconds (fig. 12.18).

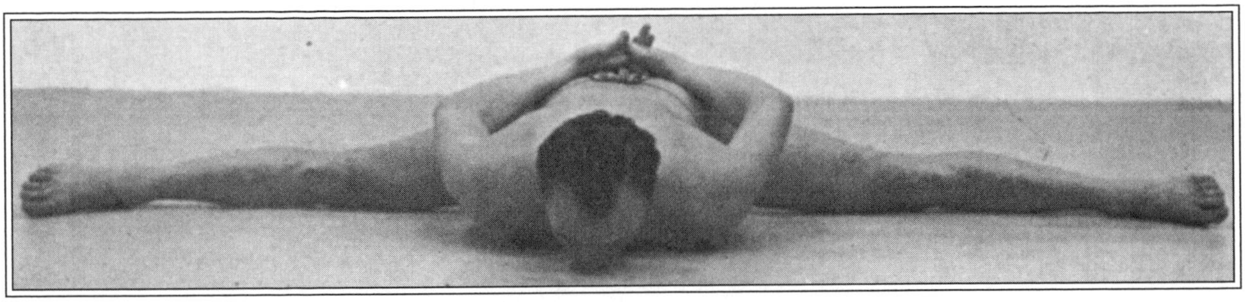

Fig. 12.18. Head-Bend Posture (Nataśirāsana)

3. Return to step 1.

Breathing: Normal until the posture is perfected and mastered. Thereafter, exhale in step 2 and inhale in step 3.

Dynamic Application: Steps 2 and 3 should be alternately executed.

Static Application: Maintain the final attitude (step 2) as instructed by a qualified Yoga teacher.

Relaxation: After completion of the exercise, dynamic or static, relax in the sitting position with the legs extended forward and the arms by the sides.

Points of Note: Same as for Forward Head-Bend Posture.

Head-Bend Lotus Posture

1. Assume Lotus Posture (fig. 20.2) with the hands clasped behind the back, the body erect.
2. Bend the body forward and downward until the forehead touches the ground. Maintain the final attitude for a few seconds (fig. 12.19).
3. Return to step 1.

Breathing: Exhale in step 2 and inhale in step 3.

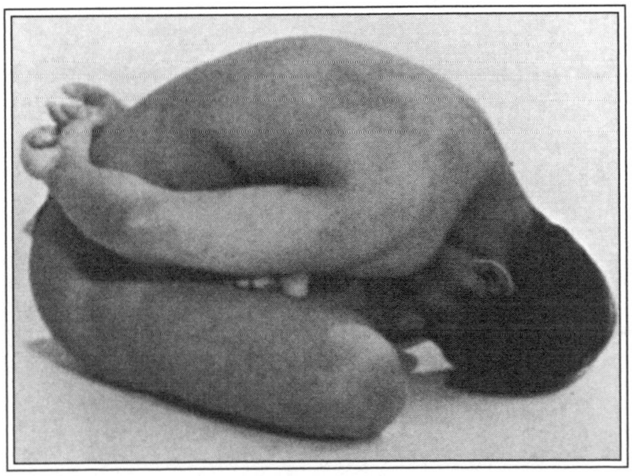

Fig. 12.19. Head-Bend Lotus Posture (Yoga-mudrā)

Dynamic Application: Steps 2 and 3 should be alternately executed.

Static Application: Maintain the final attitude (step 2) as instructed by a qualified Yoga teacher.

Relaxation: After completion of the exercise, dynamic or static, relax either in Lotus Posture or in the sitting position with the legs extended forward and the hands resting on the thighs.

Forward Body-Bend Posture

1. Sit with the legs extended sideward, the body erect, the arms stretched overhead.
2. Bend the body forward and downward until the trunk, head, and arms touch the ground. Maintain the final attitude for a few seconds (fig. 12.20).
3. Return to step 1.

Breathing: Exhale in step 2 and inhale in step 3.

Dynamic Application: Steps 2 and 3 should be alternately executed.

Static Application: Maintain the final attitude (step 2) as instructed by a qualified Yoga teacher.

Relaxation: After completion of the exercise, dynamic or static, relax in the sitting position with the legs extended forward and the hands resting on the thighs.

Points of Note: This is an advanced exercise. It requires extraordinary relaxation of the hamstring muscles and full flexibility at the hip joints to be able to extend the legs sideward. The beginner should try to go as far as possible.

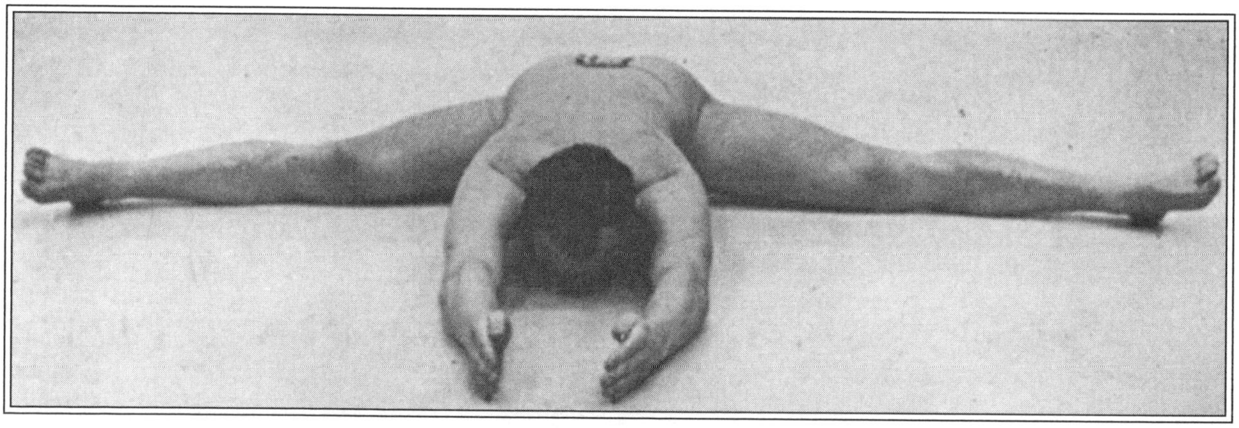

Fig. 12.20. Forward Body-Bend Posture (Praṇatāsana)

Foot-Hand Posture

1. Assume standing position with the heels together, the arms by the sides.
2. Bend the trunk forward and downward and at the same time extend the arms downward and hold either the big toes or all the toes of both feet with the hands. Finally, bend the head until the forehead touches the knees. The legs should be kept perfectly straight throughout the exercise. Maintain the final attitude for a few seconds (fig. 12.21a).
3. Return to step 1.

Breathing: Exhale in step 2 and inhale in step 3.

Dynamic Application: Steps 2 and 3 should be alternately executed.

Static Application: Maintain the final attitude (step 2) as instructed by a qualified Yoga teacher.

Relaxation: After completion of the exercise, dynamic or static, relax in Standing Posture.

Points of Note: After the movement is mastered, the head can be brought between the knees and projected beyond the legs (fig. 12.21b). This requires great flexibility of the hip joints and relaxation of the hamstring muscles.

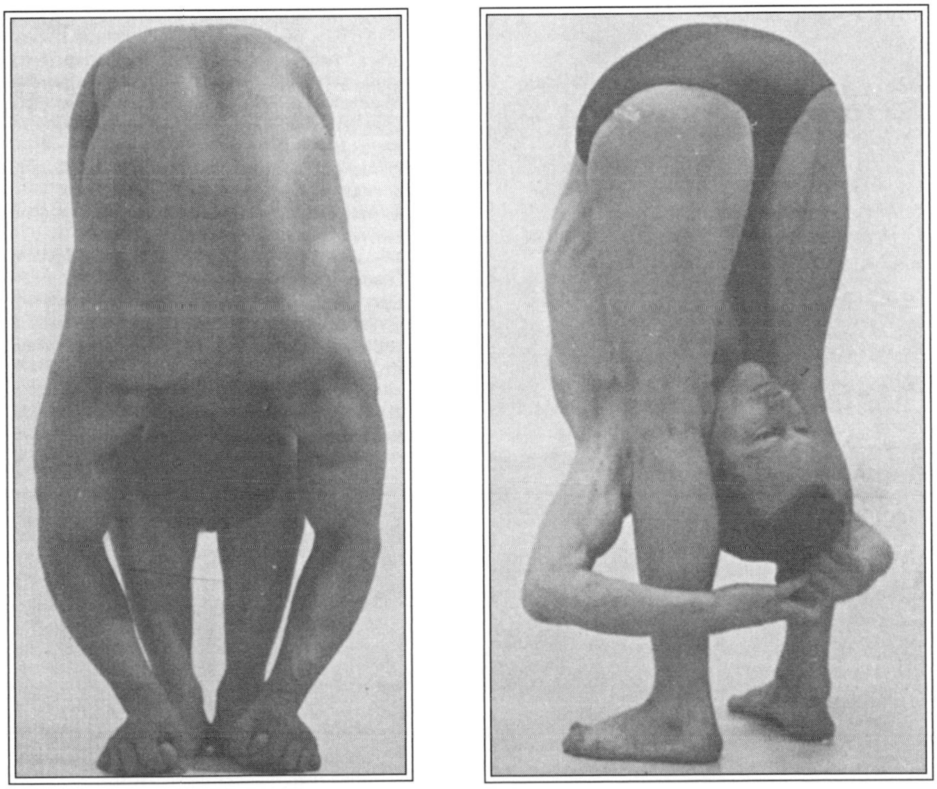

Fig. 12.21. a) Foot-Hand Posture (Pāda-hastāsana)
b) Foot-Hand Posture, Last Step (Pāda-hastāsana)

Lateral Trunk-Bend Posture Exercise

The principal muscles employed in lateral trunk-bend posture exercise are the sacrospinalis group (thoracic and lumbar portions), quadratus lumborum, obliquus externus abdominis, and obliquus internus abdominis. They are helped by the semispinalis dorsi, intertransversales, levatores costarum, rectus abdominis, psoas major, psoas minor, and latissimus dorsi. The spinal and abdominal muscles are alternately contracted and relaxed and stretched in the exercises presented here. The mind should be concentrated on the contracting muscles (spinal and abdominal). In these lateral trunk-bend posture exercises the dorso-lumbar junction and the lumbar spine are especially involved in the movements. So special concentration on these parts may be applied while exercising.

Torsion also occurs in these parts of the spine but twisting the body while doing the exercises should be avoided as much as possible. There is a strong tendency to twist the trunk in Hip-Bend Posture and Moon Posture. The increased flexibility and muscular control will enable a student to perform these exercises correctly.

Half-Moon Posture

1. Assume standing position with the heels together, the arms extended overhead and the palms facing each other.
2. Bend the trunk from the hips laterally to the left side as much as possible. The legs should be kept straight and the position of the arms and feet unchanged during the exercise. Avoid twisting the body. Maintain the final position for a few seconds (fig. 12.22).
3. Return to step 1.
4. Bend the trunk in a similar manner to the right side.
5. Return to step 1.

Breathing: Either normal, or exhalation in steps 2 and 4 and inhalation in steps 3 and 5.

Dynamic Application: There are two forms: (a) From step 2 to 3; now halt for a brief period, then recommence the movement from step 4 to 5. Continue in this manner. (b) The continuous movement from 2 to 3, then 4 to 5. Breathing normal.

Static Application: Maintain the final attitude (steps 2 and 4) as instructed by a qualified Yoga teacher.

Relaxation: After completion of the exercise, dynamic or static, relax in Standing Posture.

Hip-Bend Posture

1. Assume standing position with heels together, arms extended overhead and the palms facing each other.
2. Bend the trunk from the hips laterally to the left side until it is horizontal or almost horizontal.

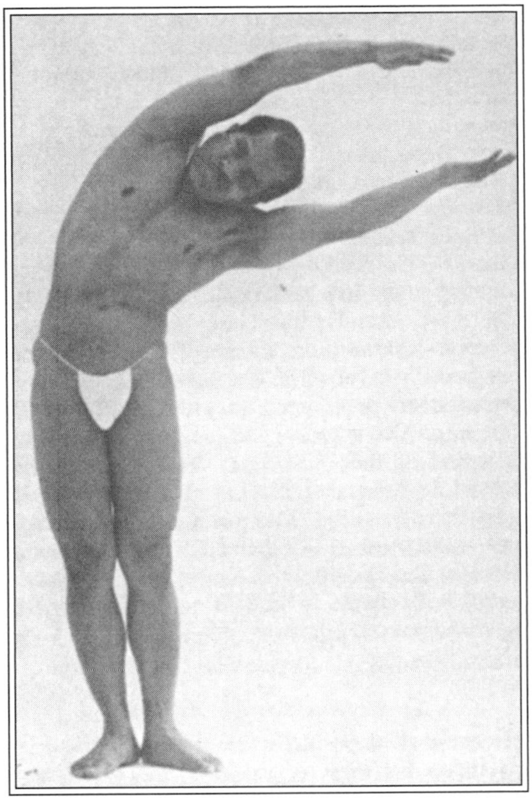

Fig. 12.22. Half-Moon Posture (Ardha Candrāsana)

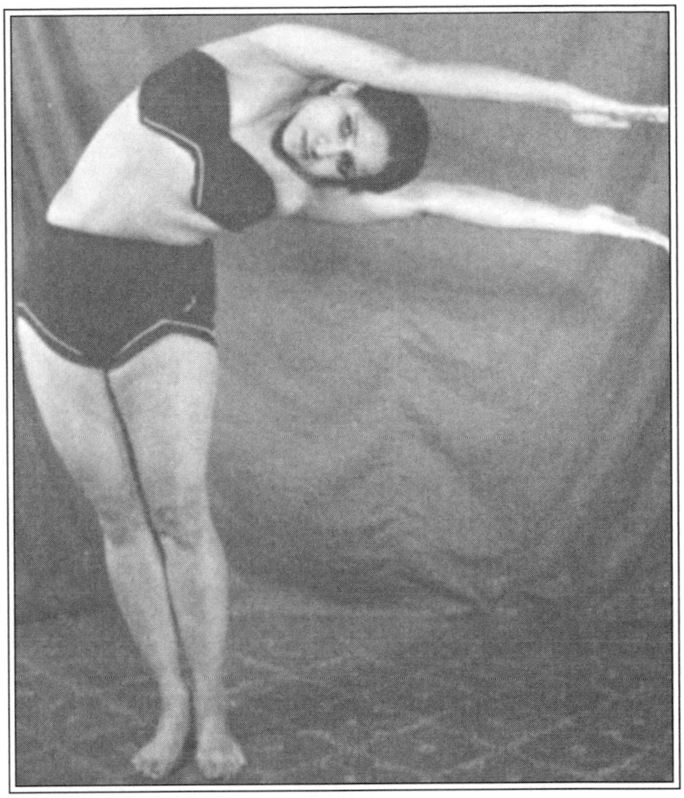

Fig. 12.23. Hip-Bend Posture (Nitambāsana)

Keep the legs straight and the position of the arms and feet unaltered during the exercise. Avoid twisting the body. Maintain the final attitude for a few seconds (fig. 12.23).

3. Return to step 1.
4. Bend the trunk in a similar manner to the right side.
5. Return to step 1.

Breathing: As in Half-Moon Posture.

Dynamic Application: As in Half-Moon Posture.

Static Application: Maintain the final attitude (steps 2 and 4) as instructed by a qualified Yoga teacher.

Relaxation: In Standing Posture, after completion of the exercise.

Points of Note: This exercise improves the flexibility of the hip joints to a remarkable extent.

Moon Posture

1. Assume standing position with the legs far apart, the arms overhead.
2. Bend the trunk from the hips laterally to the right until you are able to hold the right ankle with your right hand, the right arm being extended downward and the left passing above the head, the left forearm bent at the elbow and projecting downward. Keep the legs perfectly straight and avoid twisting the body. Maintain the final position for a few seconds (fig. 12.24).
3. Return to step 1.
4. Bend the trunk in a similar manner to the left side.
5. Return to step 1.

Breathing: As in Half-Moon Posture.

Dynamic Application: As in Half-Moon Posture.

Static Application: Maintain the final attitude (steps 2 and 4) as instructed by a qualified Yoga teacher.

Relaxation: In Standing Posture, after completion of the exercise.

Points of Note: This exercise develops the flexibility of the hip joints to a remarkable degree.

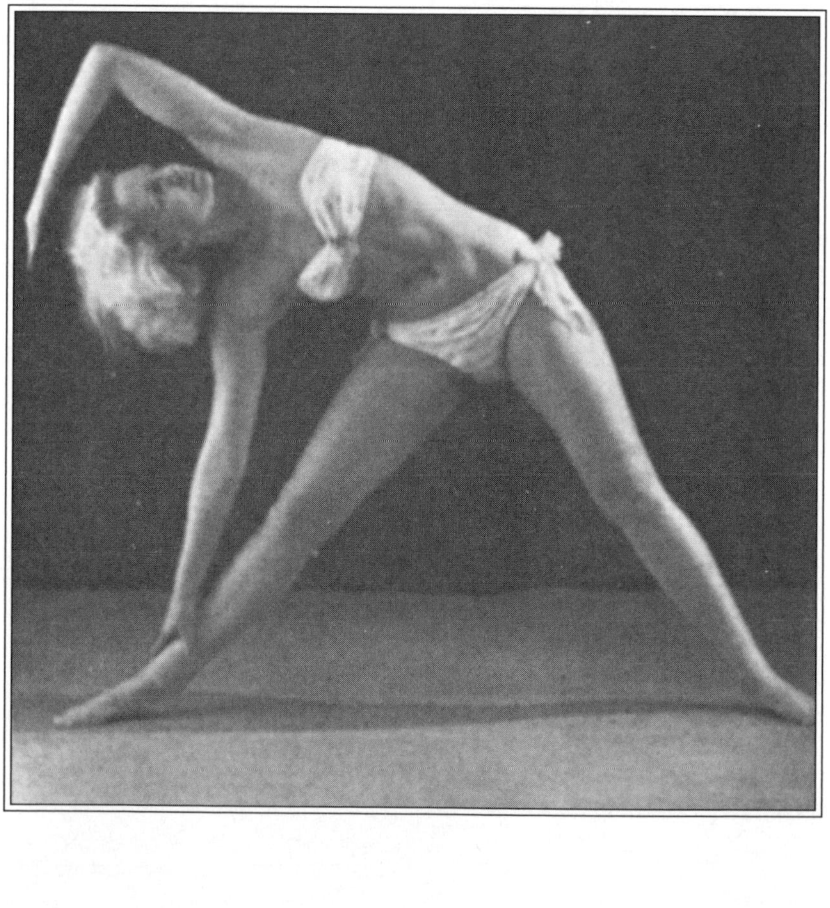

Fig. 12.24. Moon Posture (Candrāsana)

Trunk-Twist Posture Exercise

The principal muscles involved in trunk-twist posture exercise are the sacrospinalis (thoracic and lumbar portions), semispinalis dorsi, multifidus, rotatores, levatores costarum, obliquus externus abdominis, and obliquus internus abdominis. In cooperation with one another, the spinal and abdominal muscles take part in these four forms of exercise; some are contracting, while others are relaxing and stretching. The spinal muscles (except the sacrospinalis) and the obliquus externus abdominis of the left side and the sacrospinalis (thoracic and lumbar portions) and the obliquus internus abdominis of the right side are contracted in the trunk-twist posture exercise when done to the right and vice versa.

In the trunk-twist posture exercise the thoracic spine is principally involved. The movement is very limited in the lumbar spine. The twisting movement is associated with a slight lateral flexion to the same side. It is a very common tendency to go beyond this point. This should be carefully avoided. Concentration is on the spinal muscles, particularly of the thoracic region, and the abdominal muscles.

Twist Posture

1. Sit erect with the legs extended in front and far apart, the hands folded at the chest.
2. Twist the trunk to the left as much as possible without changing the position of the legs and without raising them off the floor. Avoid lateral flexion as much as possible. Maintain the final attitude for a few seconds (fig. 12.25).

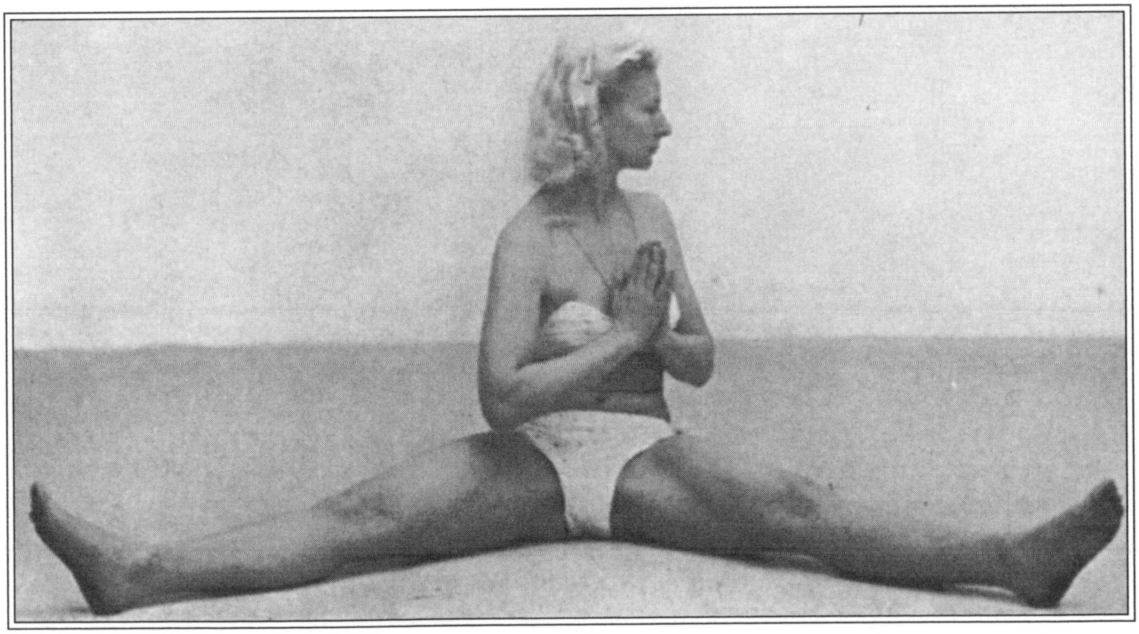

Fig. 12.25. Twist Posture (Vakrāsana)

3. Return to step 1.
4. Twist the trunk in a similar manner to the right.
5. Return to step 1.

Breathing: Either normal, or inhalation in steps 2 and 4 and exhalation in steps 3 and 5.

Dynamic Application: Either do steps 2 and 3, halt, and then do steps 4 and 5, or do continuous movement from 2 to 3 and 4 to 5, with normal breathing.

Static Application: Maintain the final attitude (steps 2 and 4) as instructed by a qualified Yoga teacher.

Relaxation: After completion of the exercise, dynamic or static, relax in the sitting position with the legs extended forward and the arms by the sides.

Points of Note: This exercise can also be performed in the standing position with the hands folded at the chest.

Modified Spinal-Twist Posture

1. Sit erect with the legs extended in front.
2. Put the right heel against the perineum, bending the leg at the knee with the right thigh on the ground. Now bring the left leg to the right side of the right knee with the left knee elevated and the left foot placed flat on the ground and close to the right side of the right knee. Then twist the body to the left as much as possible, placing the right armpit firmly against the left side of the elevated knee with the right arm extended downward, holding the left big toe with the right hand. Swing the left arm to the right side behind the back and place the left hand on the right groin. Finally twist the head to the left side, bringing the chin in line with the left shoulder. Maintain the final attitude for a few seconds (fig. 12.26).
3. Return to step 1.
4. Twist the body in a similar manner to the right.
5. Return to step 1.

Breathing: Normal.

Dynamic Application: Steps 2 and 3 and 4 and 5 should be alternately executed.

Static Application: Maintain the final attitude (steps 2 and 4) as instructed by a qualified Yoga teacher.

Relaxation: In the sitting position with the legs extended forward and the arms by the sides, after completion of the exercise.

Points of Note: Attention should be given to the twisting of the body to the maximum limit. The latissimus dorsi muscle comes into play in this exercise.

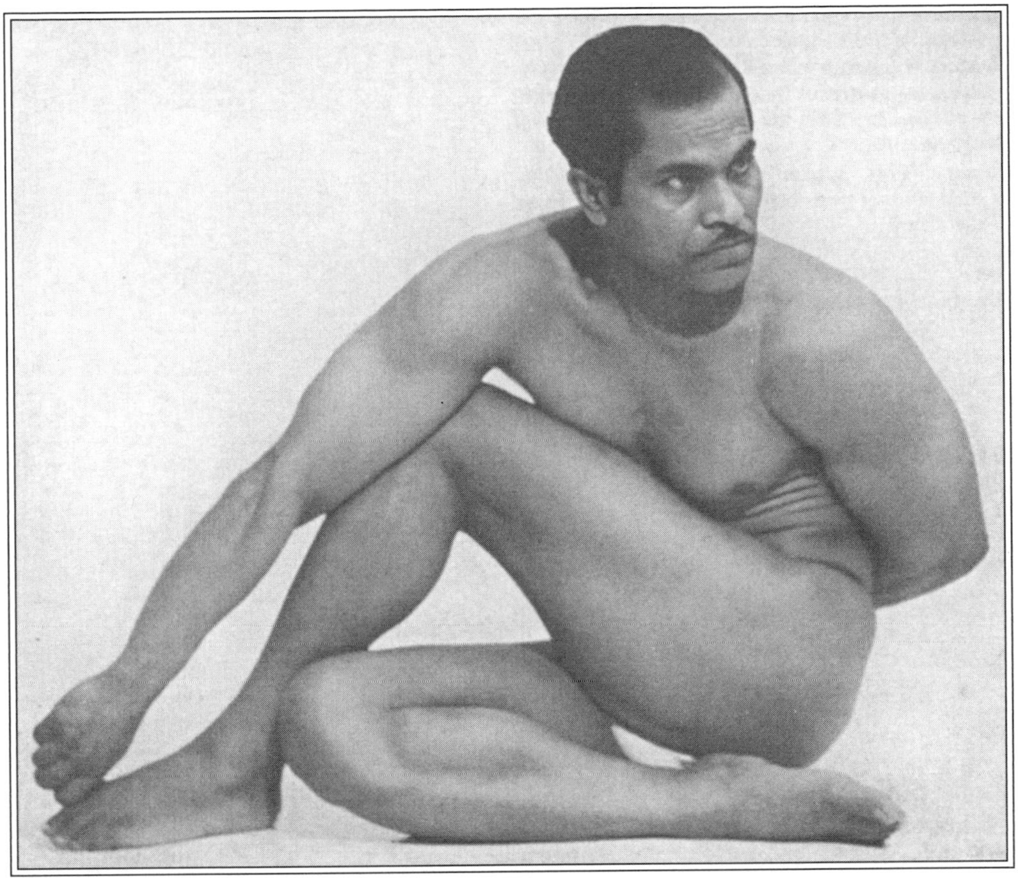

Fig. 12.26. Modified Spinal-Twist Posture (Ardha Matsyendrāsana)

Ankle-Hold Modified Spinal-Twist Posture

1. Sit erect with the legs extended in front.
2. Put the left heel against the perineum, bending the leg at the knee, with the left thigh on the ground. Now bring the right leg to the left side of the left thigh and place the right foot flat on the ground close to the left hip, with the right knee elevated. Then twist the body to the right as much as possible, placing the left armpit firmly against the right side of the elevated knee with the left arm extended downward, holding the left knee by the left hand. Swing the right arm to the left side behind the back and hold the right ankle with the right hand. Finally twist the head to the right, bringing the chin in line with the right shoulder. Maintain the final attitude for a few seconds (figs. 12.27 and 12.28 on page 132).
3. Return to step 1.
4. Twist the body in a similar manner to the left side.
5. Return to step 1.

Breathing: Normal.

Dynamic Application: Steps 2 and 3 and 4 and 5 should be alternately executed.

Static Application: Maintain the final attitude (steps 2 and 4) as instructed by a qualified Yoga teacher.

Relaxation: In the sitting position with the legs extended forward and the arms by the sides, after completion of the exercise.

Points of Note: Same as for Modified Spinal-Twist Posture.

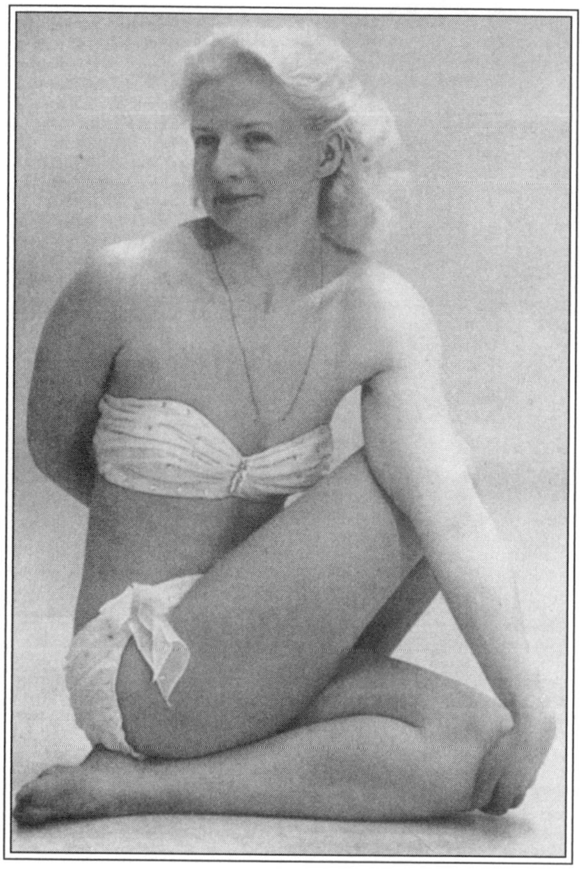

Fig. 12.27. Ankle-Hold Modified Spinal-Twist Posture, Front View (Baddha Ardha Matsyendrāsana)

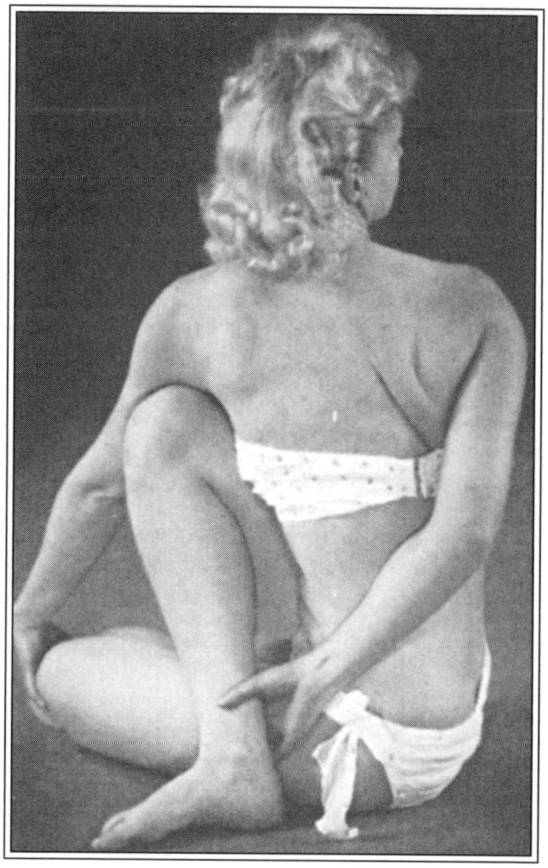

Fig. 12.28. Ankle-Hold Modified Spinal-Twist Posture, Back View (Baddha Ardha Matsyendrāsana)

Spinal-Twist Posture

1. Sit erect with the legs extended in front.
2. Place the left foot on the right hip joint with the help of your hands, the left heel pressing against the abdomen and the left thigh on the floor. Now bring the right leg to the left

side of the left knee with the right knee elevated and the right foot placed flat on the floor close to the left side of the left knee. Then twist the body as much as possible to the right side, placing the left armpit firmly against the right side of the elevated knee with the left arm extended downward, holding the right big toe with the left hand. Swing the right arm to the left side behind the back and grasp the heel of the left foot with the right hand. Finally, twist the head to the right side, bringing the chin in line with the right shoulder. Maintain the final attitude for a few seconds (fig. 12.29).

3. Return to step 1.
4. Twist the body in a similar manner to the left side.
5. Return to step 1.

Breathing: Normal.

Dynamic Application: Steps 2 and 3 and 4 and 5 should be alternately executed.

Static Application: Maintain the final attitude (steps 2 and 4) as instructed by a qualified Yoga teacher.

Relaxation: In the sitting position with the legs extended in front and the arms by the sides, after completion of the exercise.

Points of Note: The latissimus dorsi muscle comes strongly into play in this exercise. This is an advanced spinal exercise. Spinal-Twist Posture transformed into Ankle-Hold Spinal-Twist Posture causes full contraction of those muscles involved in Spinal-Twist Posture. A student is advised to practice this exercise for greater muscular development (fig. 12.30).

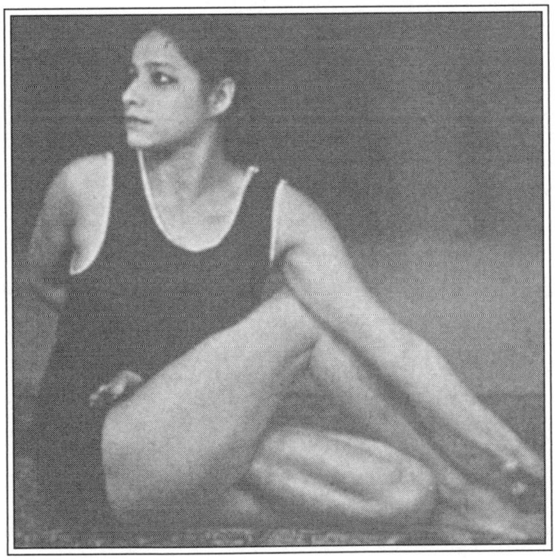

Fig. 12.29. Spinal-Twist Posture (Matsyendrāsana)

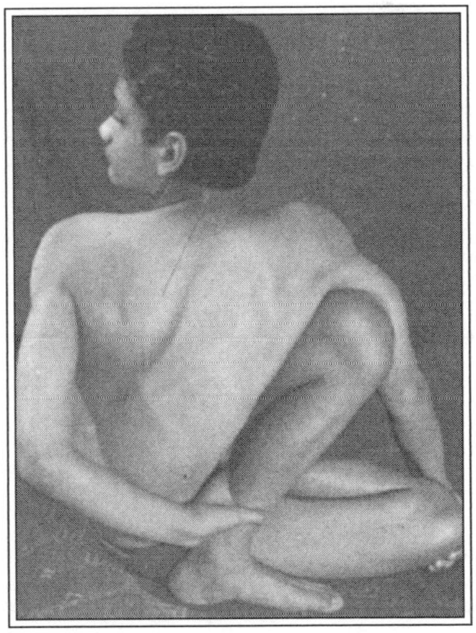

Fig. 12.30. Ankle-Hold Spinal-Twist Posture, Back View (Baddha Matsyendrāsana)

Sideward Head-Bend Posture

1. Sit erect with the legs extended in front and far apart, the hands clasped behind the back.
2. Now twist the body to the left and bend the head to the floor close to the outer side of the left leg, without changing the position of the legs and without raising them off the floor. Maintain the final attitude for a few seconds (fig. 12.31).
3. Return to step 1.
4. Twist the body and bend the head in a similar manner to the right side.
5. Return to step 1.

Breathing: Normal.

Dynamic Application: Steps 2 and 3 and 4 and 5 should be alternately executed.

Static Application: Maintain the final attitude (steps 2 and 4) as instructed by a qualified Yoga teacher.

Relaxation: In the sitting position with the legs extended in front and the arms by the sides, after completion of the exercise.

Points of Note: This exercise is actually a combination of the twisting and the lateral bending movements.

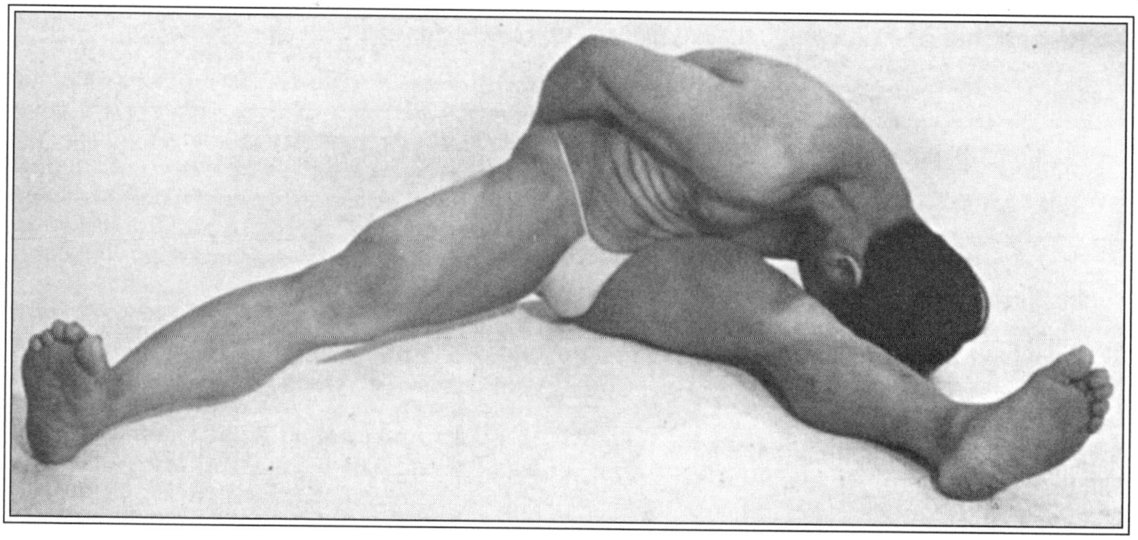

Fig. 12.31. Sideward Head-Bend Posture (Parśva Bhūnamanāsana)

Supplementary Spinal Posture Exercise

In this exercise, concentration is on the spinal and back muscles.

Fish Posture

1. Assume Lotus Posture (fig. 20.2).
2. Lie on your back, lifting the knees vertically at the same time.
3. Lower the legs on to the floor and arch the spine as much as possible by placing the elbows by your sides on the floor and bending the head backward in such a way as to cause the crown of the head to rest on the floor. Finally, extend the arms and hold the big toes or all the toes with the hands. Now the trunk is supported by the vertex and the buttocks. Maintain the final attitude for a few seconds (fig. 12.32).
4. Return to step 2.

Breathing: Normal.

Dynamic Application: Steps 3 and 4 should be alternately executed.

Static Application: Maintain the final attitude (step 3) as instructed by a qualified Yoga teacher.

Relaxation: In Corpse Posture, after completion of the exercise.

Points of Note: This is a posterior trunk-bend posture exercise more suitable for static application. It causes the stretching of the neck and therefore its practice is very useful after all contractile neck movements and Shoulder-Stand Posture.

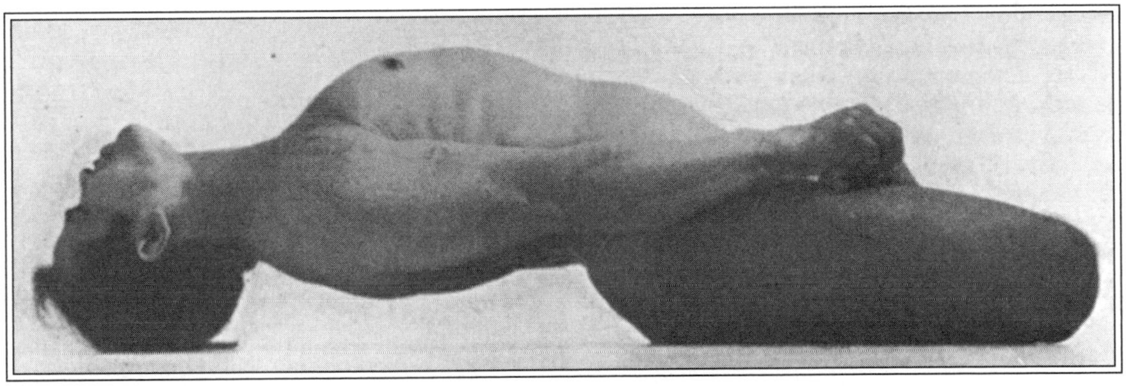

Fig. 12.32. Fish Posture (Matsyāsana)

13
Neck Posture Exercise

Neck posture exercise is an inseparable part of spinal exercise, which involves the cervical spine and the muscles connected to it. It consists of anterior, posterior, and lateral neck-bend posture exercise and neck-twist posture exercise.

In anterior neck-bend posture exercise, the sternocleidomastoideus, platysma, longus capitis and colli, rectus capitis anterior and latcralis, scalenus anterior, medius, and posterior, and the supra- and infrahyoid muscles are involved. In the posterior neck-bend posture exercises, the sacrospinalis (cervical part), semispinalis capitis and cervicis, splenius capitis and cervicis, multifidus (cervical part), interspinalis (cervical part), the suboccipitals and trapezius (upper) are brought into play.

The following muscles are involved in lateral neck-bend posture exercise: the scalenus anterior, medius, and posterior, splenius capitis and cervicis, rectus capitis lateralis, sacrospinalis (cervical part), semispinalis (cervical part), intertransversarii, longus colli, suboccipitals, and sternocleidomastoideus. The sacrospinalis (cervical part), semispinaliscapitis, splenius capitis and cervicis, multifidus (cervical part), suboccipitals, and sternocleidomastoideus are involved in neck-twist posture exercise. The mind should be concentrated on the contracting muscles.

In various posture exercises flexion, extension, lateral flexion, and rotation of the cervical spine (neck) take place. In most of the posture exercises the neck movement is combined with the movements of the other parts of the body. When the neck movements are isolated from movements of other parts of the body, they are termed voluntary-contraction neck motion. Voluntary-contraction neck motion consists of four main neck exercises: neck flexion exercise, neck extension exercise, lateral neck flexion exercise, and neck rotation exercise. These may be called preliminary neck exercise. The advanced form of neck exercise in which the muscles are more powerfully brought into play is found in some special neck posture exercises. Both the preliminary and advanced exercises are presented here. In all of these exercises, concentration is on the neck muscles.

Preliminary and Advanced Neck Exercises

Neck Flexion-Extension

1. Assume Accomplished Posture (fig. 20.1) with the arms by the sides.
2. Bend the head forward until the chin touches the top of the sternum (breast bone), voluntarily contracting the neck muscles.
3. From step 2 return to step 1 without contracting the neck muscles and then bend the head backward to some extent.

Breathing: Normal.

Relaxation: In Accomplished Posture, after completion of the exercise.

Points of Note: This exercise can also be done in Standing Posture. It is not a posture exercise but a contraction exercise.

Neck Rotation

1. Assume Accomplished Posture (fig. 20.1) with the arms by the sides.
2. Twist the head to the right and left, contracting the neck muscles.

Breathing: Normal.

Relaxation: In Accomplished Posture, after completion of the exercise.

Points of Note: As in Neck Flexion-Extension.

Lateral Neck Flexion

1. Assume Accomplished Posture (fig. 20.1) with the arms by the sides.
2. Bend the head laterally toward the right and left shoulders alternately.

Breathing: Normal.

Relaxation: In Accomplished Posture, after completion of the exercise.

Points of Note: As in Neck Flexion-Extension.

Neck Posture

1. Assume a kneeling position with the hands on the floor. Now bend the head to the floor and support the body on the head and toes of both feet with the face inward, hips well up, the hands behind the back.
2. Bend the head backward and forward (fig. 13.1 on page 138).

Breathing: Normal.

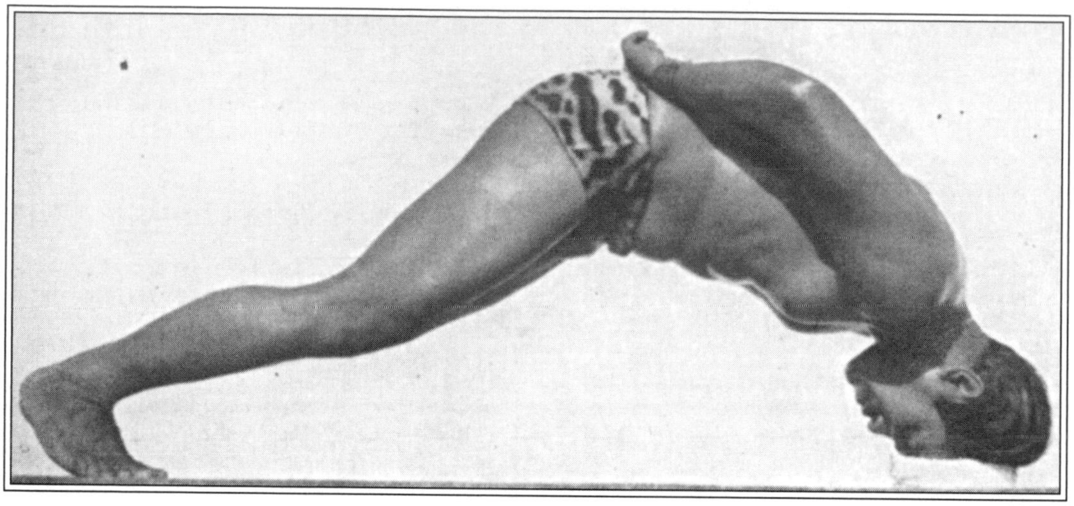

Fig. 13.1. Neck Posture (Grīvāsana)

Relaxation: In Prone Posture or Corpse Posture, after completion of the exercise.

Points of Note: This is an advanced neck exercise. When utilizing it as a static exercise, do only step 1. The head should rest on a thick cushion.

Neck-Bridge Posture

1. Assume a supine position with the forearms crossed at the chest and the heels drawn to the buttocks, bending the legs at the knees.
2. Raise the body upward into a bridge position, supporting it on the head and feet. Maintain the final attitude for a few seconds (fig. 13.2).
3. Lower the body to step 1.

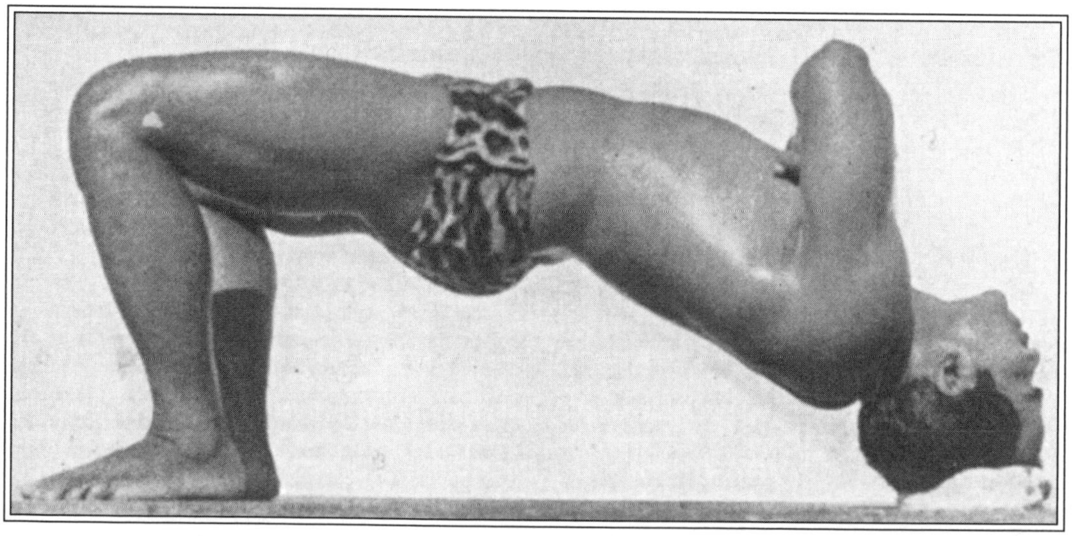

Fig. 13.2. Neck-Bridge Posture (Kandharāsana)

Breathing: Inhale in step 2 and exhale in step 3.

Dynamic Application: Steps 2 and 3 should be alternately executed.

Static Application: Maintain the final attitude (step 2) as instructed by a qualified Yoga teacher.

Relaxation: In Corpse Posture, after completion of the exercise.

Points of Note: This is an advanced neck exercise.

Supplementary Neck Posture Exercise

Chin Lock (Jālandhara Bandha)

1. Assume a folded-leg posture.
2. Bend the head forward and downward and place the chin tightly against the top of the sternum (breast bone). Maintain the final attitude for a few seconds.
3. Return to step 1.

Breathing: Normal.

Dynamic Application: Not necessary.

Static Application: Maintain the final attitude (step 2) as instructed by a qualified Yoga teacher.

Relaxation: In a folded-leg posture, after completion of the exercise.

Points of Note: This is essentially for static application.

14

Abdominal Posture Exercise

In Yoga the right abdominal development is a most important factor. It is associated with breath control and internal purificatory processes and is a great help in prolonged concentration postures when it is necessary to maintain the abdominal viscera in the correct position, thus protecting them from being subject to direct gravitational stress. Abdominal protuberance is mainly due to abdominal muscular weakness, which also causes lumbar lordosis and an anterior pelvic displacement.

Abdominal exercise increases the tone and strength of the abdominal muscles and prevents abdominal protuberance and fat accumulation in the abdominal and pelvic regions. Inactive blood accumulating in the abdominal area is forced into general circulation. A high order of functional efficiency of the alimentary canal depends to a very great extent upon abdominal development.

Abdominal Exercise Classified

In Haṭha Yoga abdominal exercise is divided into two groups: abdominal posture exercise and abdominal control exercise. The abdominal posture exercise is subdivided into trunk-raise posture exercise, pelvis-raise posture exercise, trunk-leg-raise posture exercise, and leg-raise posture exercise. The trunk-raise posture exercise, again, is classified into anterior trunk-raise posture exercise, oblique trunk-raise posture exercise, and lateral trunk-raise posture exercise. Trunk-leg-raise posture exercise is classified into anterior trunk-leg-raise posture exercise and lateral trunk-leg-raise posture exercise.

Anterior Trunk-Raise Posture Exercise

Anterior trunk-raise posture exercise consists of two parts: trunk flexion on the pelvis and pelvis flexion on the thighs. First flexion of the trunk takes place, in which the sternum and the pubis are approximated. In the trunk flexion movement the rectus abdominis and the obiquus internus abdominis are chiefly brought into play. The exercise is completed by flexion of the pelvis on the thighs, which is accomplished by the hip flexors. Just before the beginning of the flexion of the pelvis, the obliquus externus abdominis comes into play. In these exercises, concentration is on the abdominal muscles, especially the rectus abdominis.

Spine Posture

1. Assume a supine position with the arms extended overhead, the heels together, the head between the arms.
2. Raise the body slowly to a sitting position, first by raising the head, then the shoulders, and then the entire trunk. The whole range of movement is continuous, slow, and without any jerk. The head should remain between the arms during the movement (fig. 14.1).
3. From the sitting position return to step 1.

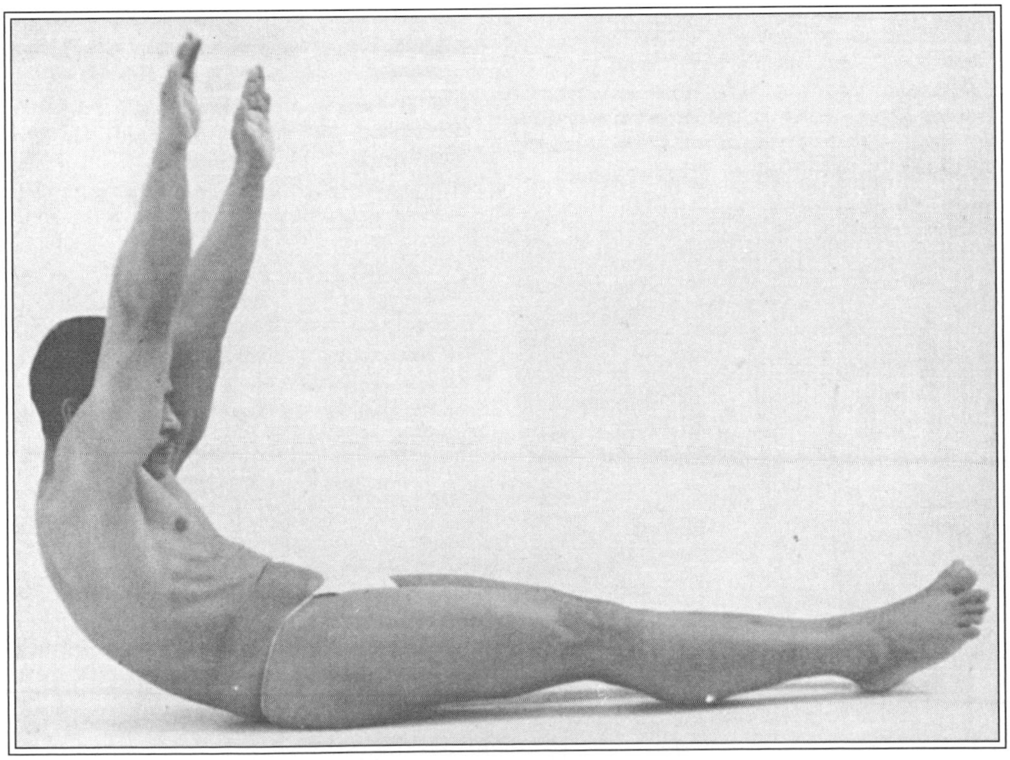

Fig. 14.1. Spine Posture (Merudaṇḍāsana)

Breathing: Either normal, or inhalation in step 3 and exhalation in step 2.

Dynamic Application: Steps 2 and 3 should be alternately executed.

Static Application: Maintain the trunk attitude just at the point when flexion of the pelvis on the thighs commences, at the point when the seventh cervical vertebral region is raised about 8 inches off the floor.

Relaxation: In Corpse Posture, after completion of the exercise.

Spine Posture with Hands Clasped behind Head

1. Assume a supine position with the hands clasped behind the head, the heels together.
2. Raise the body slowly to a sitting position in a continuous movement without any jerk. The position of the hands should not change and the legs should not be lifted off the floor during the movement (fig. 14.2).
3. From the sitting position return to step 1.

Breathing: Either normal, or inhalation in step 3 and exhalation in step 2.

Dynamic Application: Steps 2 and 3 should be alternately executed.

Static Application: Maintain the trunk attitude at the point when flexion of the pelvis on the thighs is initiated (see fig. 14.2).

Relaxation: In Corpse Posture, after completion of the exercise.

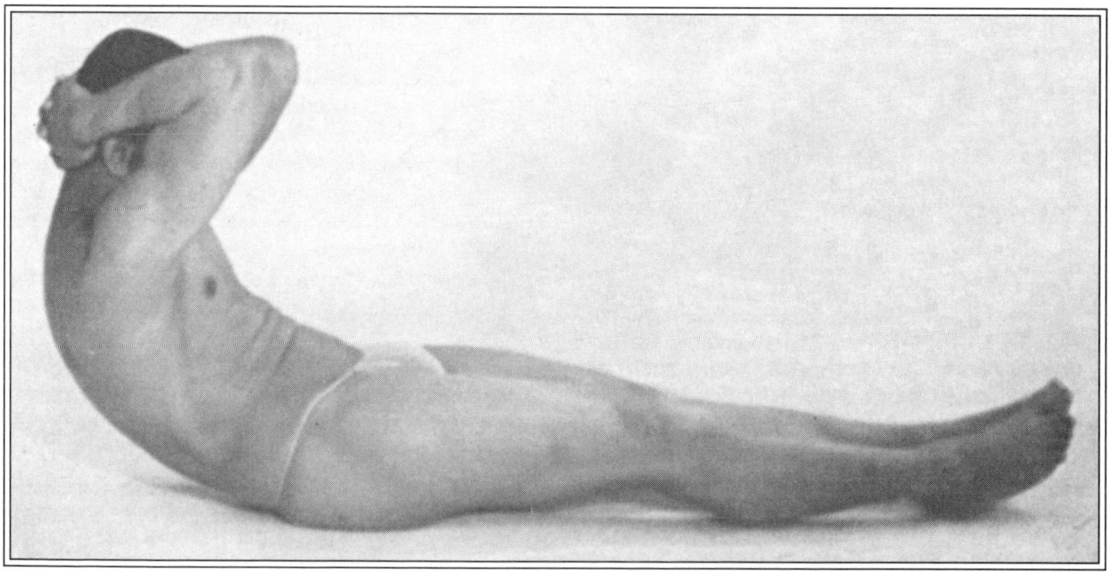

Fig. 14.2. Spine Posture with Hands Clasped behind Head
(Śirahasta Merudaṇḍāsana)

Spine Posture with Forearms Locked behind Head

1. Assume a supine position with the forearms locked behind the head, the heels together.
2. Raise the trunk slowly to a sitting position in a continuous movement without any jerk. The position of the forearms should not change and the legs should not be lifted off the floor during the movement (fig. 14.3).
3. From the sitting position return to step 1.

Breathing: Either normal, or inhalation in step 3 and exhalation in step 2.

Dynamic Application: Steps 2 and 3 should be alternately executed.

Static Application: Maintain the trunk attitude at the point when flexion of the pelvis on the thighs is initiated (see fig. 14.3).

Relaxation: In Corpse Posture, after completion of the exercise.

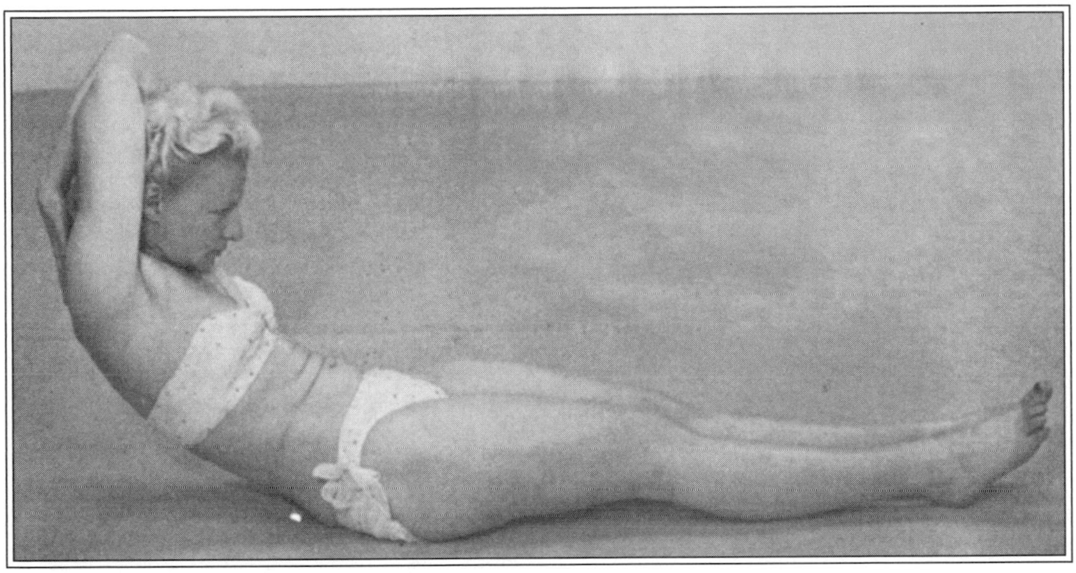

Fig. 14.3. Spine Posture with Forearms Locked behind Head (Śirabāhu Merudaṇḍasana)

Risen Balance Posture

1. Assume Lotus Posture (fig. 20.2).
2. Lie on your back with legs placed on the floor, arms extended upward.
3. Raise the body slowly to a sitting position without jerk (fig. 14.4 on page 144).
4. From the sitting position return to step 2.

Breathing: Normal.

Dynamic Application: Steps 3 and 4 should be alternately executed.

Static Application: Not suitable.

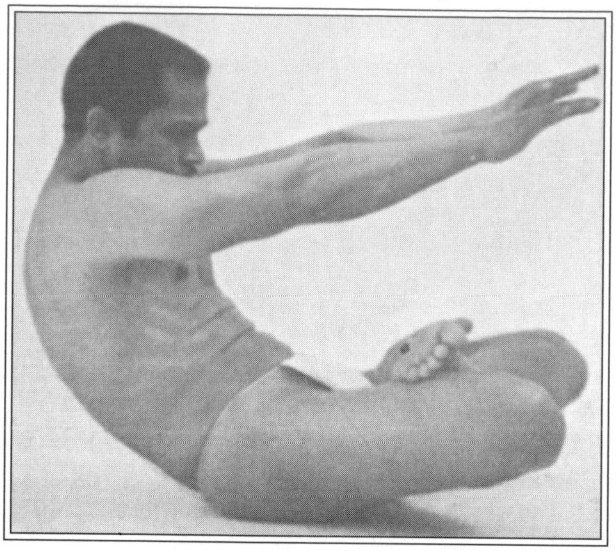

Fig. 14.4. Risen Balance Posture (Utthita Tolāngulāsana)

Relaxation: In Corpse Posture, after completion of the exercise.

Points of Note: This is an advanced form of abdominal exercise designed to strengthen the abdominal muscles to a high degree.

Oblique Trunk-Raise Posture Exercise

In oblique trunk-raise posture exercise the obliquus externus abdominis and obliquus internus abdominis come strongly into action. Concentration is on the obliquus externus abdominis.

Oblique Spine Posture

1. Assume a supine position with arms extended overhead, heels together, and the head between the arms.
2. Raise the body slowly to a sitting position while twisting it to the right. The movement should be diagonal, continuous, and without any jerk. The head should remain between the arms and the legs should not be lifted off the floor during the movement (fig. 14.5).
3. From the sitting position return to step 1.
4. Raise the body to a sitting position in a similar way (step 2) to the left.
5. Return to step 1.

Breathing: Normal, or inhale in steps 3 and 5 and exhale in steps 2 and 4.

Dynamic Application: Steps 2 and 3 and 4 and 5 should be alternately executed.

Static Application: Not suitable.

Relaxation: In Corpse Posture, after completion of the exercise.

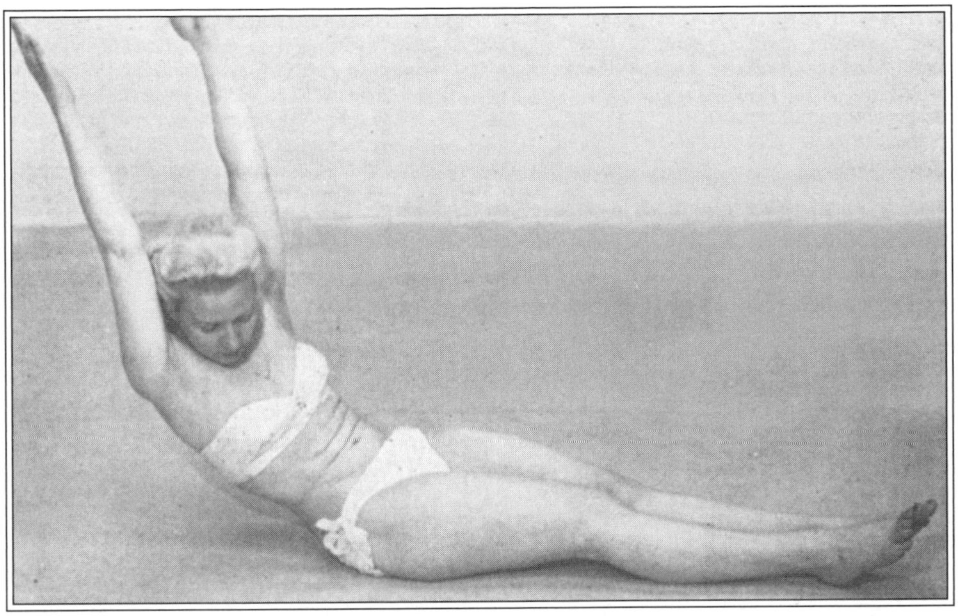

Fig. 14.5. Oblique Spine Posture (Pārśvavakra Merudaṇḍāsana)

Oblique Spine Posture with Hands Clasped behind Head

1. Assume a supine position with the hands clasped behind the head, the heels together.
2. Raise the body slowly to a sitting position while twisting it to the right. The movement should be diagonal, continuous, and without any jerk. The positions of the hands should remain unchanged and the legs should not be lifted off the floor during the movement (fig. 14.6).
3. From the sitting position return to step 1.
4. Raise the body to a sitting position in a similar way (step 2) to the left.
5. Return to step 1.

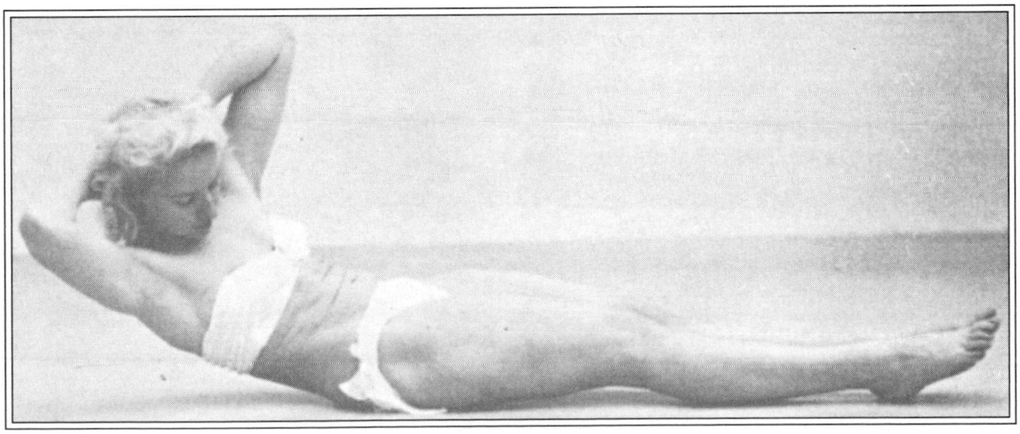

Fig. 14.6. Oblique Spine Posture with Hands Clasped behind Head
(Pārśvavakra Śirahasta Merudaṇḍāsana)

Breathing: Normal, or inhale in steps 3 and 5 and exhale in steps 2 and 4.
Dynamic Application: Steps 2 and 3 and 4 and 5 should be alternately executed.
Static Application: Not suitable.
Relaxation: In Corpse Posture, after completion of the exercise.

Oblique Spine Posture with Forearms Locked behind Head

1. Assume a supine position with the forearms locked behind the head, the heels together.
2. Raise the body slowly to a sitting position while twisting it to the right. The movement should be diagonal, continuous, and without any jerk. The positions of the forearms should remain unchanged and the legs should not be lifted off the floor during the movement (fig. 14.7).
3. From the sitting position return to step 1.
4. Raise the body to a sitting position in a similar way (step 2) to the left.
5. Return to step 1.

Breathing: Normal, or inhale in steps 3 and 5 and exhale in steps 2 and 4.
Dynamic Application: Steps 2 and 3 and 4 and 5 should be alternately executed.
Static Application: Not suitable.
Relaxation: In Corpse Posture, after completion of the exercise.

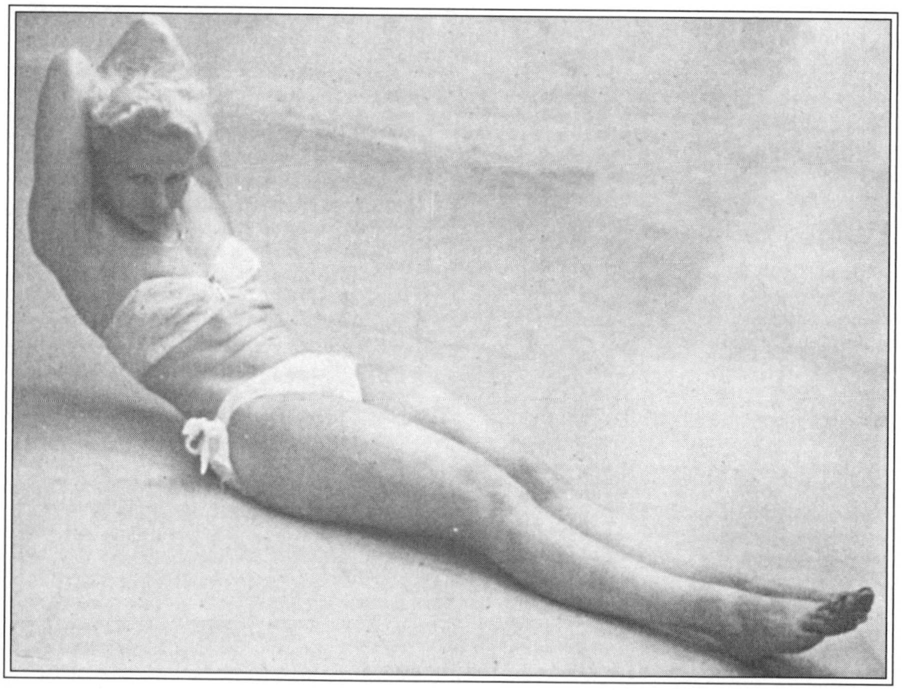

Fig. 14.7. Oblique Spine Posture with Forearms Locked behind Head (Pārśvavakra Śirabāhu Merudaṇḍāsana)

Lateral Trunk-Raise Posture Exercise

In the lateral trunk-raise posture exercise the obliquus externus abdominis and obliquus internus abdominis are brought into action. Concentration is on both.

Lateral Spine Posture

1. Assume a right side-lying position with the trunk, pelvis, and legs in a straight line, the left arm extended downward along the left side and on the left thigh, the right forearm locked behind the right side of the head.
2. Raise the head and the trunk laterally until the whole trunk is lifted off the floor. The locked forearm will be raised along with the head. The movement is to be executed slowly and without raising the legs off the floor.
3. Return to step 1.
4. Assume left side-lying position in the same manner as in step 1.
5. Raise the trunk laterally in a similar way (fig. 14.8).
6. Return to step 4.

Breathing: Normal.

Dynamic Application: Steps 2 and 3 should be alternately executed. The same applies to steps 5 and 6.

Static Application: Not suitable.

Relaxation: In Corpse Posture, after completion of the exercise.

Points of Note: Avoid twisting the body as much as possible while raising the trunk. This is an advanced exercise requiring powerful muscular contraction. It is desirable to practice this exercise at first with the legs supported or stabilized by an assistant.

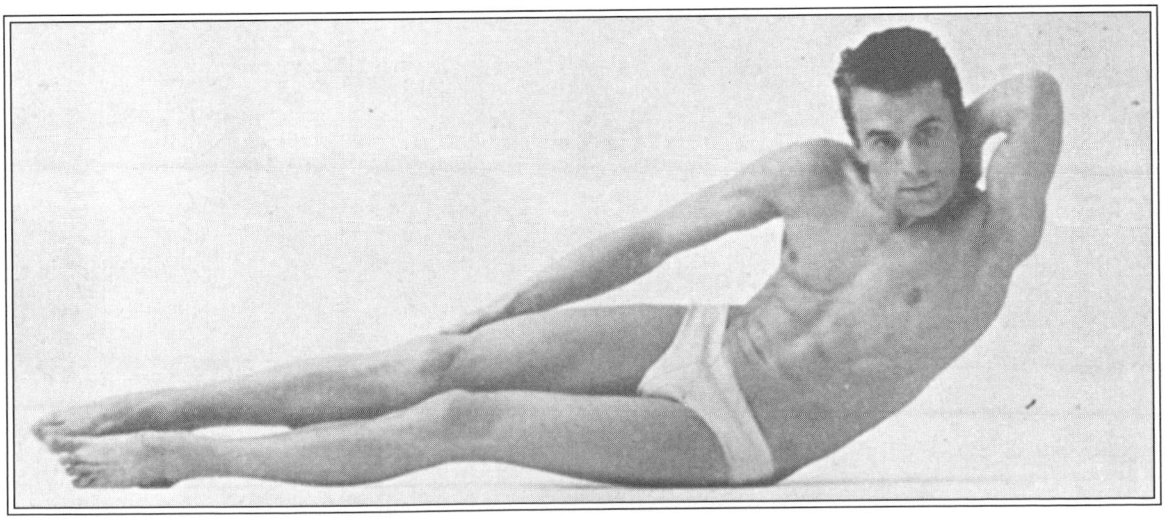

Fig. 14.8. Lateral Spine Posture (Utthitapārśva Merudaṇḍāsana)

Pelvis-Raise Posture Exercise

In pelvis-raise posture exercise the rectus abdominis is principally brought into play. Concentration is on the abdominal muscles, especially the rectus abdominis.

Plow Posture

1. Assume a supine position with the legs extended, the feet together, the arms extended by the sides.
2. Slowly raise the legs, pelvis, and trunk, stage by stage, until the body is vertical. Do not stop at this point but rather continue the movement by carrying the legs beyond the head and making the toes touch the floor. The whole range of movement—from raising the legs off the floor to touching the floor beyond the head with the toes—should be continuous, without any break at any step. The movement should be done without any jerk and the legs should be kept close to each other and unbent throughout the movement. After the toes touch the floor, try to push the toes still further from the head. Maintain the final attitude for a few seconds (fig. 14.9).
3. Return to step 1 without any jerky movement and without bending the legs.

Breathing: Normal, or exhale in step 2 and inhale in step 3.

Dynamic Application: Steps 2 and 3 should be alternately executed.

Static Application: Maintain the final attitude (step 2) as instructed by a qualified Yoga teacher.

Relaxation: In Corpse Posture, after completion of the exercise.

Points of Note: Before commencing the leg raising flatten the lumbar spine on the floor and maintain the connection until the lumbar spine is raised off the floor. In returning, when the lumbar spine comes to the floor, flatten it and maintain it till the legs are lowered on the floor.

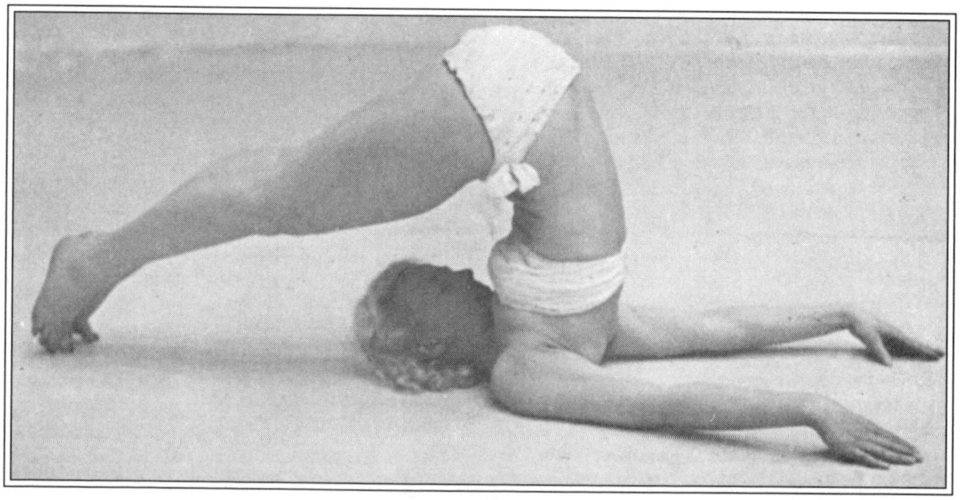

Fig. 14.9. Plow Posture (Halāsana)

Plow Posture with Forearms Locked behind Head

1. Assume a supine position with the legs extended, feet together, the forearms locked behind the head.
2. Slowly raise the legs, pelvis, and trunk as in Plow Posture (fig. 14.10).
3. Return to step 1 without any jerky movement and without bending the legs.

Breathing: Normal.

Dynamic Application: Steps 2 and 3 should be alternately executed.

Static Application: Maintain the final attitude (step 2) as instructed by a qualified Yoga teacher.

Relaxation: In Corpse Posture, after completion of the exercise.

Points of Note: As in Plow Posture.

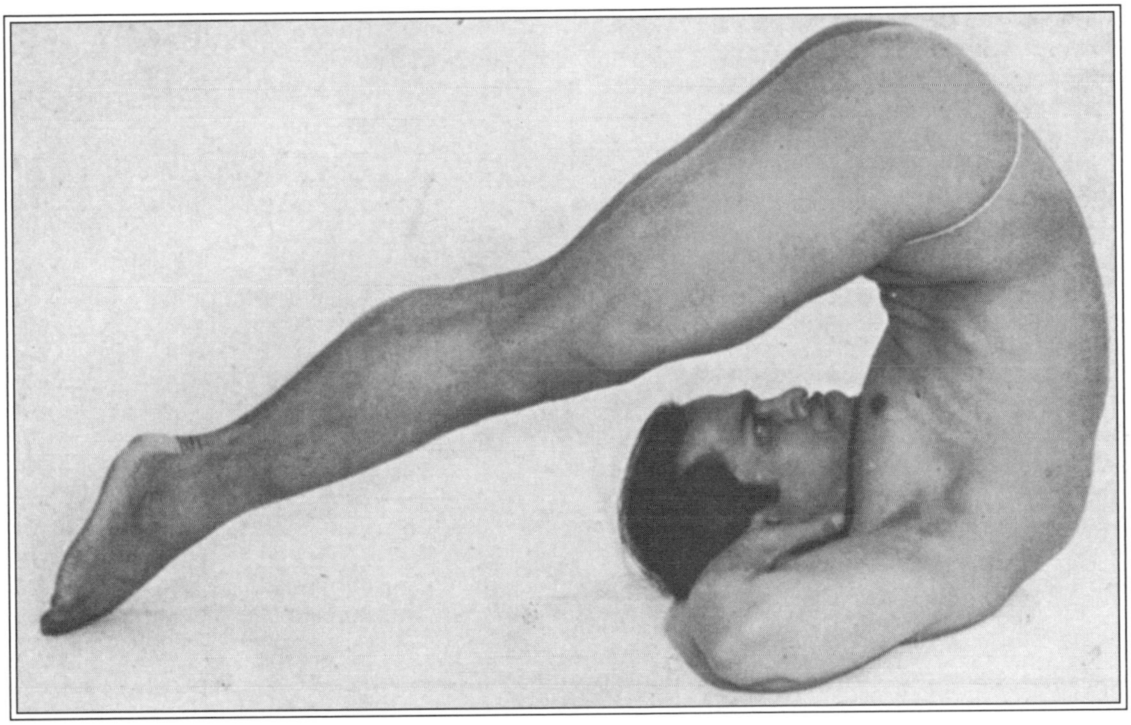

Fig. 14.10. Plow Posture with Forearms Locked behind Head (Śirabāhu Halāsana)

Ear-Pressing Posture

1. Assume a supine position with the legs extended, feet together, the arms extended by the sides.
2. Slowly raise the legs, pelvis, and trunk, step by step, until the body is vertical. Then bend the knees downward to touch the ears with the legs extended beyond the head and the toes placed on the floor. Maintain the final attitude for a few seconds (fig. 14.11).
3. Return slowly to step 1.

Breathing: Normal.

Dynamic Application: Steps 2 and 3 should be alternately executed.

Static Application: Maintain the final attitude (step 2) as instructed by a qualified Yoga teacher.

Relaxation: In Corpse Posture, after completion of the exercise.

Points of Note: As in Plow Posture.

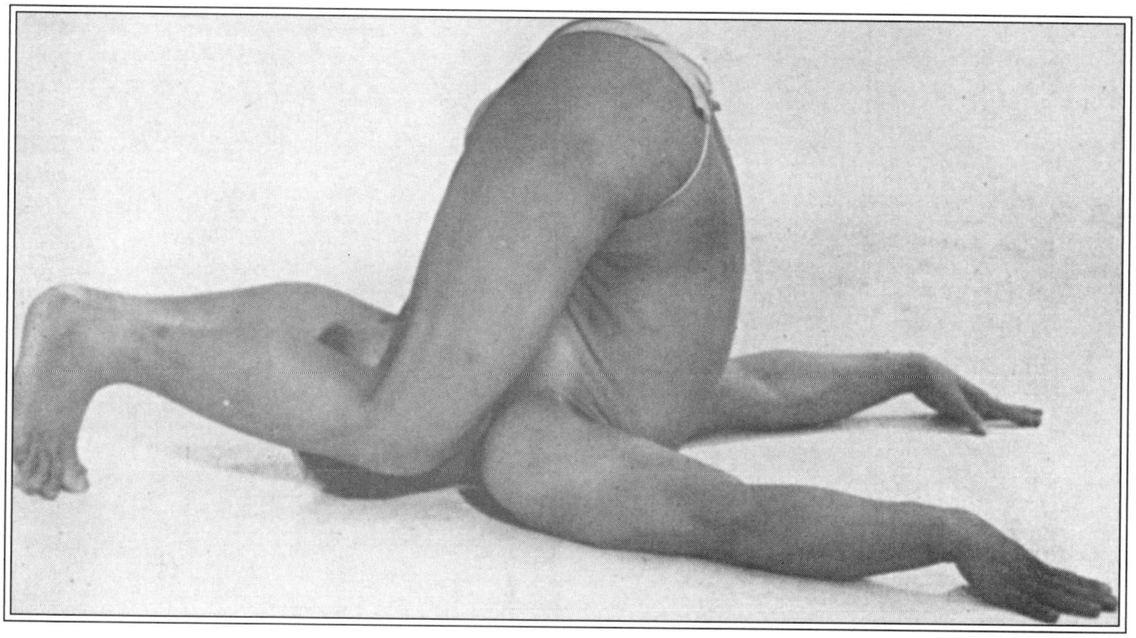

Fig. 14.11. Ear-Pressing Posture (Karṇapīḍanāsana)

Risen Back Posture

1. Assume Lotus Posture (fig. 20.2).
2. Lie down with the arms extended by the sides, the folded legs down on the floor with the thighs placed on the floor.
3. Raise the legs, pelvis, and the trunk without any jerk until the body is almost vertical, supported on the arms. Maintain the final attitude for a few seconds (fig. 14.12).

4. Return to step 2.

Breathing: Normal.

Dynamic Application: Steps 3 and 4 should be alternately executed.

Static Application: Maintain the final attitude (step 3) as instructed by a qualified Yoga teacher.

Relaxation: In Corpse Posture, after completion of the exercise.

Points of Note: This is an advanced abdominal exercise.

Lotus-Plow Posture

1. Assume Lotus Posture (fig. 20.2).
2. Lie down with the arms extended by the sides, the folded legs down on the floor with the thighs placed on the floor.
3. Raise the legs, pelvis, and trunk until the body is almost vertical as in Risen Back Posture.
4. Lower the knees down to the shoulders. Maintain the final attitude for a few seconds (fig. 14.13).
5. Return to step 3.

Breathing: Normal, or exhale in step 4 and inhale in step 5.

Dynamic Application: Steps 4 and 5 should be alternately executed.

Static Application: Maintain the final attitude (step 4) as instructed by a qualified Yoga teacher.

Relaxation: In Corpse Posture, after completion of the exercise.

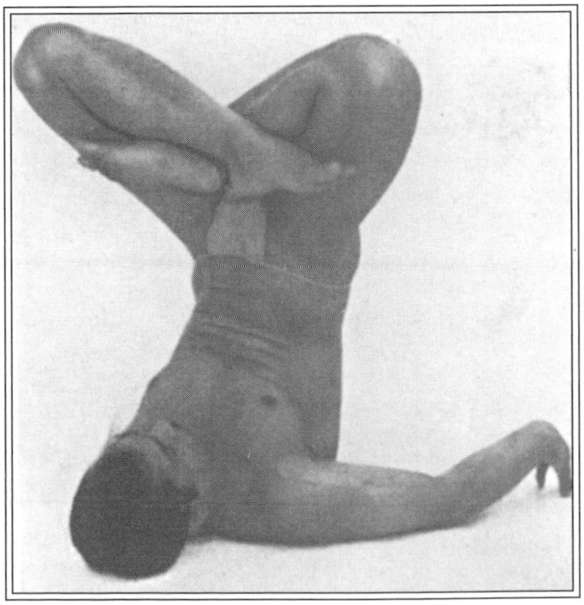

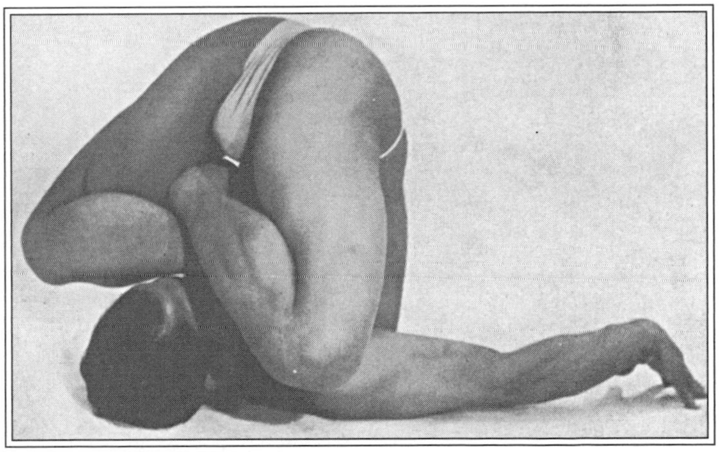

Left: Fig. 14.12. Risen Back Posture (Utthita Pṛiṣṭhāsana)

Above: Fig. 14.13. Lotus-Plow Posture (Natajānu Pṛiṣṭhāsana)

Leg-Raise Posture Exercise

Leg-raise posture exercise is actually hip flexion. The leg raising is accomplished by the hip flexors. The role of the rectus abdominis is to flatten the lumbar spine by exerting and maintaining an upward pull on the pelvis against the downward pull of the leg. The rectus abdominis is assisted by the obliquus externus abdominis and obliquus internus abdominis. When the abdominal muscles are weak, hyperextension of the lumbar spine takes place and the abdominal muscles are in a stretched state. This is an unfavorable condition for the abdominal muscles.

If hyperextension of the lumbar spine cannot be prevented during double leg raising exercise, the abdominal muscular strength should be first increased by trunk raising exercise. However, when the hyperextension is controlled, leg-raise posture exercise becomes very helpful in abdominal development. In fact, leg-raising posture exercise is the supplementary abdominal exercise, and when both trunk-raise and leg-raise exercises are combined, very satisfactory results are obtained. The leg-raising exercises are contraindicated in cases of lordosis. Concentration is on the abdominal muscles.

Risen Leg Posture

1. Assume a supine position with the legs extended, feet together, the arms extended by the sides.
2. Raise both legs simultaneously to a perpendicular position. Maintain the final attitude for a few seconds (fig. 14.14).

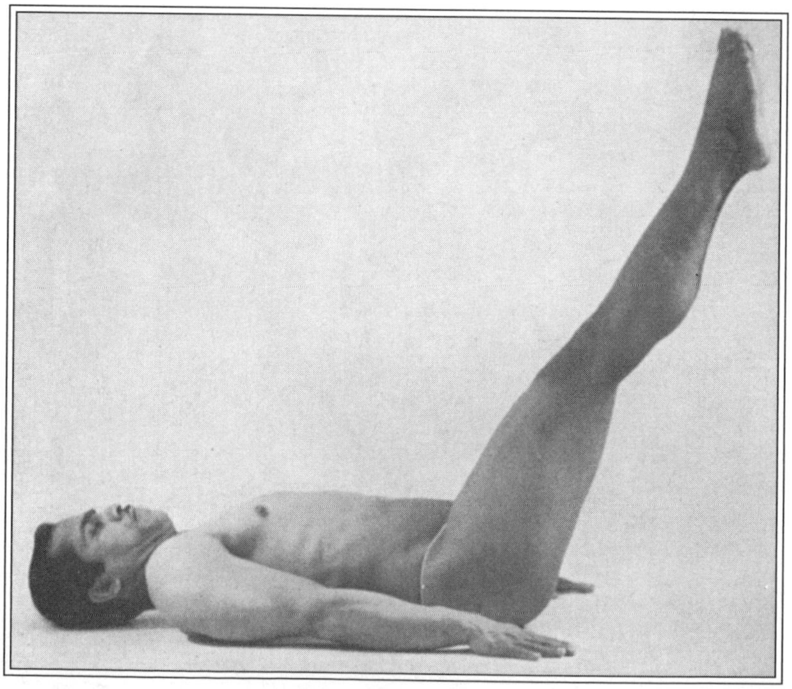

Fig. 14.14. Risen Leg Posture (Utthita Dvipādāsana)

3. Return to step 1.

Breathing: Normal, or inhale in step 2 and exhale in step 3.

Dynamic Application: Steps 2 and 3 should be alternately executed.

Static Application: Unsuitable.

Relaxation: In Corpse Posture, after completion of the exercise.

Points of Note: The lumbar spine should be kept flattened during the leg-raising movement. In leg raising the hip flexors are brought into play. But when this exercise is employed for abdominal development, the mind should be concentrated on the abdominal muscles.

When it is not possible to flatten the lumbar spine during this exercise, the abdominal muscles should first be strengthened by other abdominal exercises to gain this ability. The Single Risen Leg Posture, in which one leg is raised instead of both legs at a time, should be practiced first.

Sideward Leg-Motion Posture

1. Assume a supine position with the legs extended, feet together, arms extended by the sides.
2. Raise the legs simultaneously to a perpendicular position and move them slowly to the right and left until the feet almost touch the floor, keeping the legs straight and the feet together (fig. 14.15).
3. Return to step 1 after completion of the exercise.

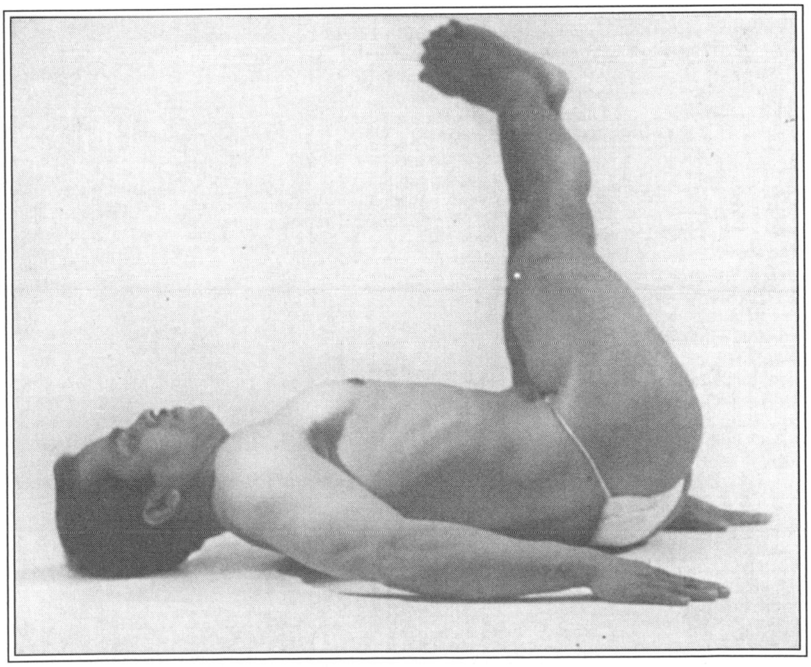

Fig. 14.15. Sideward Leg-Motion Posture (Pārśva Pāda-cālanāsana)

Breathing: Normal.

Dynamic Application: Step 2.

Static Application: Not suitable.

Relaxation: In Corpse Posture, after completion of the exercise.

Right-Angle Leg Posture

1. Assume a supine position with the legs extended, feet together, the arms by the sides, the hands on the waist.
2. Raise the legs simultaneously to a perpendicular position.
3. Lower the right leg to the floor at right angle to the body slowly from the perpendicular position and raise it again to the perpendicular position. Keep the leg straight throughout the movement (fig. 14.16).
4. The same movement with the left leg.

Breathing: Normal, or inhale when lowering the leg and exhale when raising it.

Dynamic Application: Steps 3 and 4.

Static Application: Not suitable.

Relaxation: In Corpse Posture, after completion of the exercise.

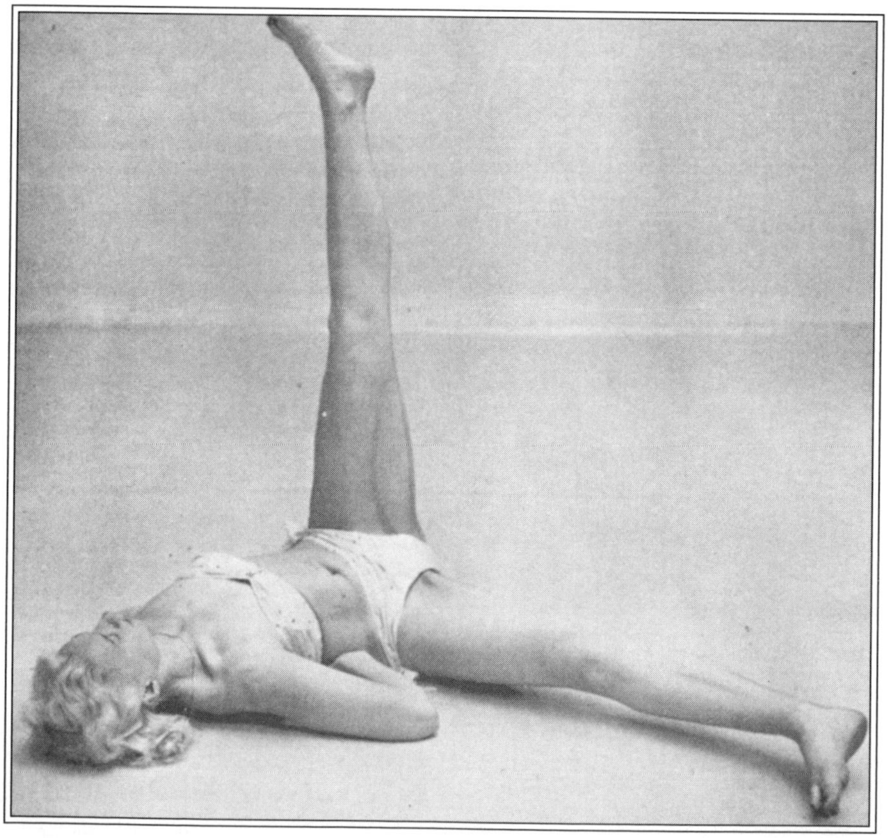

Fig. 14.16. Right-Angle Leg Posture (Natapādāsana)

Anterior Trunk-Leg-Raise Posture Exercise

In anterior trunk-leg-raise posture exercise the abdominal muscles are actively employed, and concentration is on those muscles.

Head-Knee Spine Posture

1. Assume a supine position with the hands clasped behind the head, the legs extended, feet together.
2. Raise the head and the trunk to a point at which the region of the seventh cervical vertebra is from 6 to 8 inches from the floor and at the same time bring the left knee to the forehead by bending at the knee. Maintain the final attitude for a few seconds (fig. 14.17).
3. Return to step 1.
4. Same movement (step 2) with the right leg.
5. Return to step 1.

Breathing: Normal.

Dynamic Application: Steps 2 and 3 and 4 and 5 should be alternately executed.

Static Application: The final attitude (steps 2 and 4) should be maintained as instructed by a qualified Yoga teacher.

Relaxation: In Corpse Posture, after the exercise is over.

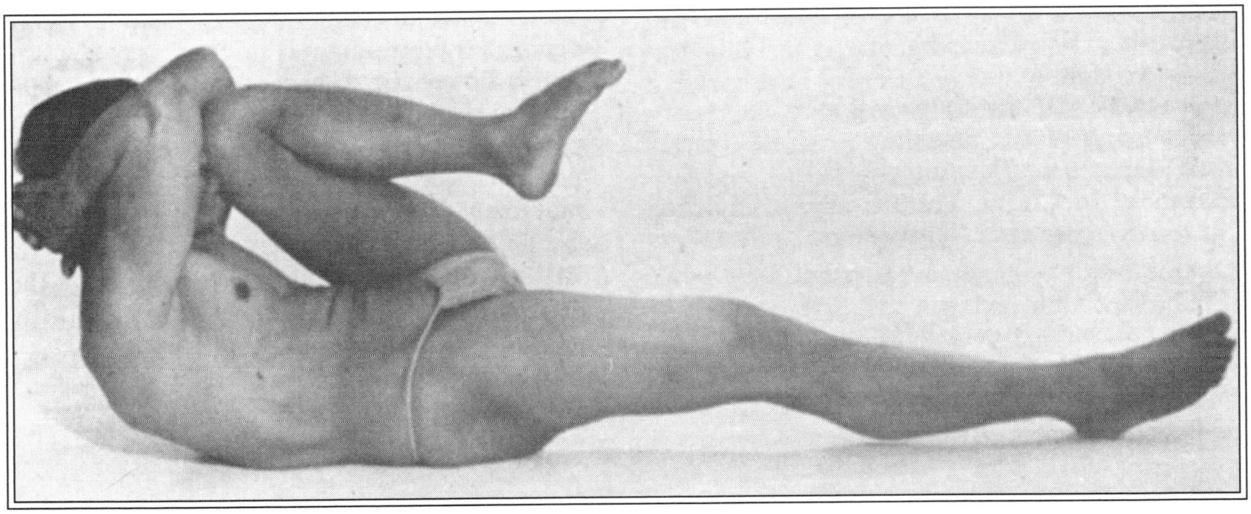

Fig. 14.17. Head-Knee Spine Posture (Jānuśira Merudaṇḍāsana)

Knee-Touching Spine Posture

1. Assume a supine position with the legs extended, feet together, arms extended over the head.
2. Raise the legs and at the same time the trunk and the arms slowly until the legs and the trunk are almost vertical. At this stage hold the toes with the hands and touch the knees with the forehead. Maintain the final attitude for a few seconds. There should be no jerk and the legs should be kept straight during the exercise (fig. 14.18).
3. Return to step 1.

Breathing: Normal.

Dynamic Application: Steps 2 and 3 should be alternately executed.

Static Application: Maintain the final attitude (step 2) as instructed by a qualified Yoga teacher.

Relaxation: In Corpse Posture, after completion of the exercise.

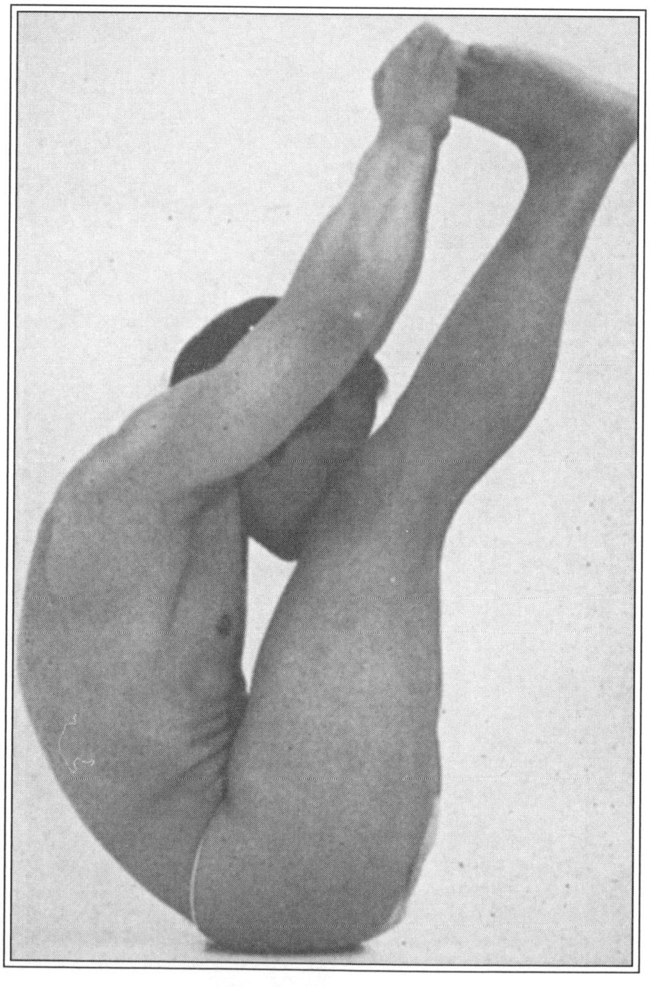

Fig. 14.18. Knee-Touching Spine Posture (Bhālaspṛiṣṭajānu Merudaṇḍāsana)

Pillow Posture

1. Assume a supine position with the legs extended, feet together, arms by the sides.
2. Raise the left leg and bring it toward the head. Now with the help of the hands place the left foot behind the neck, at the same time raising the head and the trunk quite high. The body will now remain on the buttocks, lower part of the trunk, and right leg. Maintain the final attitude for a few seconds (fig. 14.19).
3. Return to step 1.
4. Perform the movement with the right leg in a similar manner (step 2).
5. Return to step 1.

Breathing: Normal.

Dynamic Application: Steps 2 and 3 and 4 and 5 should be alternately executed.

Static Application: Maintain the final attitude (steps 2 and 4) as instructed by a qualified Yoga teacher.

Relaxation: In Corpse Posture, after completion of the exercise.

Points of Note: This is an advanced abdominal exercise requiring great relaxation of the hamstring muscles for the necessary flexion of the hip joint.

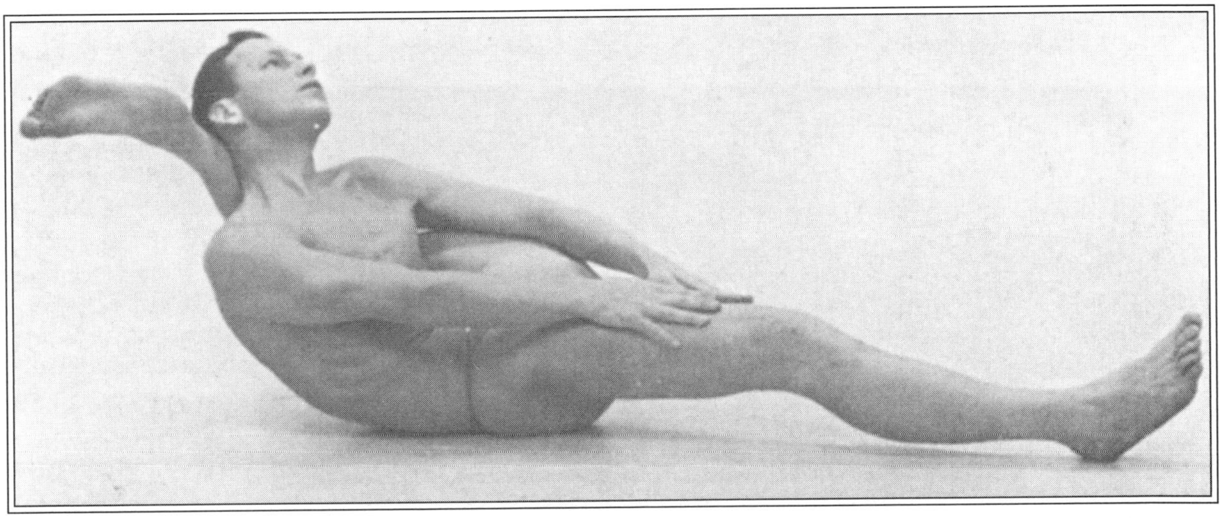

Fig. 14.19. Pillow Posture (Upādhānāsana)

Lateral Trunk-Leg-Raise Posture Exercise

In lateral trunk-leg-raise posture exercise the abdominal muscles are actively employed, and concentration is on those muscles.

Toe-Hold Lateral Spine Posture

1. Assume right side-lying position with the trunk, pelvis, and legs in a straight line, the left arm extended downward along the left side and on the left thigh, the right forearm locked behind the right side of the head.
2. Raise the head and the trunk laterally until the trunk is lifted off the floor as much as possible. The locked forearm should be raised along with the head. During the head and trunk raising, the left leg should also be raised to a perpendicular position and the left toes should be held with the left hand by extending the left arm upward. Maintain the final attitude for a few seconds (fig. 14.20).
3. Return to step 1.
4. Assume left side-lying position in the same manner (step 1).
5. Perform the movement in a similar manner (step 2).
6. Return to step 4.

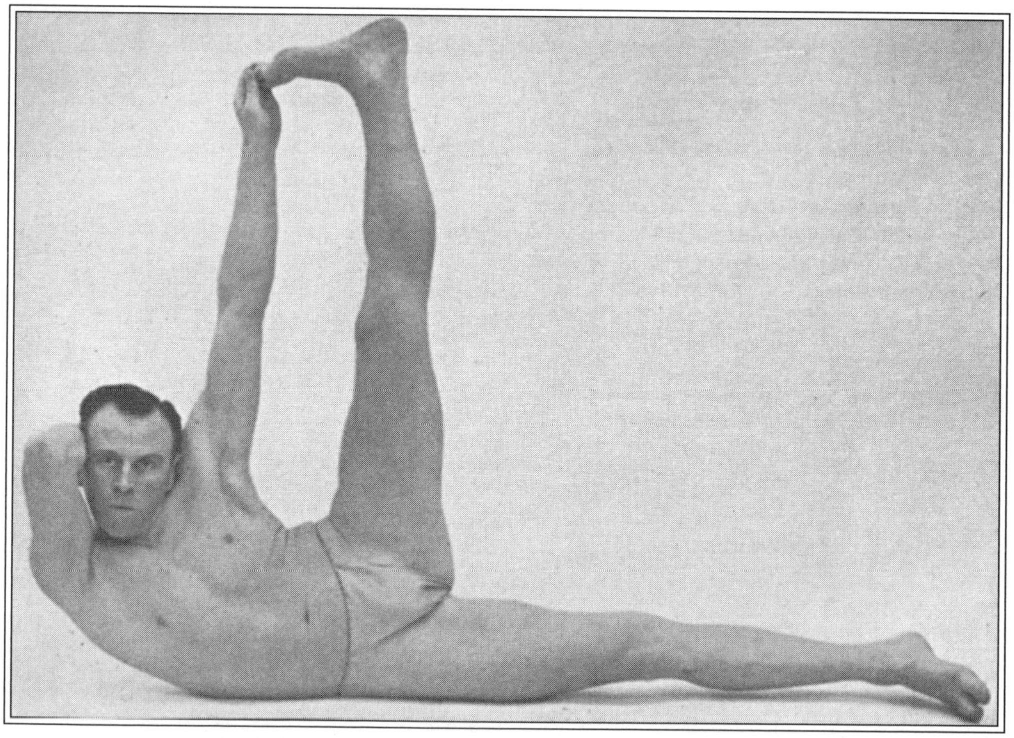

Fig. 14.20. Toe-Hold Lateral Spine Posture (Baddhānguli Pārśva Merudaṇḍāsana)

Breathing: Normal.

Dynamic Application: Steps 2 and 3 and 5 and 6 should be alternately executed.

Static Application: Maintain the final attitude (steps 2 and 5) as instructed by a qualified Yoga teacher.

Relaxation: In Corpse Posture, after completion of the exercise.

Points of Note: Avoid twisting the body as much as possible when raising the trunk. This is an advanced exercise. In order to gain strength first practice this exercise with the support of the disengaged arm.

Supplementary Abdominal Posture Exercise

Concentration is on the abdominal muscles in these exercises.

Risen Right-Angle Posture

1. Sit with the legs extended in front, the arms by the sides, the palms on the ground.
2. Raise the buttocks and the legs simultaneously off the floor, keeping the legs straight and supporting the body on the hands. Maintain the attitude for a few seconds (fig. 14.21).
3. Return to step 1.

Breathing: Normal.

Dynamic Application: Steps 2 and 3 should be alternately executed.

Static Application: Not suitable.

Relaxation: In Corpse Posture, after completion of the exercise.

Points of Note: This is an advanced abdominal exercise.

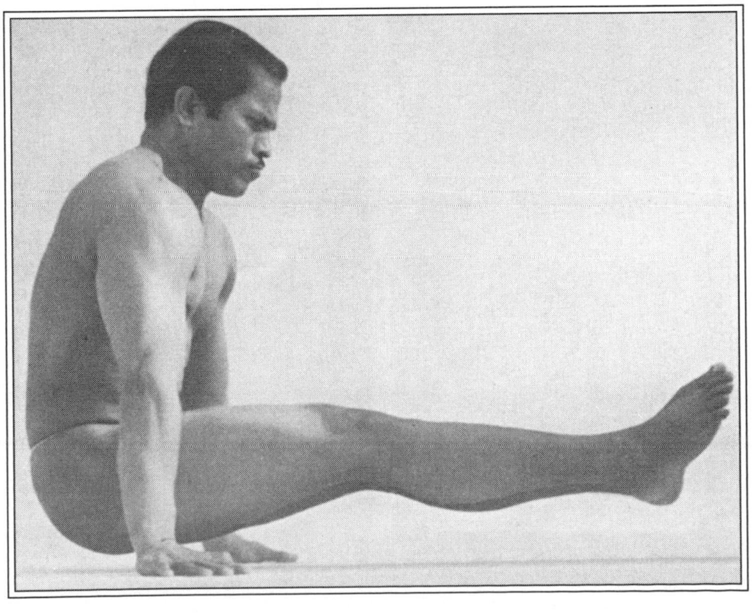

Fig. 14.21. Risen Right-Angle Posture (Utthita Samakoṇāsana)

Bent-Knee Inverse Lotus Posture

1. Assume Inverse Lotus Posture (fig. 19.4).
2. Lower the knees down to the elbows. Maintain the final attitude for a few seconds (fig. 14.22).
3. Return to step 1.

Breathing: Normal, or exhale when lowering the knees and inhale when raising them.

Dynamic Application: Steps 2 and 3 should be alternately executed.

Static Application: Maintain the final attitude (step 2) as instructed by a qualified Yoga teacher.

Relaxation: In Corpse Posture, after completion of the exercise.

Points of Note: This is also a balance and inverse-body posture. Concentration is on the rectus abdominis especially.

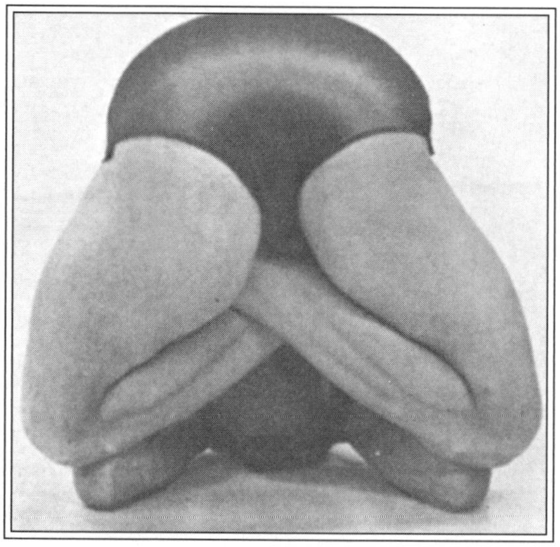

Fig. 14.22 Bent-Knee Inverse Lotus Posture (Natajānu Ūrdhva Padmāsana)

Abdominal Control Exercise

Abdominal Retraction (Uḍḍīyāna) and Straight Muscle Exercise (Naulī) are the most important of all abdominal control exercises. Full control over the abdominal muscles is attained by the practice of these two exercises. The alimentary canal is also profoundly influenced by them. Abdominal Retraction is the best exercise for the transversus abdominis and Straight Muscle Exercise for the isolation and full control of the rectus abdominis. In Abdominal Retraction concentration is on the retraction. In Straight Muscle Exercise concentration is on the isolated abdominis.

Abdominal Retraction (Uḍḍīyāna)

1. Stand with the heels either together or a few inches apart. It is more convenient for beginners to bend the body slightly forward with the legs slightly bent at the knees. When better control is gained, the body may be kept erect. The hands are either on the thighs or the arms by the sides.
2. Relax the abdomen completely. Now exhale fully and at the end of exhalation hold the breath. During the exhalation breath suspension, try to draw the abdomen inward and upward as much as possible by a muscular effort with the concentration of the mind. This will result in the concave appearance of the abdomen. Maintain this abdominal state for a few seconds (fig. 14.23).
3. Relax the abdomen and inhale.

Breathing: As stated above (step 2).

Dynamic Application: Steps 2 and 3 should be alternately executed.

Static Application: Maintain the retracted abdomen (step 2) as instructed by a qualified Yoga teacher.

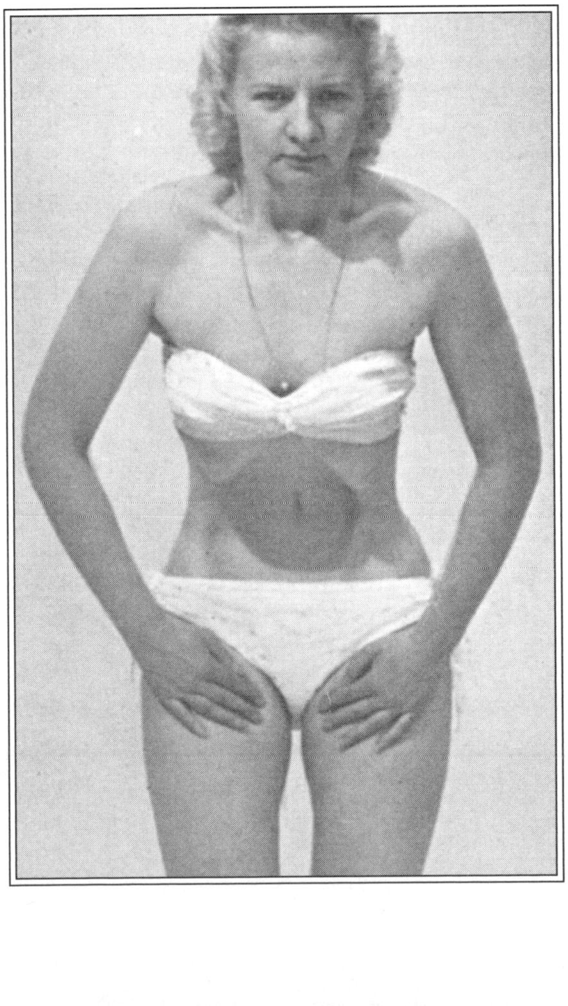

Fig. 14.23. Abdominal Retraction (Uḍḍīyāna)

Relaxation: In Standing Posture, after completion of the exercise.

Points of Note: This exercise should be performed when the stomach is empty. The best time is in the morning after toilet and oral cleansing. The next best time is in the evening, before dinner. If there is an accumulation of fat beyond the normal limit, it should be reduced by general and abdominal posture exercises, restricted diet, fasting, and other appropriate measures. This exercise can also be performed in any folded-leg posture.

Straight Muscle Exercise (Naulī)

1. Stand with the heels either together or a few inches apart, the legs either straight or slightly bent at the knees, the body bent forward, and the hands on the thighs.
2. Relax the abdomen completely. Now exhale fully; at the end of exhalation hold the breath. During the exhalation breath suspension first perform Abdominal Retraction and then mentally visualize the rectus abdominis and cause it to stand out against the collapsed abdomen by pressing strongly on the thighs with the hands and by skillfully making a forward-downward abdominal thrust. Concentrate your mind fully on the process. Maintain the isolated rectus abdominis for a few seconds (fig. 14.24).
3. Relax the abdomen and inhale.

Breathing: As stated above (step 2).

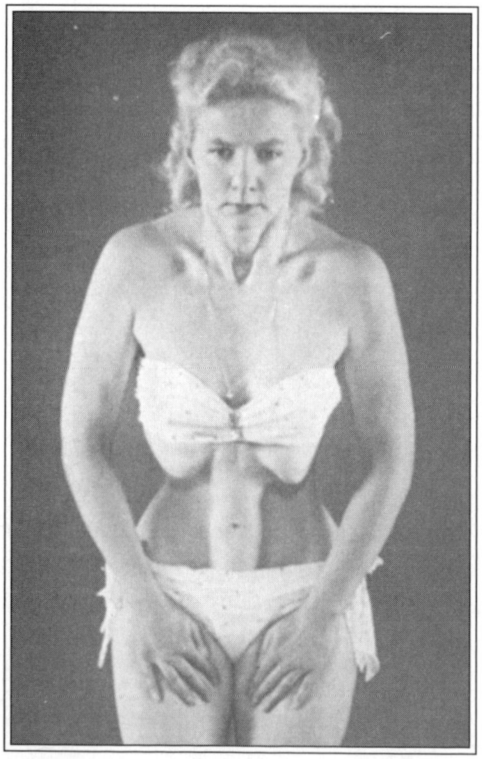

Fig. 14.24. Straight Muscle Exercise, Central Isolation (Naulī)

Dynamic Application: Steps 2 and 3 should be alternately executed.

Static Application: Maintain the isolated rectus abdominis (step 2) as instructed by a qualified Yoga teacher.

Relaxation: In Standing Posture, after completion of the exercise.

Points of Note: After the central isolation of the rectus abdominis is mastered, the right and the left isolation can be practiced. In right isolation the rectus abdominis is made to stand out on the right side of the abdomen. In a similar way it is made to stand out on the left side in left isolation. The unilateral isolation consists of two processes. In one, both recti are brought to the side (fig. 14.25). In another, the right rectus abdominis is isolated and made to stand out on the right side of the abdomen while keeping the left rectus abdominis relaxed. In a similar manner the left rectus abdominis is made to stand out on the left side (fig. 14.26). In the standing position (step 1), the skillful application of right-hand pressure will cause the right isolation and left-hand pressure left isolation. When sufficient control is gained, the rectus abdominis may be moved from the right to the left and vice versa. Finally, the rectus abdominis may be rolled in all possible directions.

Please also refer to points of note under Abdominal Retraction.

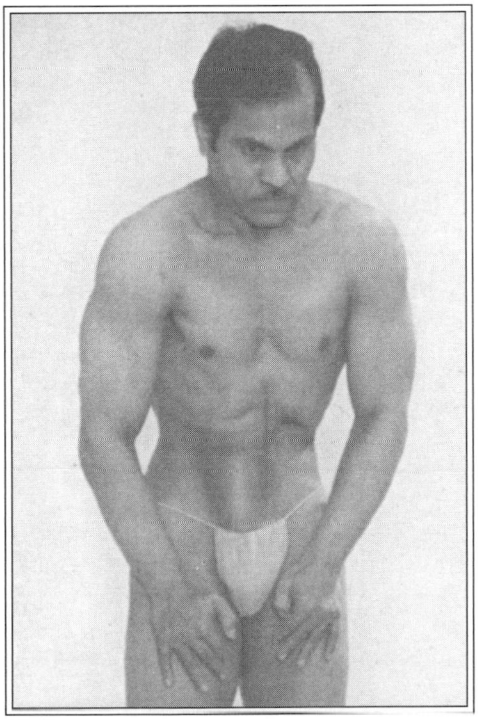

Fig. 14.25. Straight Muscle Exercise, unilateral isolation, making both recti stand on the right side (Naulī)

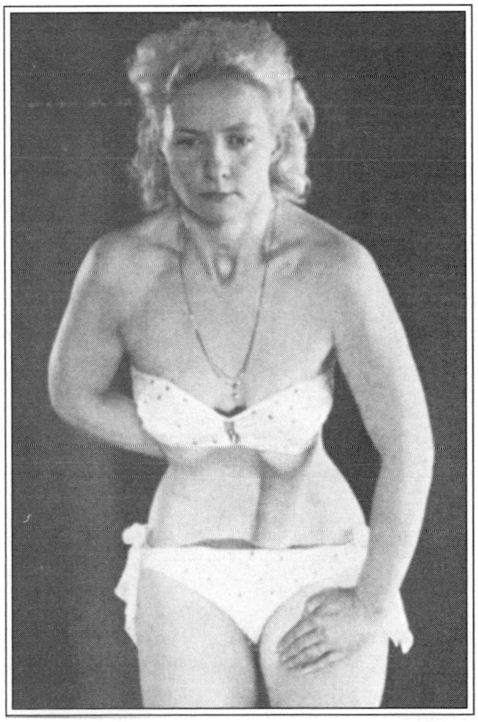

Fig. 14.26. Straight Muscle Exercise, unilateral isolation, making left rectus stand on the left side (Naulī)

15

Pelvic Posture and Control Exercise

The pelvic and the perineal muscles are exercised, strengthened, and controlled by pelvic exercise. It is closely associated with sex efficiency and control. Pelvic exercise is subdivided into pelvic posture exercise and pelvic control exercise.

Pelvic Posture Exercise

Concentration during the pelvic posture exercises is on the pelvic and perineal region.

Pelvis-Raise Posture

1. Sit with the legs extended in front, heels together, the arms by the sides.
2. Raise the pelvis and the trunk as high as you can while supporting yourself on your hands and feet. Maintain the final attitude for a few seconds (fig. 15.1).
3. Return to step 1.

Breathing: Normal, or inhale in step 2 and exhale in step 3.

Dynamic Application: Steps 2 and 3 should be alternately executed.

Static Application: Maintain the final attitude (step 2) as instructed by a qualified Yoga teacher.

Relaxation: In the sitting position (step 1), after completion of the exercise.

Points of Note: Certain leg movements are executed in the final attitude of this exercise. They are called Pelvis-Raise Posture exercise. Some of the exercises are as follows:

- Raising one leg to a perpendicular position and lowering it.

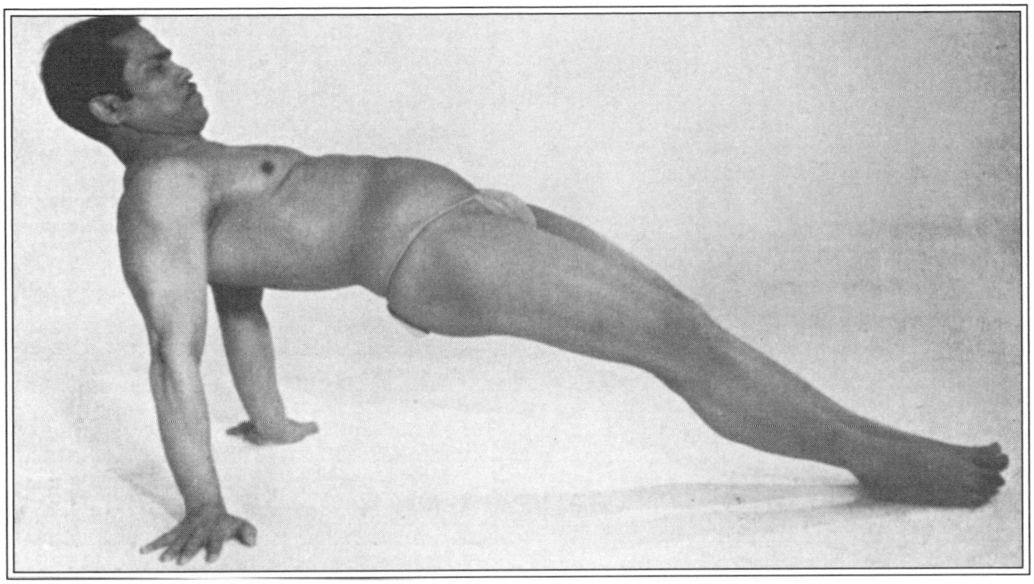

Fig. 15.1. Pelvis-Raise Posture (Kaṭikāsana)

- Lowering one leg from the perpendicular position sideward to the floor.
- Lowering one leg from the perpendicular position sideward to the floor to the opposite side.
- Bringing the knee to the chest.

Arm-Head Posture

1. Sit with the left leg bent and folded, the thigh on the lower leg, the left foot under the left buttock, the right knee elevated, the arms by the sides.
2. Insert the right arm under the right knee and lift it to the right side of the head and then clasp the hands behind the neck. Maintain the final attitude for a few seconds (fig. 15.2 on page 166).
3. Return to step 1.
4. Sit in the same way (step 1) with the right leg folded.
5. Raise the left knee in a similar manner (step 2).
6. Return to step 4.

Breathing: Normal.

Dynamic Application: Steps 2 and 3 and 5 and 6 should be alternately executed.

Static Application: Maintain the final attitude (steps 2 and 5) as instructed by a qualified Yoga teacher.

Relaxation: In the sitting position with the legs extended forward and the arms by the sides, after completion of the exercise.

Single Foot-Head Posture

1. Sit erect with the right heel set against the perineum.
2. With the help of the hands place the left leg across the neck by making the left thigh stand in a slanting manner. Now remove the hands from the left leg. Maintain the final attitude for a few seconds (fig. 15.3).
3. Return to step 2.
4. Sit with the left heel set against the perineum.
5. Place the right leg across the neck in a similar manner (step 2).
6. Return to step 4.

Breathing: Normal.

Dynamic Application: Steps 2 and 3 and 5 and 6 should be alternately executed.

Static Application: Maintain the final attitude (steps 2 and 5) as instructed by a qualified Yoga teacher.

Relaxation: In the sitting position with the legs extended forward and the arms by the sides, after completion of the exercise.

Points of Note: This exercise develops the flexibility of the hip joints and causes relaxation, to a great extent, of the hamstring muscles.

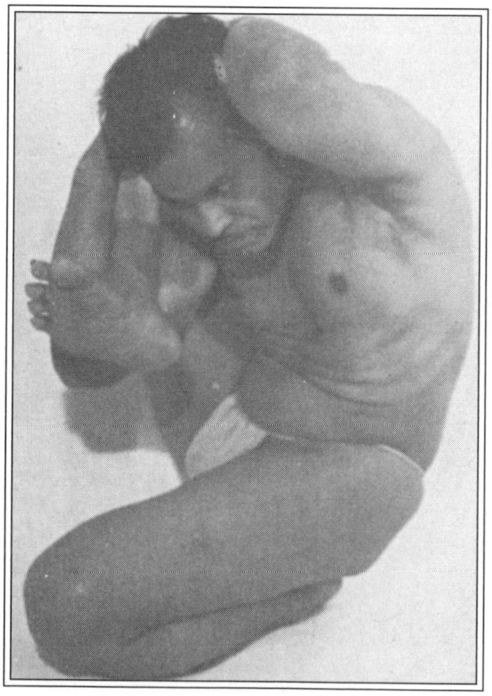

Fig. 15.2. Arm-Head Posture (Bhuja Śirāsana)

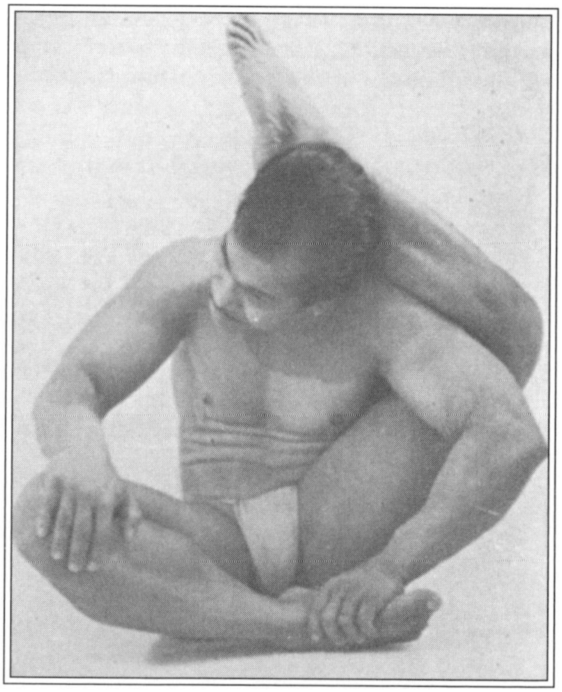

Fig. 15.3. Single Foot-Head Posture (Ekapāda Śirāsana)

Double Foot-Head Posture

1. Sit erect with the legs extended forward.
2. Place both legs with the ankles crossed at the back of the neck with the help of the hands. This can be done with one leg at a time or both legs together. Then remove the hands from the legs and either keep the arms extended across the thighs or the hands folded at the chest. Maintain the final attitude for a few seconds (fig. 15.4).
3. Return to step 1.

Breathing: Normal.

Dynamic Application: Steps 2 and 3 should be alternately executed.

Static Application: Maintain the final attitude (step 2) as instructed by a qualified Yoga teacher.

Relaxation: In the sitting position with the legs extended forward and the arms by the sides, after completion of the exercise.

Points of Note: As in Single Foot Head Posture.

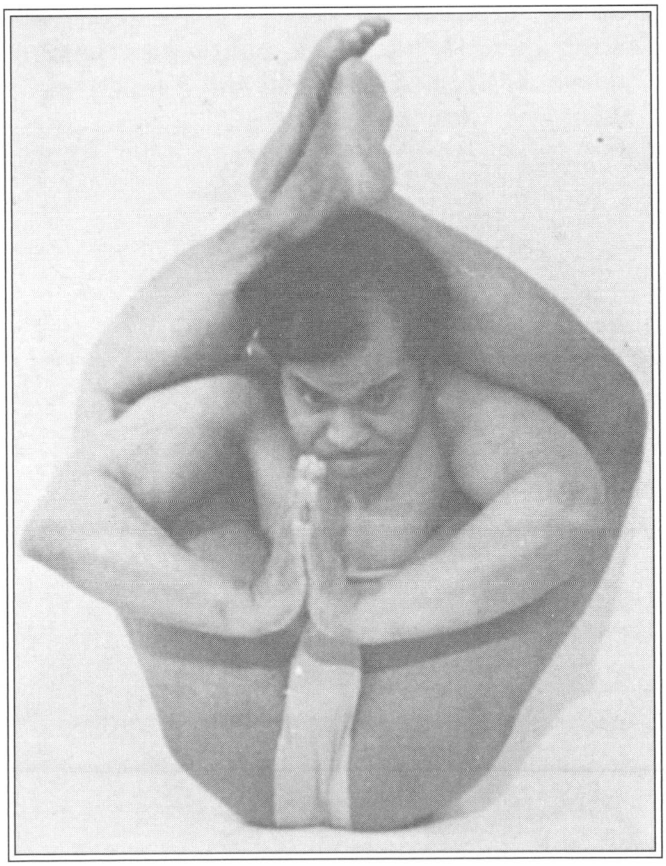

Fig. 15.4. Double Foot-Head Posture (Dvipāda Śirāsana)

Single Foot-Head Head-Knee Posture

1. Sit erect with the legs extended in front, the arms by the sides. Then place the right leg behind the neck as in Single Foot-Head Posture, keeping the left leg stretched forward.
2. Bend the body forward and downward, hold the toes of the left foot with both hands and bring the head down to the left knee, keeping the left leg straight. Maintain the final attitude for a few seconds (fig. 15.5).
3. Return to step 1.
4. Sit with the left leg placed behind the neck as in step 1.
5. Bend the body to the right leg as in step 2.
6. Return to step 4.

Breathing: Normal.

Dynamic Application: Steps 2 and 3 and 5 and 6 should be alternately executed.

Static Application: Maintain the final attitude (steps 2 and 5) as instructed by a qualified Yoga teacher.

Relaxation: In the sitting position with the legs extended forward and the arms by the sides, after completion of the exercise.

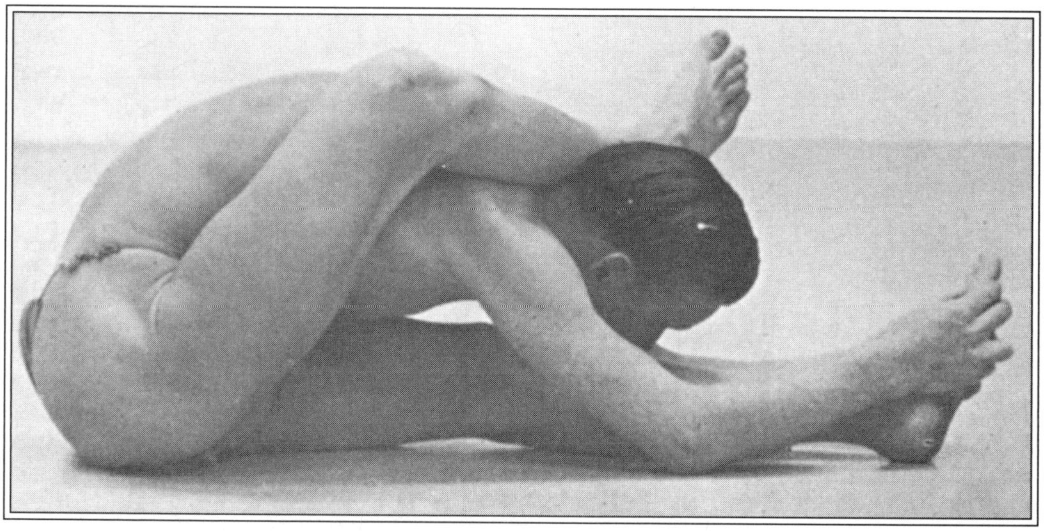

Fig. 15.5. Single Foot-Head Head-Knee Posture
(Ekapāda-śira Jānuśirāsana)

One-Leg Pillar Posture

1. Sit erect with the left leg extended in front, the right heel set against the perineum, the arms by the sides, the palms on the floor.
2. Slowly raise the left leg upward by applying a downward pressure with the hands until it is vertical, keeping the leg straight and without bending the body backward too much. There should be no jerk in the movement. Maintain the final attitude for a few seconds (fig. 15.6).
3. Return to step 1.
4. Sit with the right leg extended, the left heel against the perineum.
5. Slowly raise the right leg as in step 2.
6. Return to step 4.

Breathing: Normal, or inhale when raising the leg, exhale when lowering it.

Dynamic Application: Steps 2 and 3 and 5 and 6 should be alternately executed.

Static Application: Maintain the final attitude (steps 2 and 5) as instructed by a qualified Yoga teacher.

Relaxation: In the sitting position with the legs extended forward and the arms by the sides, after completion of the exercise.

Points of Note: This exercise requires relaxation of the hamstring muscles and flexibility of the hip joint to a remarkable extent. Regular practice of the exercise will develop them.

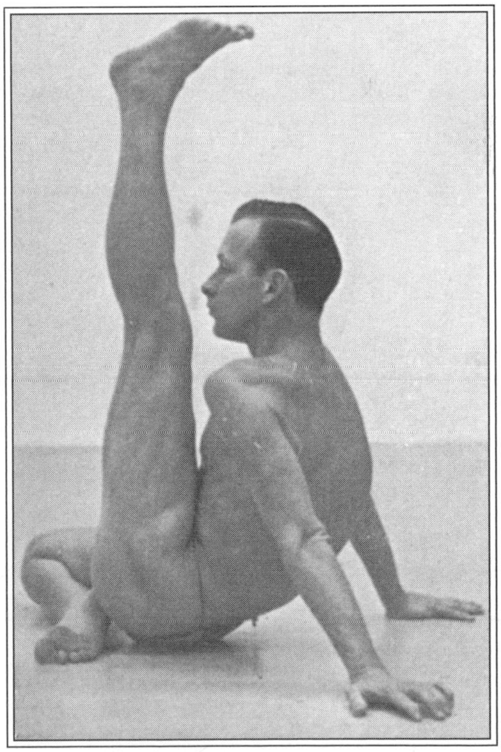

Fig. 15.6. One-Leg Pillar Posture
(Ekapāda Stambhāsana)

Pillar Posture

1. Sit erect with the legs extended in front, the heels together, the arms by the sides, the palms on the floor.
2. Slowly raise both legs upward until they are vertical by applying a downward pressure with the hands. The legs should be kept straight, the body should not be bent backward too much, and there should not be any jerk during the movement. Maintain the final attitude for a few seconds (fig. 15.7).
3. Return to step 1.

Breathing: Normal, or inhale when raising the legs and exhale when lowering them.

Dynamic Application: Steps 2 and 3 should be alternately executed.

Static Application: Maintain the final attitude (step 2) as instructed by a qualified Yoga teacher.

Relaxation: In the sitting position with the legs extended forward and the arms by the sides, after completion of the exercise.

Points of Note: As in One-Leg Pillar Posture.

Noose Posture

1. Assume a supine position with the legs extended, the feet together, the arms by the sides.
2. Raise both legs and, with the help of the hands, place them with the ankles crossed at the back of the neck, while raising the head, shoulders, and the pelvis from the floor. Then remove the hands from the legs, and either keep the arms extended across the thighs or the hands folded at the hip region. Maintain the attitude for a few seconds (fig. 15.8).

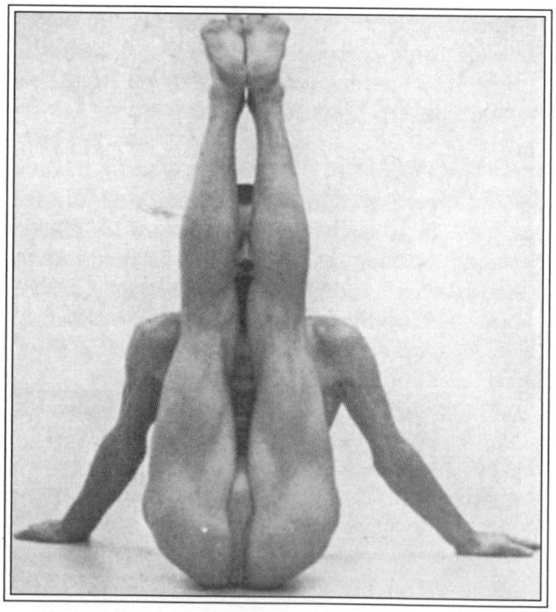

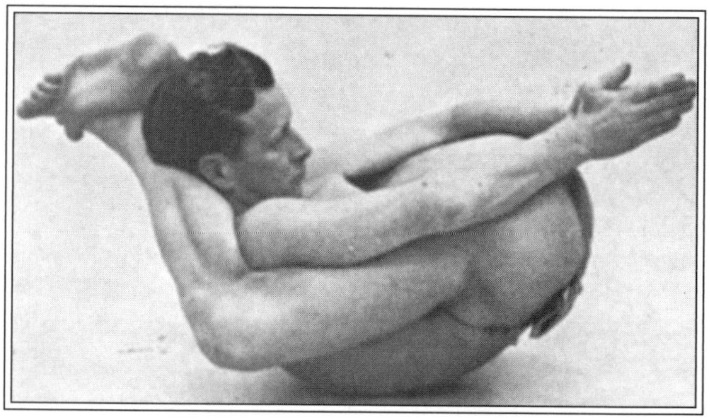

Left: Fig. 15.7. Pillar Posture (Stambhāsana)

Above: Fig. 15.8. Noose Posture (Pāśini-mudrā)

3. Return to step 1.

Breathing: Normal.

Dynamic Application: Steps 2 and 3 should be alternately executed.

Static Application: Maintain the final attitude (step 2) as instructed by a qualified Yoga teacher.

Relaxation: In Corpse Posture, after completion of the exercise.

Points of Note: As in One-Leg Pillar Posture.

Supplementary Pelvic Posture Exercise

Happy Posture

1. Sit erect with the legs extended in front, the arms by the sides.
2. Place the heels against the perineum with the soles together, the toes extending toward the front, the knees bent on the floor, and the hands of the extended arms on the knees. Maintain the final attitude for a few seconds (fig. 15.9).
3. Return to step 1.

Breathing: Normal.

Dynamic Application: Not suitable.

Static Application: Maintain the final attitude (step 2) as instructed by a qualified Yoga teacher.

Relaxation: In the sitting posture with the legs extended in front and the hands resting on the knees or joined in the lap, after completion of the exercise.

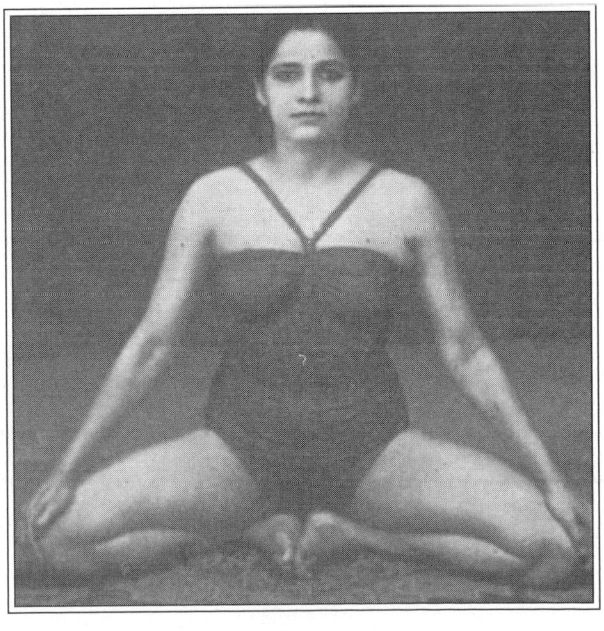

Fig. 15.9. Happy Posture (Bhadrāsana)

Sideward Leg-Stretch Posture

1. Sit erect with the legs extended in front, the arms by the sides.
2. Bring the legs to the sides and keep them extended sideward. Keep them perfectly straight and on the floor. Extend the arms sideward and place the hands on the knees. Maintain the final attitude for a few seconds (fig. 15.10).
3. Return to step 1.

Breathing: Normal.

Dynamic Application: Steps 2 and 3 should be alternately executed.

Static Application: Maintain the final attitude (step 2) as instructed by a qualified Yoga teacher.

Relaxation: In the sitting position with the legs extended in front and the hands resting on the thighs, after completion of the exercise.

Points of Note: As in One-Leg Pillar Posture.

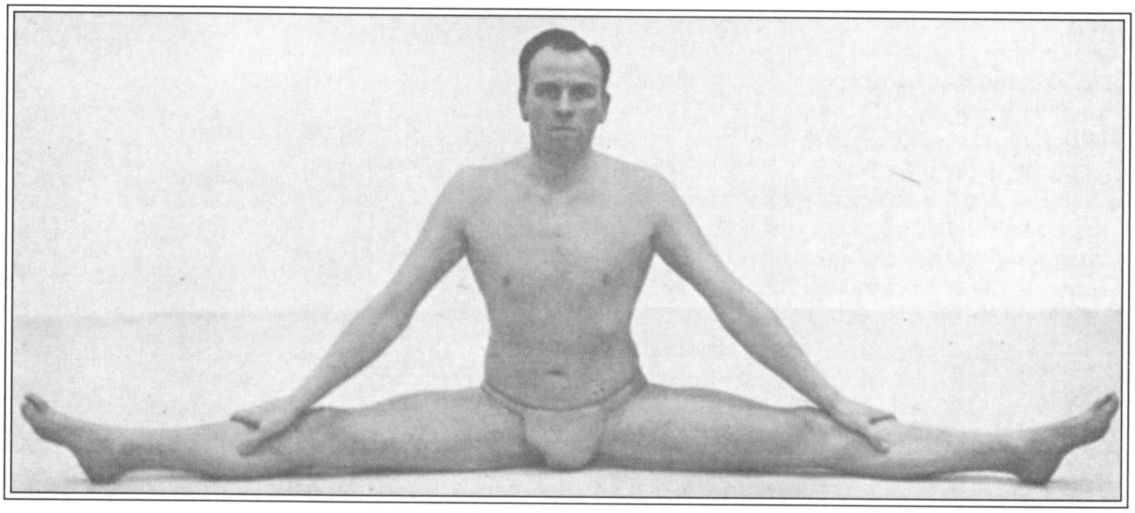

Fig. 15.10. Sideward Leg-Stretch Posture (Pādaprasāraṇāsana)

Backward-Forward Leg-Stretch Posture

1. Sit erect with the legs extended in front, the arms by the sides.
2. Bring the left leg to the back and extend it backward, keeping the right leg extended forward. Both legs are now almost in a straight line, unbent at the knees and on the floor. Keep the hands folded at the chest. Maintain the attitude for a few seconds (fig. 15.11).
3. Return to step 1.
4. Reverse the position of the legs.
5. Return to step 1.

Breathing: Normal.

Dynamic Application: Steps 2 and 3 and 4 and 5 should be alternately executed.

Static Application: Maintain the final attitude (steps 2 and 4) as instructed by a qualified Yoga teacher.

Relaxation: In the sitting position with the legs extended in front and the arms by the sides, after completion of the exercise.

Points of Note: As in One-Leg Pillar Posture.

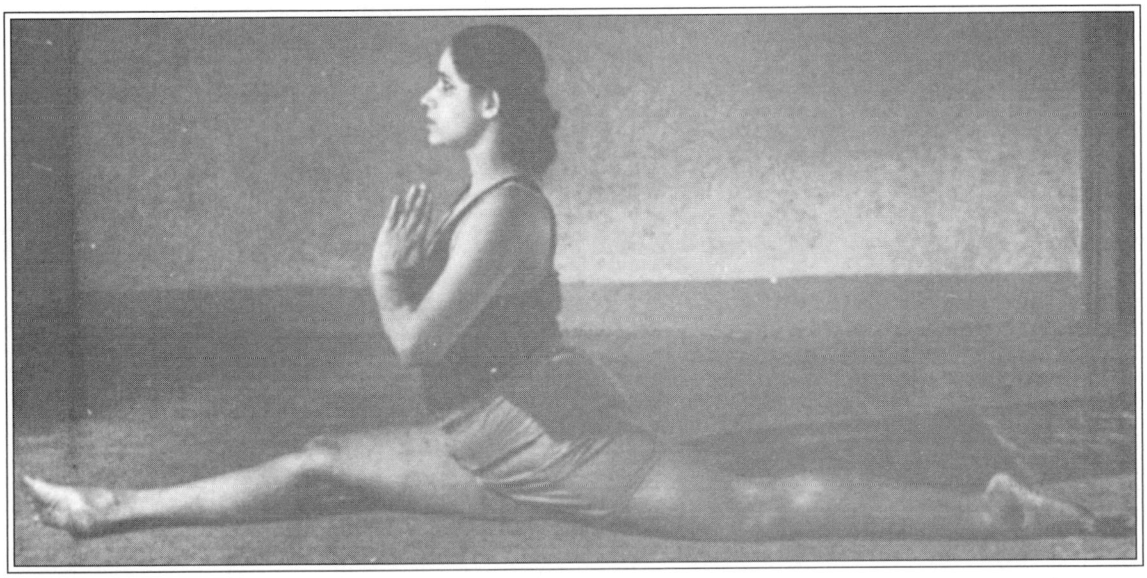

Fig. 15.11. Backward-Forward Leg-Stretch Posture (Hanumadāsana)

Pelvic Control Exercise

Concentration in pelvic control exercise is on the anal contraction and relaxation.

Anal Exercise (Aśvinī Mudrā)

1. Sit in Accomplished Posture (fig. 20.1) or Pleasant Posture (fig. 20.3).
2. Contract the anus in such a way as to cause an inward movement of the anal region as well as the genital region.
3. After the contractile movement, relax the anus. The relaxation will be a passive act. Do not force the anus out during relaxation.

Breathing: Normal.

Dynamic Application: The volitional and active anal contraction and volitional but passive anal relaxation should be alternately executed.

Static Application: None.

Relaxation: Fully relax the pelvic region in Accomplished Posture, Pleasant Posture, or in a sitting posture with the legs extended in front and the arms by the sides, after completion of the exercise.

Points of Note: Before doing this exercise the bladder and the bowels should be evacuated. The best time to practice this exercise is in the morning. The next best time is in the evening. The colon should be generally maintained as healthy and clean by internal baths, laxative diet, and other hygienic measures.

Anal Lock (Mūla Bandha)

1. Sit in Accomplished Posture (fig. 20.1) or Pleasant Posture (fig. 20.3).
2. Contract the anus volitionally and powerfully as in the Anal Exercise, and retain the anal contraction as instructed by a qualified Yoga teacher.
3. After retention relax the anus. Do not force the anus out during relaxation.

Breathing: Normal.

Dynamic Application: None.

Static Application: Anal contraction should be retained as instructed by a qualified Yoga teacher.

Relaxation: As in Anal Exercise.

Points of Note: As in Anal Exercise.

16

Pectoral Limb Posture Exercise

The pectoral limb muscles are the muscles concerned in the movements of the arm at the shoulder joint (scapulohumeral articulation), the shoulder girdle (acromioclavicular and sternoclavicular articulations), the forearm at the elbow and radio-ulnar joints, and the wrist and fingers. Special exercises have been developed in Yoga for the exercise of the muscles of these joints. These are contraction exercises. However, the pectoral limb muscles can be exercised in a more general but effective manner by the posture exercises presented here. In these exercises concentration is either on the trapezius muscle or on the arm muscles, especially the triceps.

Risen Lotus Posture

1. Assume Lotus Posture (fig. 20.2) with the arms by the sides and the palms on the floor.
2. Raise the body (the buttocks, thighs, and knees) off the floor, supporting it on the palms. Maintain the final attitude for a few seconds. During the movement and the maintenance of the attitude, contract the trapezius volitionally (fig. 16.1).
3. Return to step 1.

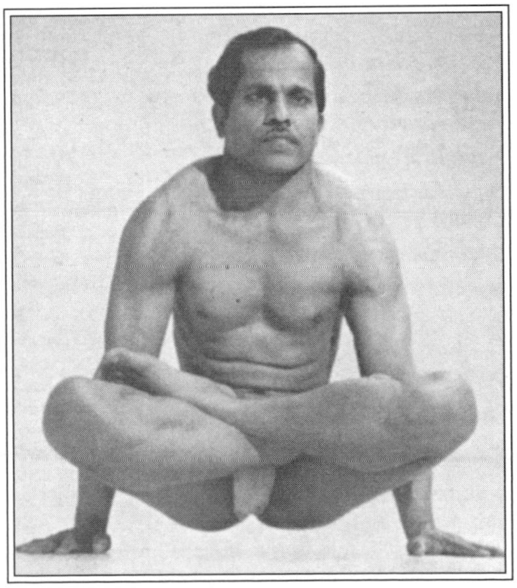

Fig. 16.1. Risen Lotus Posture (Utthita Padmāsana)

Breathing: Normal.

Dynamic Application: Steps 2 and 3 should be alternately executed.

Static Application: Maintain the final attitude (step 2) as instructed by a qualified Yoga teacher.

Relaxation: In Lotus Posture or the sitting position with the legs extended forward and the arms by the sides, after completion of the exercise.

Points of Note: Concentration is on the trapezius muscle.

Cock Posture

1. Assume Lotus Posture (fig. 20.2).
2. Insert the right arm into the space formed between the right thigh and calf and push the hand and wrist through the thigh and calf. In a similar manner bring the left hand and wrist through. Now place the palms on the floor, close to each other, and raise the body (the buttocks, thighs, and knees) off the floor. Maintain the final attitude for a few seconds. During the upward movement of the body and the maintenance of the attitude, contract the trapezius volitionally (fig. 16.2).
3. Return to step 1.

Breathing: Normal.

Dynamic Application: Steps 2 and 3 should be alternately executed.

Static Application: Maintain the final attitude (step 2) as instructed by a qualified Yoga teacher.

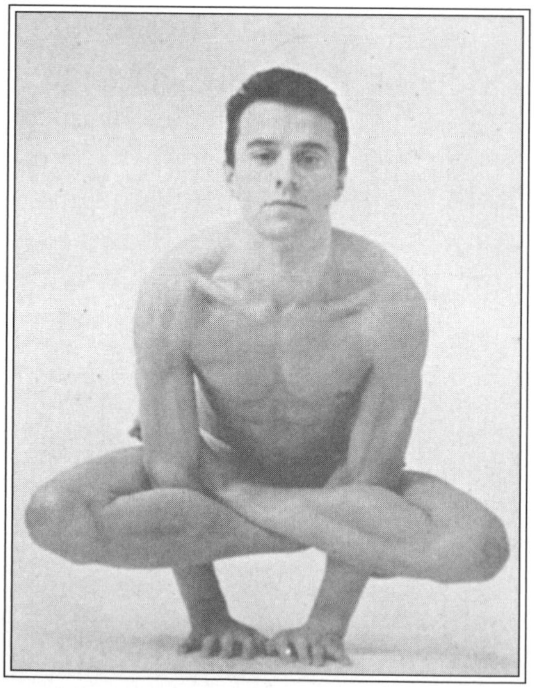

Fig. 16.2. Cock Posture (Kukkuṭāsana)

Relaxation: As in Risen Lotus Posture.

Points of Note: Concentration is on the trapezius muscle.

One-Arm Cock Posture

1. Assume Lotus Posture (fig. 20.2).
2. Insert the right arm into the space formed between the body and ankles and push the hand and wrist through. Now place the right palm on the floor and raise the body off the floor by supporting it on the right arm. Maintain the final attitude for a few seconds. During the movement and the maintenance of the attitude, contract the trapezius volitionally (fig. 16.3).
3. Return to step 1.
4. In a similar manner (step 2) raise the body on the left arm.
5. Return to step 1.

Breathing: Normal.

Dynamic Application: Steps 2 and 3 and 4 and 5 should be alternately executed.

Static Application: Maintain the final attitude (steps 2 and 4) as instructed by a qualified Yoga teacher.

Relaxation: As in Risen Lotus Posture.

Points of Note: This is an advanced exercise requiring powerful muscular action, especially of the shoulder region, and also balance. Concentration is on the trapezius muscle.

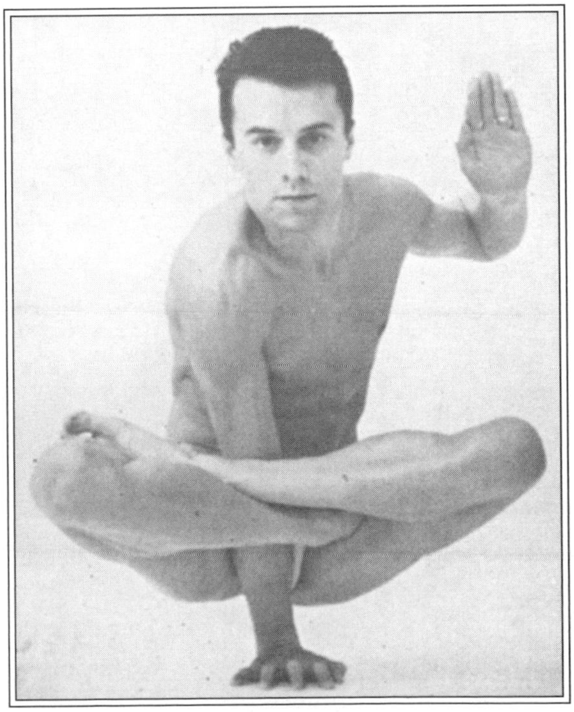

Fig. 16.3. One-Arm Cock Posture (Ekahasta Kukkuṭāsana)

Four-Point Posture

1. Assume a prone position with the palms placed flat on the floor by the shoulders, the fingers facing forward, and with the toes on the floor.
2. Raise the body off the floor supporting it on the palms and toes and keeping it straight.
3. Press the body up to full arms' length. Maintain the final attitude for a few seconds (fig. 16.4).
4. Return to step 2, keeping the body straight.

Breathing: Inhale in step 3 and exhale in step 4.

Dynamic Application: Steps 3 and 4 should be alternately executed.

Static Application: Maintain the final attitude (step 3) as instructed by a qualified Yoga teacher.

Relaxation: In Prone Posture, after completion of the exercise.

Points of Note: In this exercise concentration is especially on the triceps, pectoralis major, and serratus anterior. For the special development of the pectoralis major, the hands should be placed far apart instead of keeping them at the shoulder width. Gradually the distance between the hands may be made greater by placing them farther and farther apart.

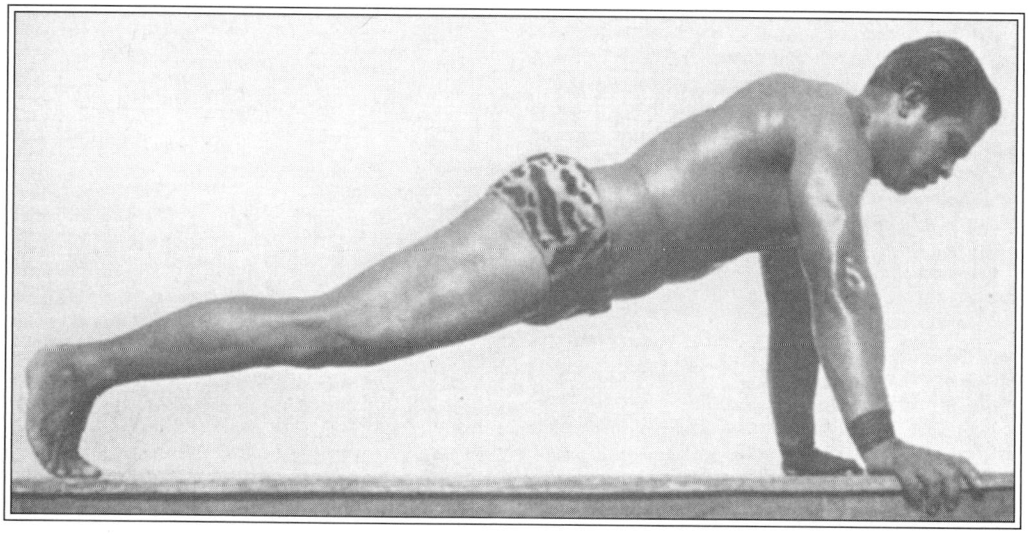

Fig. 16.4. Four-Point Posture (Catuṣpādāsana)

Three-Footed Posture

1. Assume a prone position with the palms placed flat on the floor by the shoulders. Press the body up to full arms' length.
2. Bring the right arm behind the back, supporting the body on the left arm and both feet.
3. Lower the body until the chest nearly touches the floor, by bending at the left elbow

and keeping the body straight. Now the body remains suspended on the left hand and both feet.

4. Push up the body by straightening the left arm (fig. 16.5).
5. Repeat, using the right arm.

Breathing: Exhale in step 3, inhale in step 4.

Dynamic Application: Steps 3 and 4 should be alternately executed.

Static Application: Not suitable.

Relaxation: In Prone Posture or Corpse Posture, after completion of the exercise.

Points of Note: This is an advanced exercise for developing the arm muscles, especially the triceps, which is the focus of concentration.

This exercise has two other forms:

- Keep the body supported on one arm and both legs, and grasp the elbow of the supporting arm with the other hand by bringing the arm behind the back; lower the body and touch the fingers of the supporting arm with the face by a twisting movement. Then straighten the supporting arm. Repeat and then perform the movement on the other arm.
- Keep the body supported on both arms and one leg, raising the other leg off the floor and keeping it suspended in the air, lower the body until the chest nearly touches the floor. Then push up the body by straightening the arms. Keep the non-supporting leg suspended throughout the movements. Repeat and then perform the movements while keeping the other leg suspended.

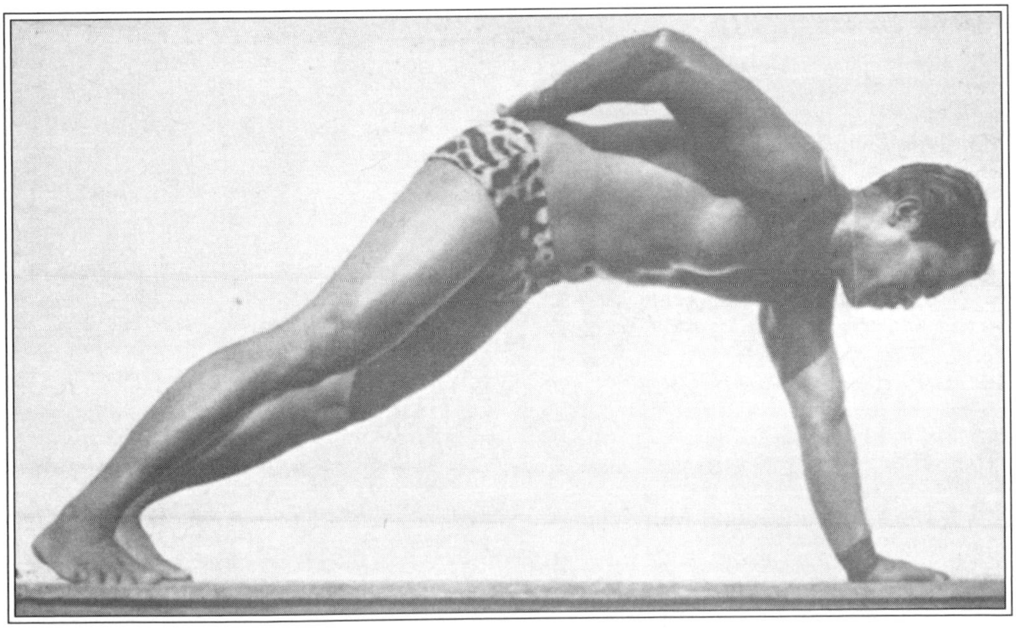

Fig. 16.5. Three-Footed Posture (Tripādāsana)

Arm-Leg Posture

1. Assume a prone position with the palms placed flat on the floor by the shoulders. Press the body up to full arms' length.
2. Bring the right arm behind the back and raise the right leg off the floor and keep it suspended, leaning on the left side and maintaining the weight of the body on the left arm and leg.
3. Lower the body by bending the left elbow until it almost touches the floor.
4. Push the body up by straightening the left arm (fig. 16.6).
5. Perform the movement in a similar manner on the opposite arm and leg.

Breathing: Exhale in step 3, inhale in step 4.

Dynamic Application: Steps 3 and 4 should be alternately executed.

Static Application: Not suitable.

Relaxation: In Prone Posture or Corpse Posture, after completion of the exercise.

Points of Note: This is an advanced exercise for developing the arm muscles, especially the triceps, which is the focus of concentration.

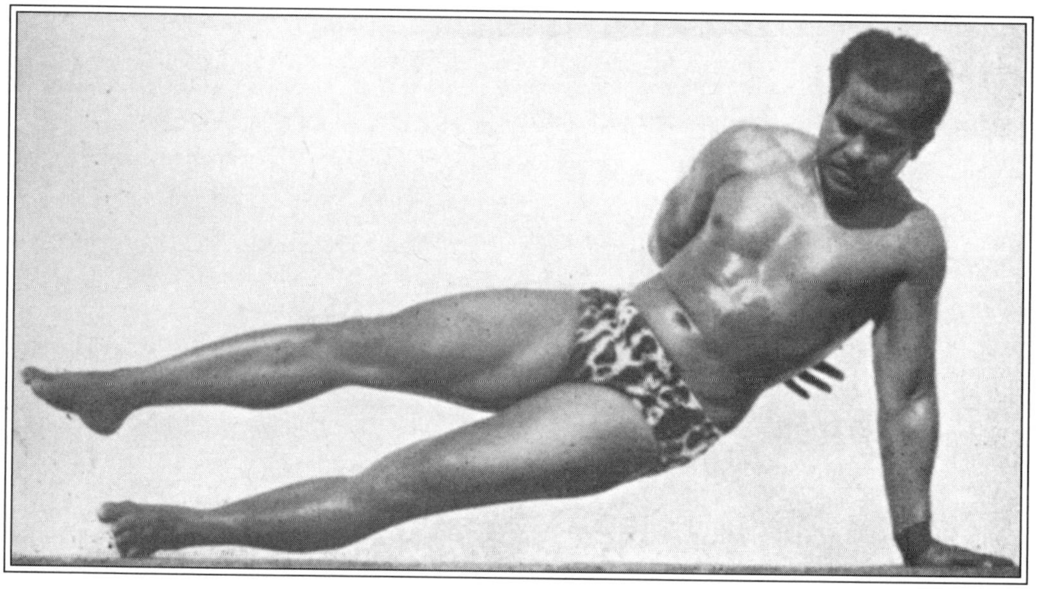

Fig. 16.6. Arm-Leg Posture (Bāhu-pādāsana)

Opposite Arm-Leg Posture

1. Assume a prone position with the palms placed flat on the floor by the shoulders. Push the body up to full arms' length.
2. Bring the left arm behind the back and raise the right leg off the floor, supporting the body on the right arm and the left leg.

3. Lower the body by bending the right elbow until it nearly touches the floor.
4. Push the body up by straightening the right arm (fig. 16.7).
5. Perform the movement in a similar manner on the left arm and the right leg.

Breathing: Exhale in step 3, inhale in step 4.

Dynamic Application: Steps 3 and 4 should be alternately executed.

Static Application: Not suitable.

Relaxation: In Prone Posture or Corpse Posture, after completion of the exercise.

Points of Note: This is an advanced exercise for developing the arm muscles, especially the triceps, which is the focus of concentration.

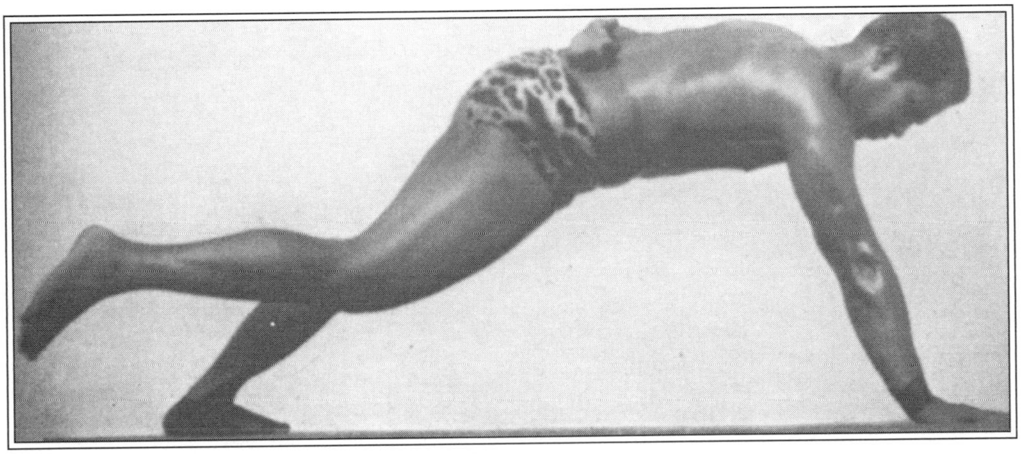

Fig. 16.7. Opposite Arm-Leg Posture (Viparīta Bāhu-pādāsana)

Arm Posture

1. Assume Squat Posture, extend the right arm in front and place the fist on the floor, about 27 inches from the right toes, and the left arm behind the back.
2. Bend the head and the body toward the right fist until the tip of the nose touches the top of the fist. This is done by bending at the right elbow, and without allowing the knees to touch the floor (fig. 16.8 on page 182).
3. Return to step 1.
4. Perform the movement in a similar manner with the left arm.

Breathing: Normal.

Dynamic Application: Steps 2 and 3 should be alternately executed.

Static Application: Not suitable.

Relaxation: In the sitting position with the legs extended in front and the arms by the sides, after completion of the exercise.

Points of Note: This is an advanced exercise for the pectoral limb muscles, especially the triceps, which is the focus of concentration.

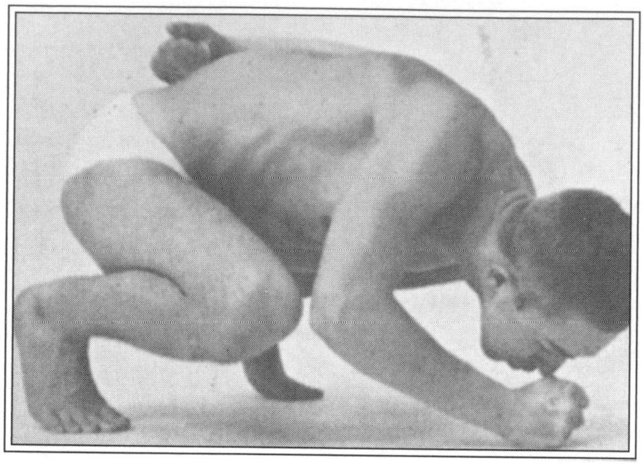

Fig. 16.8. Arm Posture (Pragaṇḍāsana)

Arm Motion

1. Assume Accomplished Posture (fig. 20.1) or Pleasant Posture (fig. 20.3) with the arms extended sideward at the shoulder level, the palms upward, the hands clenched.
2. Contract the arm muscles and simultaneously bring both fists close to the shoulders, bending at the elbows and raising the elbows high enough from the shoulder level to secure the full contraction of the biceps. Maintain the attitude for a few seconds (fig. 16.9).
3. Extend both arms simultaneously to the starting position (step 1), maintaining the contraction of the arm muscles.

Breathing: Inhale in step 2, exhale in step 3.

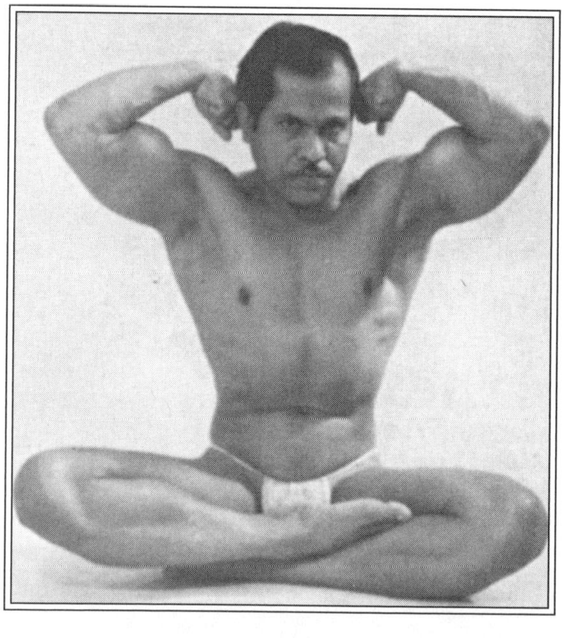

Fig. 16.9. Arm Motion (Bāhu-cāraṇā)

Dynamic Application: Steps 2 and 3 should be alternately executed.

Static Application: Not suitable.

Relaxation: In the sitting position with the legs extended forward and the arms by the sides, after completion of the exercise.

Points of Note: This exercise can also be performed in Standing Posture. It is not a posture exercise, but a contraction exercise. It is especially for the development of the biceps muscle, which is the focus of concentration. When the fists are close to the shoulders and the elbows are raised high from the shoulder level, an additional effort should be made to contract the biceps more powerfully to secure the full contraction. This additional contraction should be maintained for a few seconds before extending the arms to the starting position.

17

Pelvic Limb Posture Exercise

The muscles acting on the hip joint, the knee joint, the ankle joint, and the foot are the pelvic limb muscles. A systematized form of exercise for these muscles is included in contraction exercises. We are presenting here the posture exercise for the pelvic limb muscles. These exercises are not only important for the development of the pelvic limb muscles but for maintaining efficient circulation and heart action and increasing the vital vigor. These exercises also have especial value. They are designed to counteract the unhealthful effects of the prolonged folded-leg postures required in concentration. In the thigh and squat postures, concentration is on the thigh muscles, and in the toe postures, concentration is on the calf muscles.

Thigh Posture

1. Assume Squat Posture with the feet about 6 inches apart and the hands folded at the chest.
2. Raise the heels high and straighten the body to a standing position (fig. 17.1).
3. Lower the body to step 1.

Breathing: Inhale in step 2, exhale in step 3.
Dynamic Application: Steps 2 and 3 should be alternately executed.
Static Application: Not necessary.

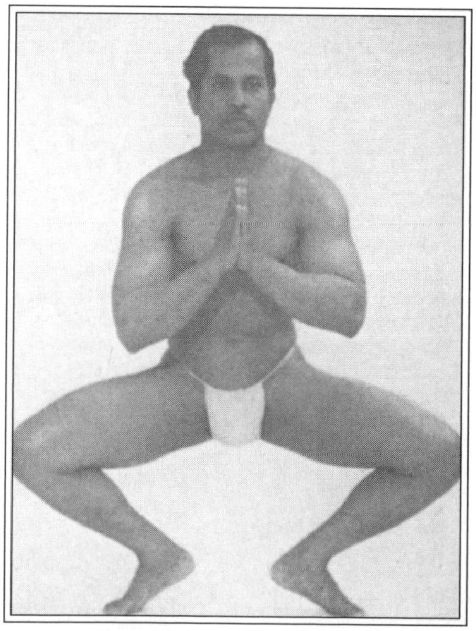

Fig. 17.1. Thigh Posture (Ūrvāsana)

Relaxation: In Standing Posture, after completion of the exercise.

Points of Note: This exercise is also called Squat Posture.

Knee-Touching Thigh Posture

1. Stand with the feet apart, the hands folded at the chest or on the hips.
2. Raise the heels high and lower the body to a squatting position, bringing the knees in contact with each other. Maintain the final attitude for a few seconds (fig. 17.2).
3. Return to step 1 by straightening the legs.

This exercise can also be performed with a short forward jump to stimulate the heart and lungs more vigorously. It is done as follows:

1. Stand with the feet together, the hands folded at the chest or on the hips.
2. Squat fully with a short forward jump, bringing the feet apart and bringing the knees in contact with each other.
3. Return to step 1 with a short backward jump.

Breathing: Exhale in step 2, inhale in step 3.

Dynamic Application: Steps 2 and 3 should be alternately executed.

Static Application: Maintain the final attitude (step 2) as per instruction.

Relaxation: In Standing Posture, after completion of the exercise.

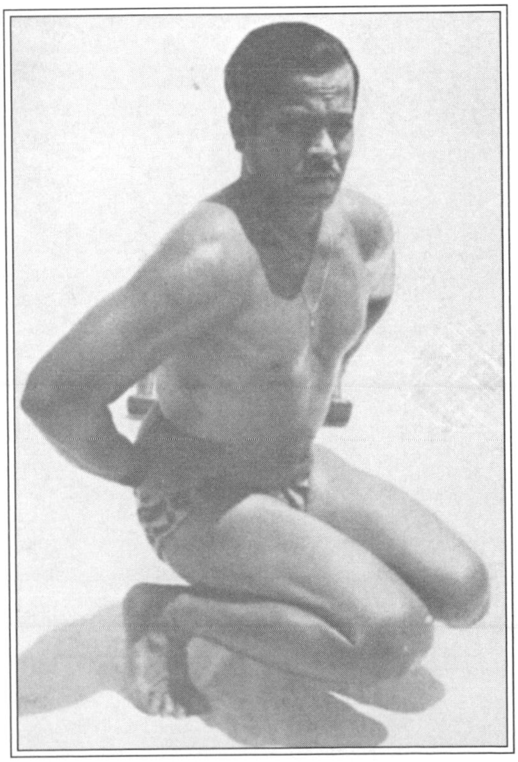

Fig. 17.2. Knee-Touching Thigh Posture (Jānuspṛiṣṭa Ūrvāsana)

Feet-Extending Thigh Posture

1. Stand with the right leg extended forward as much as possible, the hands either folded at the chest or at the waist.
2. Raise the heels off the ground and bend the right leg at the knee until you almost sit on the right heel, with the weight of the body mainly on the bent leg. The left leg should be kept straight throughout the movement. Maintain the final attitude for a few seconds (fig. 17.3).
3. Return to step 1 by straightening the right leg.
4. Perform the movement in a similar manner (steps 2 and 3) with the left leg.

Breathing: Exhale in step 2, inhale in step 3.

Dynamic Application: Steps 2 and 3 should be alternately executed.

Static Application: Maintain the final attitude (step 2) as per instruction.

Relaxation: In Standing Posture, after completion of the exercise.

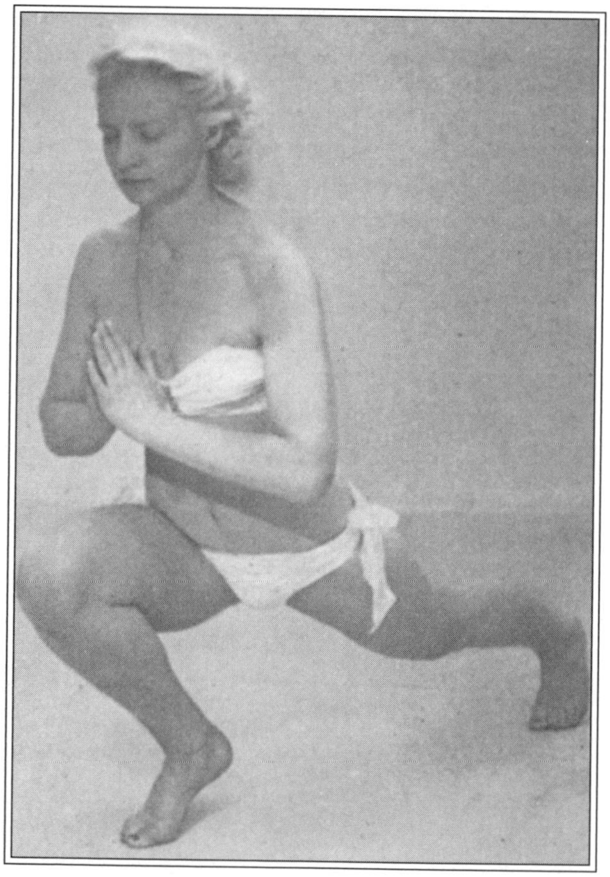

Fig. 17.3. Feet-Extending Thigh Posture (Pādaprasāraṇa Ūrvāsana)

Sideward Feet-Extending Thigh Posture

1. Stand with the legs well spread sideward, the hands either folded at the chest or at the waist.
2. Bend the right leg at the knee, raising the right heel off the floor, and sit on the elevated heel. The left leg should be kept straight throughout the movement. Maintain the final attitude for a few seconds (fig. 17.4).
3. Return to step 1 by straightening the right leg, keeping the left leg straight.
4. Perform the movement in a similar manner (steps 2 and 3) with the left leg.

Breathing: Exhale in step 2, inhale in step 3.

Dynamic Application: Steps 2 and 3 should be alternately executed moving back and forth between the right and left legs.

Static Application: Maintain the final attitude (step 2) as per instruction.

Relaxation: In Standing Posture, after completion of the exercise.

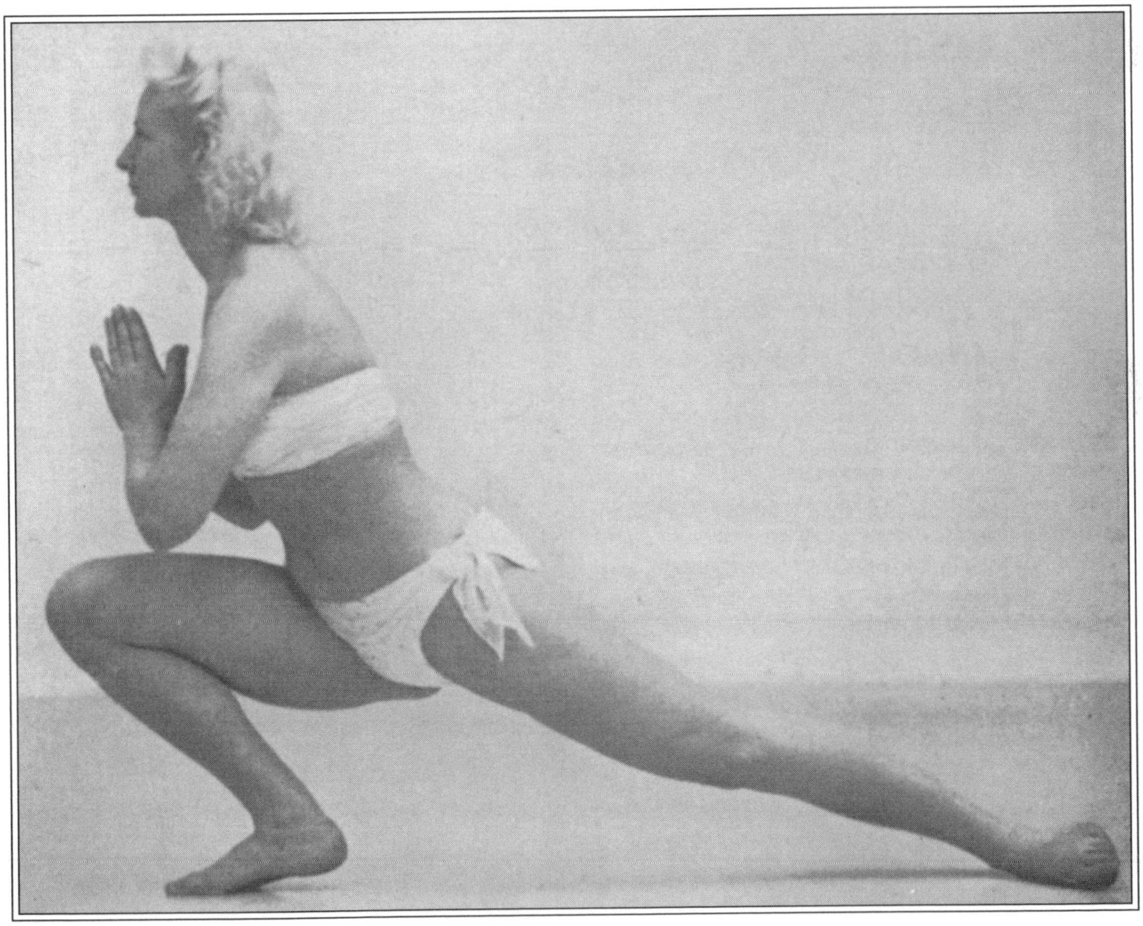

Fig. 17.4. Sideward Feet-Extending Thigh Posture (Pārśva Pādaprasāraṇa Ūrvāsana)

Leg-Raise Thigh Posture

1. Stand on the right leg with the left leg stretched forward at a right angle to the body, the hands folded at the chest.
2. Lower the body to a squatting position by bending the right leg at the knee, keeping the left leg straight. Maintain the attitude for a few seconds (fig. 17.5).
3. Return to step 1 by straightening the right leg.
4. Perform the movement in a similar manner (steps 2 and 3) with the opposite leg.

Breathing: Exhale in step 2, inhale in step 3.

Dynamic Application: Steps 2 and 3 should be alternately executed with both legs.

Static Application: Maintain the final attitude (step 2) as per instruction.

Relaxation: In Standing Posture, after completion of the exercise.

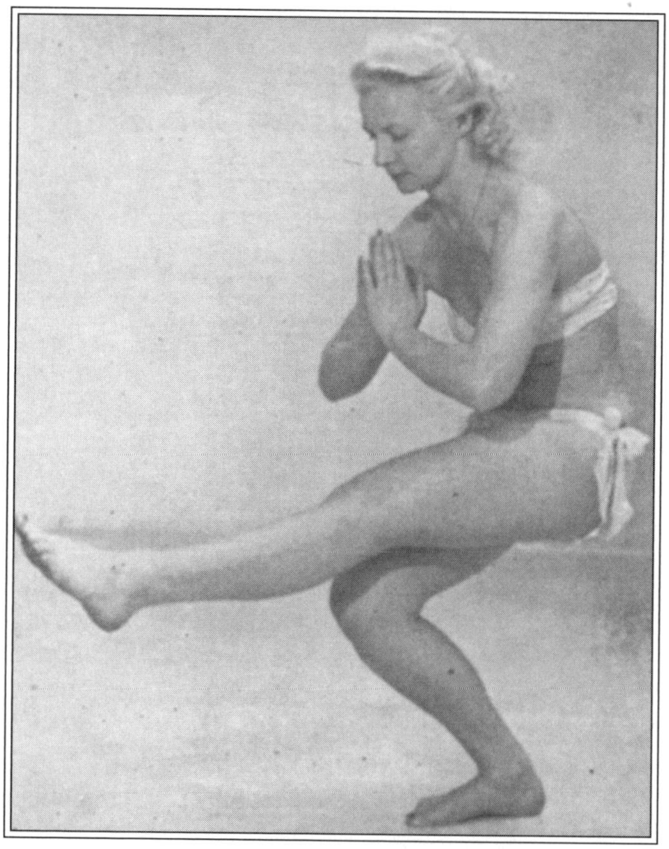

Fig. 17.5. Leg-Raise Thigh Posture (Pādotthita Ūrvāsana)

One-Legged Squat Posture

1. Assume Squat Posture with the body erect, the heels either raised or on the floor, the right foot placed on the left thigh bending at the knee, the hands either folded at the chest or at the waist.
2. Raise the body to a standing position by straightening the left leg (fig. 17.6).
3. Return to step 2 by bending the left leg at the knee.
4. Perform the movement in a similar manner (steps 2 and 3) with the opposite leg.

Breathing: Inhale in step 2 and exhale in step 3.

Dynamic Application: Steps 2 and 3 should be alternately executed with both legs.

Static Application: None.

Relaxation: In Standing Posture, after completion of the exercise.

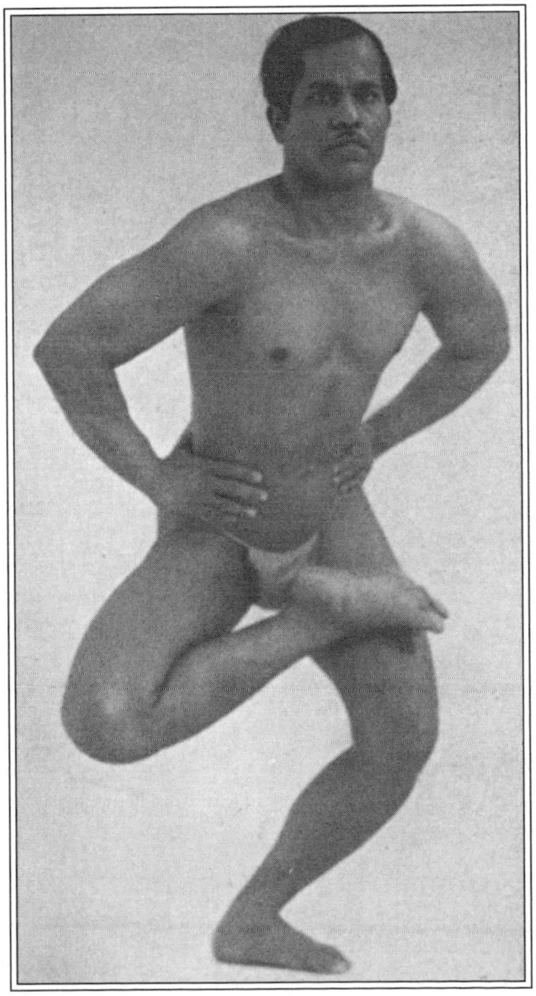

Fig. 17.6. One-Legged Squat Posture (Ekapāda Ūrvāsana)

Toe Posture

1. Assume the squatting position with the hands folded at the chest, the feet about 6 inches apart.
2. While on your toes, raise the heels as high as you can. Maintain the final attitude for a few seconds (fig. 17.7).
3. Return to step 1 by lowering the heels onto the floor.

Breathing: Normal, or inhale in step 2, exhale in step 3.

Dynamic Application: Steps 2 and 3 should be alternately.

Static Application: Maintain the final attitude (step 2) as per instruction.

Relaxation: In Standing Posture, after completion of the exercise.

Points of Note: After raising the heels to a high degree, try to raise them still further. Concentration is on the calf muscles.

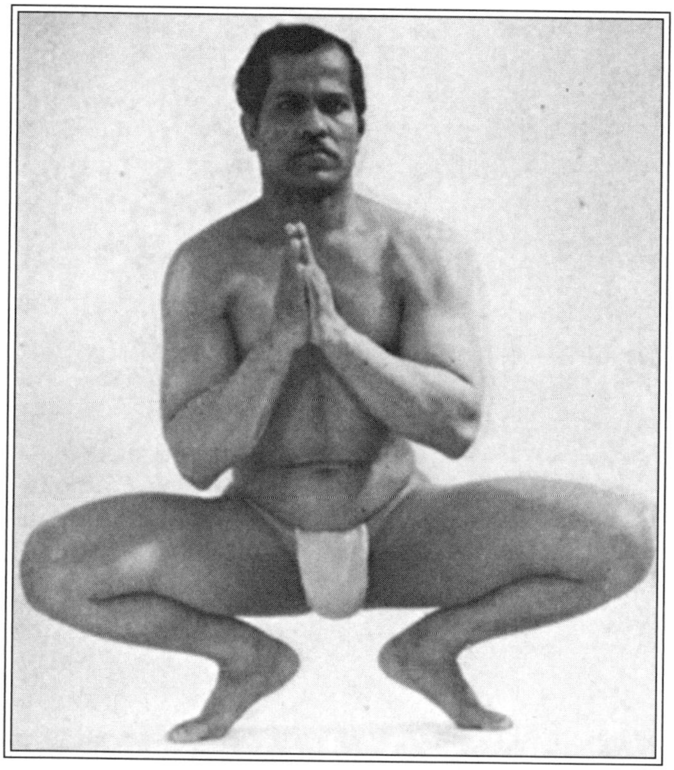

Fig. 17.7. Toe Posture (Anguṣṭhāsana)

One-Legged Toe Posture

1. Assume the squatting position, then place the right foot on the left thigh, the hands either folded at the chest or at the waist.
2. Raise the left heel as high as you can while resting on the toes. Maintain the final attitude for a few seconds (fig. 17.8).
3. Return to step 1 by lowering the left heel on the floor.
4. Perform the movement in a similar manner (steps 2 and 3) with the opposite leg.

Breathing: Normal, or inhale in step 2, exhale in step 3.

Dynamic Application: Steps 2 and 3 should be alternately executed with both legs.

Static Application: Maintain the final attitude (step 2) as per instruction.

Relaxation: In Standing Posture, after completion of the exercise.

Points of Note: This is an advanced exercise for the calf muscles. After raising the heel to a high degree, try to raise it still further. Concentration is on the calf muscles.

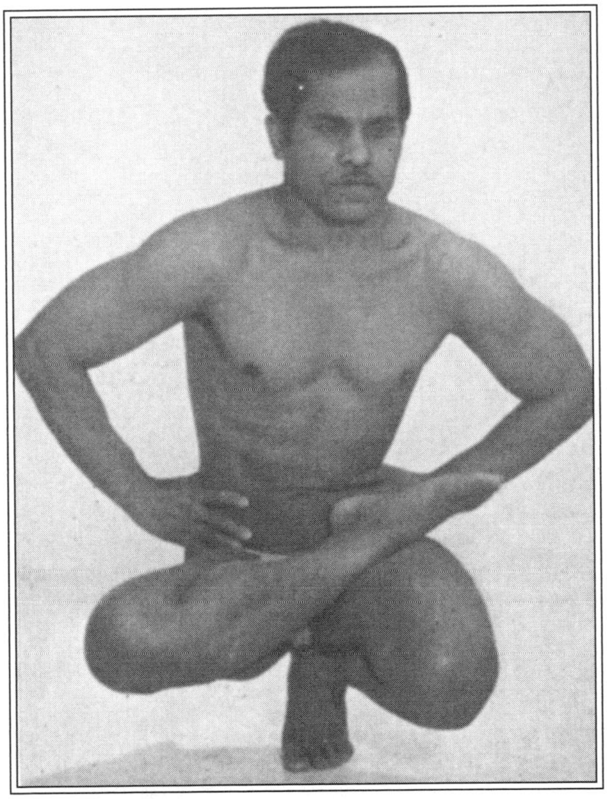

Fig. 17.8. One-Legged Toe Posture (Ekapāda Anguṣṭhāsana)

18
Balance Posture Exercise

Balance posture exercise consists of postures requiring balance. In this type of exercise the retina of the eye, the muscle spindles, the semicircular canals, the cerebellum, and the cerebral cortex are involved and educated. The nervous system is strengthened and neuromuscular control is developed. This type of exercise also plays a part in improving the general physical condition. Its special significance in Yoga is that it develops willpower and concentration. During exercise the mind should be concentrated on the movement, especially on the final attitude. The real value of the balance posture exercise lies in its static form. Dynamic form is useful in the preliminary steps when the movements are being mastered.

Eagle Posture

1. Stand erect with the heels together, the arms by the sides.
2. Raise the right leg, bring the right thigh to the left side of the left thigh by crossing it in front; the right leg encircles the left one, on which you are standing. Now bring the arms in front of the body and let one arm encircle the other, palms close to each other. Maintain the final attitude (fig. 18.1).
3. Return to step 1.
4. Perform the movement in a similar manner (steps 2 and 3) with the other leg.

Breathing: Normal.

Dynamic Application: Steps 2 and 3 should be alternately executed with both legs.

Static Application: Maintain the final attitude (step 2) as per instruction.

Relaxation: In Standing Posture, after completion of the exercise.

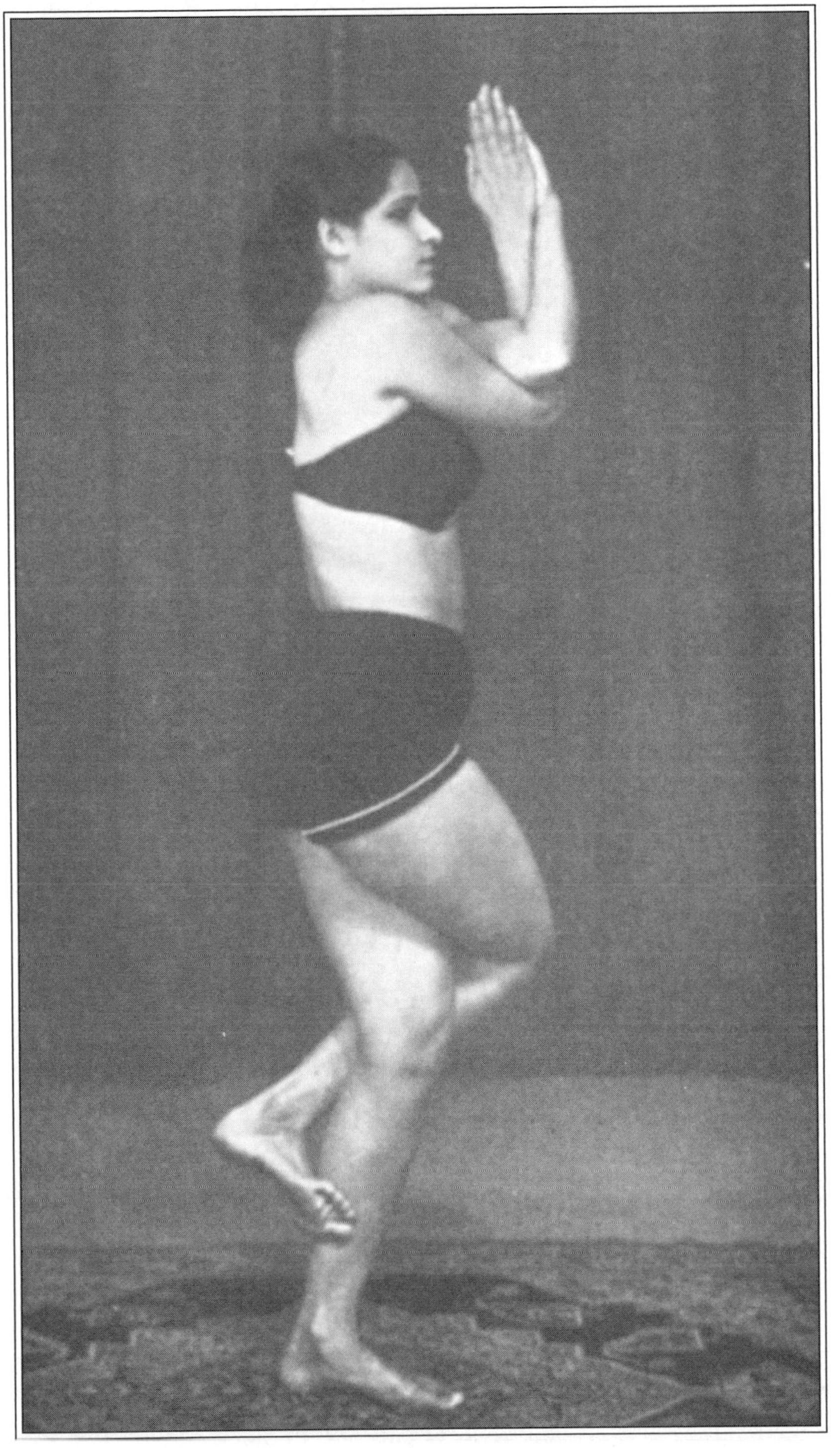

Fig. 18.1. Eagle Posture (Garuḍāsana)

Standing Head-Knee Posture

1. Stand erect with the heels together, the arms by the sides.
2. Raise the left leg forward horizontally, standing on the right leg. Then bend the body forward, hold the left toes with both hands and touch the left knee with the forehead. Maintain the final attitude (fig. 18.2).
3. Return to step 1.
4. Perform the movement in a similar manner (steps 2 and 3) with the opposite leg.

Breathing: Normal.

Dynamic Application: Steps 2 and 3 should be alternately executed with both legs.

Static Application: Maintain the final attitude (step 2) as per instruction.

Relaxation: In Standing Posture, after completion of the exercise.

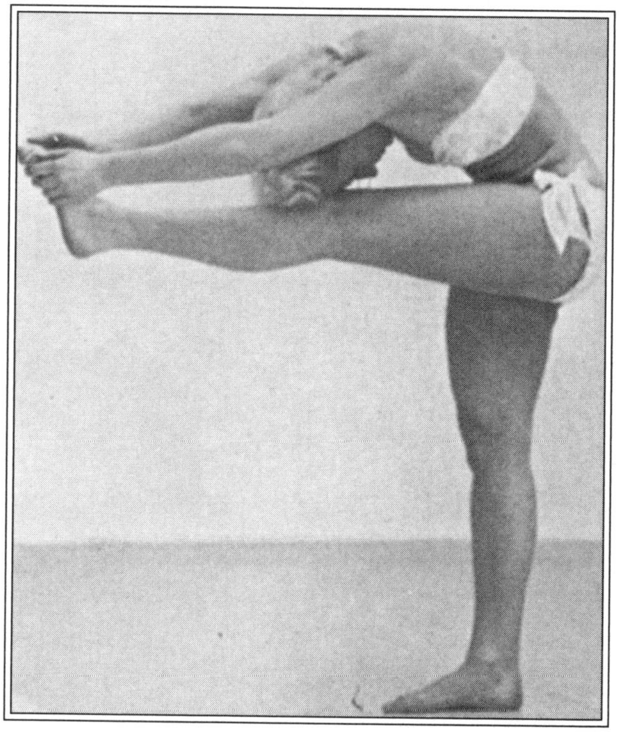

Fig. 18.2. Standing Head-Knee Posture (Uttha Jānuśirāsana)

Wing Posture

1. Stand erect with the heels together, the arms by the sides.
2. Raise the right leg sideward horizontally, standing on the left leg. Now stretch the right arm sideward and hold the right toes with the right hand. Maintain the final attitude for a few seconds (fig. 18.3).
3. Return to step 1.

4. Perform the movement in a similar manner (steps 2 and 3) with the opposite leg.

Breathing: Normal.
Dynamic Application: Steps 2 and 3 should be alternately executed with both legs.
Static Application: Maintain the final attitude (step 2) as per instruction.
Relaxation: In Standing Posture, after completion of the exercise.

Bent-Head Wing Posture

1. Stand erect with the heels together, the arms by the sides.
2. Raise the right leg sideward horizontally, standing on the left leg. Now bend the body sideward, hold the right toes with the right hand and bend the forehead to the right knee. Maintain the final attitude (fig. 18.4).
3. Return to step 1.
4. Perform the movement in a similar manner (steps 2 and 3) with the opposite leg.

Breathing: Normal.
Dynamic Application: Steps 2 and 3 should be alternately executed with both legs.
Static Application: Maintain the final attitude (step 2) as per instruction.
Relaxation: In Standing Posture, after completion of the exercise.

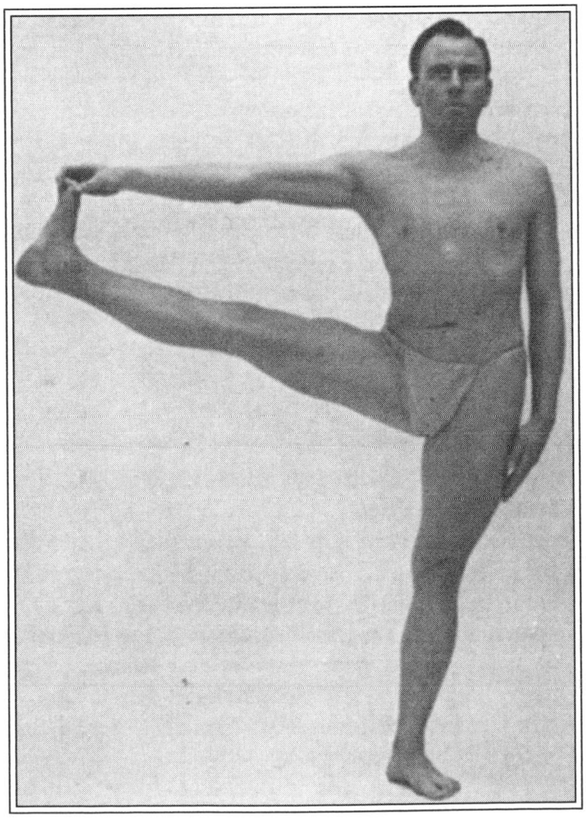

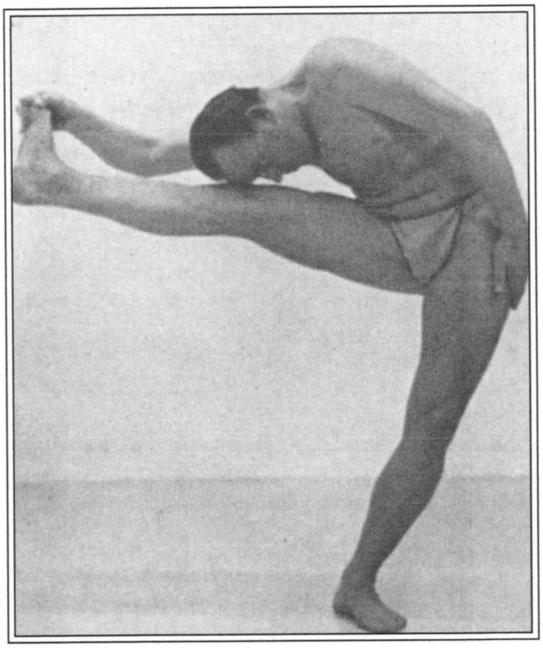

Left: Fig. 18.3. Wing Posture (Pakṣāsana)

Above: Fig. 18.4. Bent-Head Wing Posture (Nataśira Pakṣāsana)

Knee-Heel Posture

1. Stand erect with the heels together, the arms by the sides.
2. Raise the right leg and place the right foot on the left groin or the upper part of the left thigh, and keep the hands folded at the chest.
3. Raise the left heel off the floor and slowly bend the left leg at the knee, either sideward or forward, finally allowing the right knee to touch the left heel or ankle. The left heel may also be kept flat on the floor during the movement. Maintain the final attitude for a few seconds (fig. 18.5).
4. Return to step 2.
5. Perform the movement in a similar manner (steps 3 and 4) with the other leg.

Breathing: Normal.

Dynamic Application: Steps 3 and 4 should be alternately executed with both legs.

Static Application: Maintain the final attitude (step 3) as per instruction.

Relaxation: In Standing Posture, after completion of the exercise.

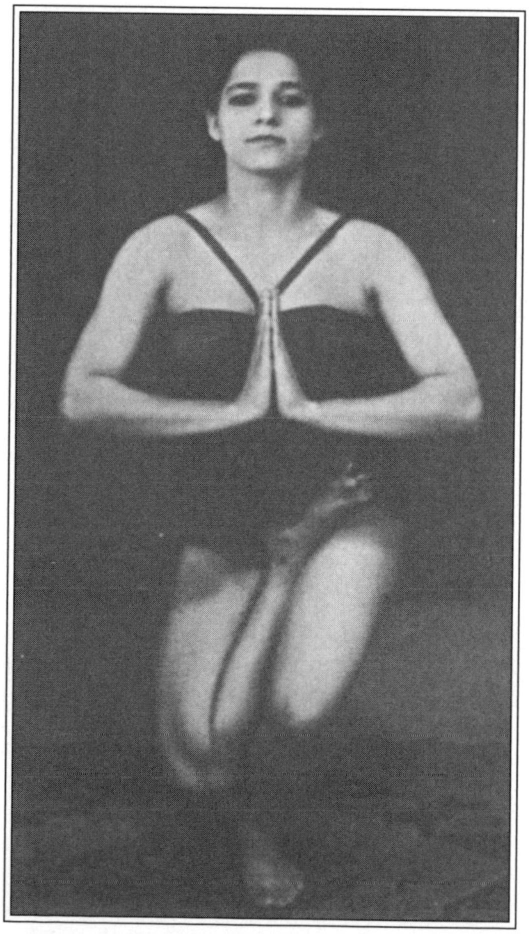

Fig. 18.5. Knee-Heel Posture (Vātāyanāsana)

Standing Single Foot-Head Posture

1. Stand erect, the heels together, the arms by the sides.
2. With the help of the hands place the left leg across the neck by making the left thigh stand almost vertically. Now remove the hands from the neck, place them on the right thigh, and try to raise the body as upright as possible, standing on the right leg. Maintain the final attitude for a few seconds (fig. 18.6).
3. Return to step 1.
4. Perform the movement in a similar manner (steps 2 and 3) with the opposite leg.

Breathing: Normal.

Dynamic Application: Steps 2 and 3 should be alternately executed with both legs.

Static Application: Maintain the final attitude (step 2) as per instruction.

Relaxation: In Standing Posture, after completion of the exercise.

Points of Note: This exercise requires relaxation of the hamstring muscles and flexibility of the hip joint to a remarkable extent. The practice of the exercise develops them.

Standing Leg-Stretch Posture

1. Stand erect with the heels together and the arms by the sides.
2. Raise the right leg almost vertically, holding the right toes with both hands and standing on the left leg. Try to make the elevated leg as vertical as possible by a backward pull of the leg with the hands. Maintain the final attitude for a few seconds (fig. 18.7).

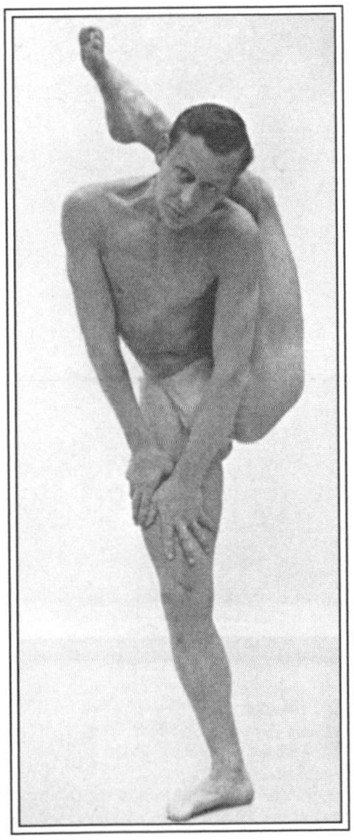

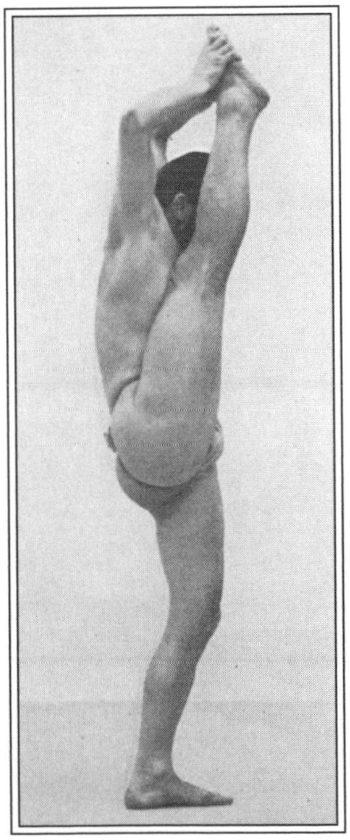

Left: Fig. 18.6. Standing Single Foot-Head Posture (Uttha Ekapāda Śirāsana)

Right: Fig. 18.7. Standing Leg-Stretch Posture (Uttha Pādaprasāraṇāsana)

3. Return to step 1.
4. Perform the movement in a similar manner (steps 2 and 3) with the opposite leg.

Breathing: Normal.
Dynamic Application: Steps 2 and 3 should be alternately executed with both legs.
Static Application: Maintain the final attitude (step 2) as per instruction.
Relaxation: In Standing Posture, after completion of the exercise.
Points of Note: As in Standing Single Foot-Head Posture.

Mountain Posture

1. Assume Lotus Posture (fig. 20.2).
2. Stand on the knees and either stretch the arms above the head or keep the hands folded at the chest. Maintain the final attitude for a few seconds (fig. 18.8).
3. Return to step 1.

Breathing: Normal.
Dynamic Application: Steps 2 and 3 should be alternately executed.
Static Application: Maintain the final attitude (step 2) as per instruction.
Relaxation: In a sitting position with the legs extended forward and the hands resting on the thighs, after completion of the exercise.

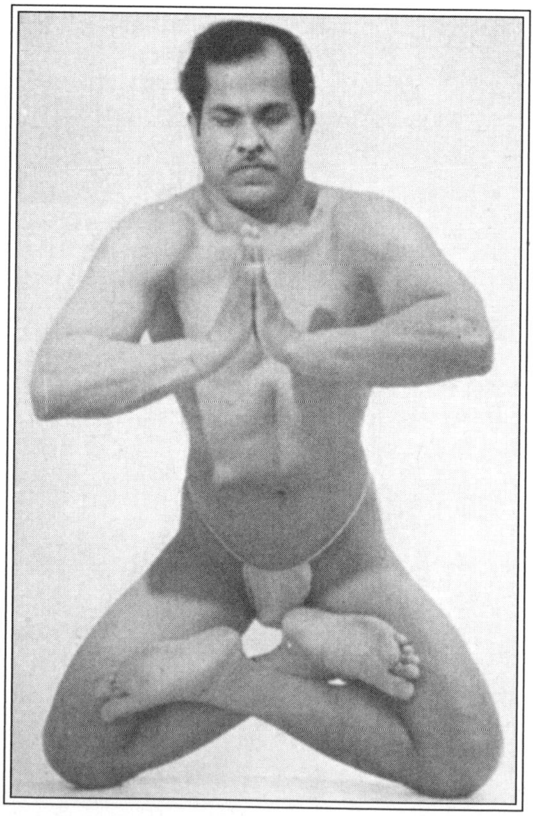

Fig. 18.8. Mountain Posture (Parvatāsana)

Peacock Posture

1. Assume a kneeling position with the knees sufficiently apart. Place the palms on the floor in front of you and between the knees with the fingers directed toward you, keeping the forearms vertical and leaning forward. The palms and forearms should be kept close to each other.
2. Bending forward, place your abdomen, just below the umbilicus, on the elbow joints, which will act as a fulcrum, and then extend the body forward and the legs backward. The whole body is thus balanced on the elbow joints. The extended legs are kept close together. Maintain the final attitude for a few seconds (fig. 18.9).
3. Return to step 1.

Breathing: Normal.

Dynamic Application: Steps 2 and 3 should be alternately executed.

Static Application: Maintain the final attitude (step 2) as per instruction.

Relaxation: In Prone Posture or Corpse Posture, after completion of the exercise.

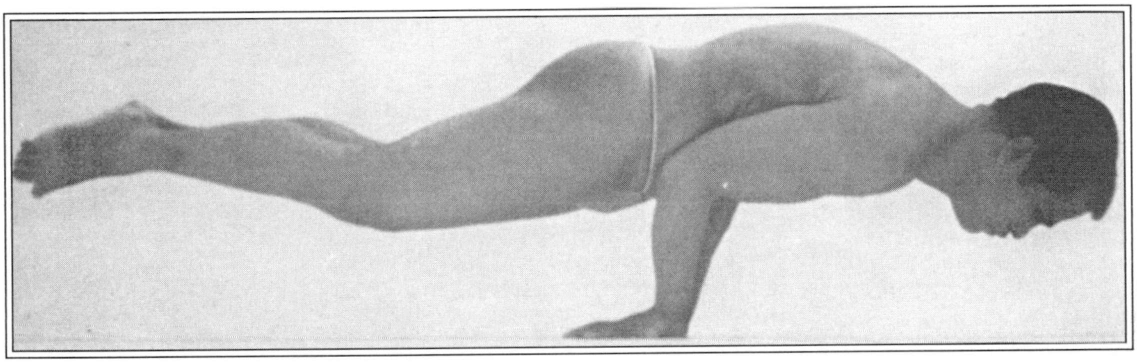

Fig. 18.9. Peacock Posture (Mayūrāsana)

Crab Posture

1. Assume a kneeling position and place the right palm on the floor in front of you with the fingers directed toward you, the right forearm vertical.
2. Bending forward, place your abdomen on the right elbow joint and extend your body forward and the legs backward, thus making the body balanced on the elevated elbow with the legs apart and the left arm suspended. Maintain the final attitude for a few seconds (fig. 18.10 on page 200).
3. Return to step 1.
4. Perform the movement in a similar manner (steps 2 and 3) with the other arm.

Breathing: Normal.

Dynamic Application: Steps 2 and 3 should be alternately executed with both arms.

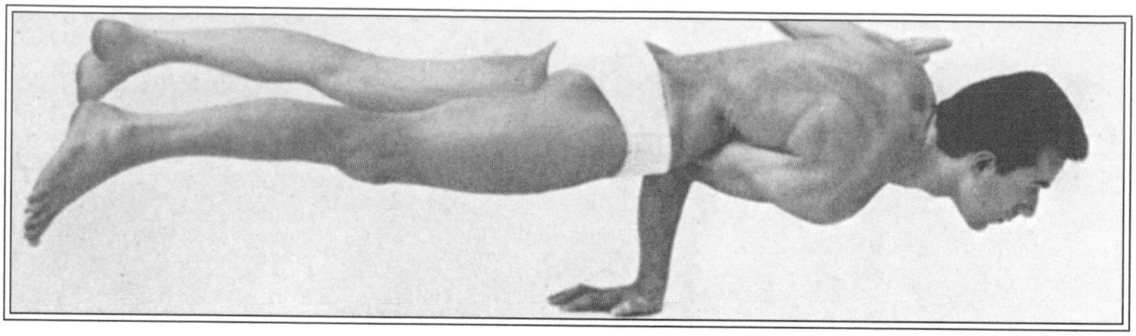

Fig. 18.10. Crab Posture (Karkaṭāsana)

Static Application: Maintain the final attitude (step 2) as per instruction.
Relaxation: In Prone Posture or Corpse Posture, after completion of the exercise.

Rolling Posture

1. Assume Lotus Posture (fig. 20.2), stand on the knees and, leaning forward, place the palms on the floor in front of you with the fingers directed toward you, the forearms vertical, the palms and forearms close together.
2. Bending forward, place your abdomen on the elbow joints and balance the body as in Peacock Posture. Maintain the final attitude for a few seconds (fig. 18.11).
3. Return to step 1.

Breathing: Normal.
Dynamic Application: Steps 2 and 3 should be alternately executed.
Static Application: Maintain the final attitude (step 2) as per instruction.
Relaxation: In Prone Posture or Corpse Posture, after completion of the exercise.

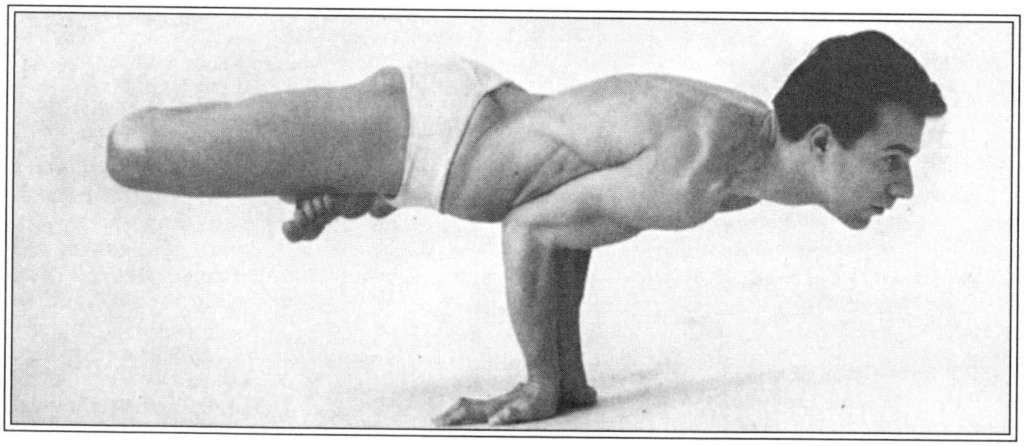

Fig. 18.11. Rolling Posture (Lolāsana)

One-Arm Rolling Posture

1. Assume Lotus Posture (fig. 20.2) and place the right palm on the floor in front of you with the fingers directed toward you, the right forearm vertical.
2. Bending forward, place your abdomen on the right elbow and balance your body as in Rolling Posture with the left arm on your back. Maintain the final attitude for a few seconds (fig. 18.12).
3. Return to step 1.
4. Perform the movement in a similar manner (step 2) with the other arm.

Breathing: Normal.
Dynamic Application: Steps 2 and 3 should be alternately executed with both arms.
Static Application: Maintain the final attitude (step 2) as per instruction.
Relaxation: In Prone Posture or Corpse Posture, after completion of the exercise.

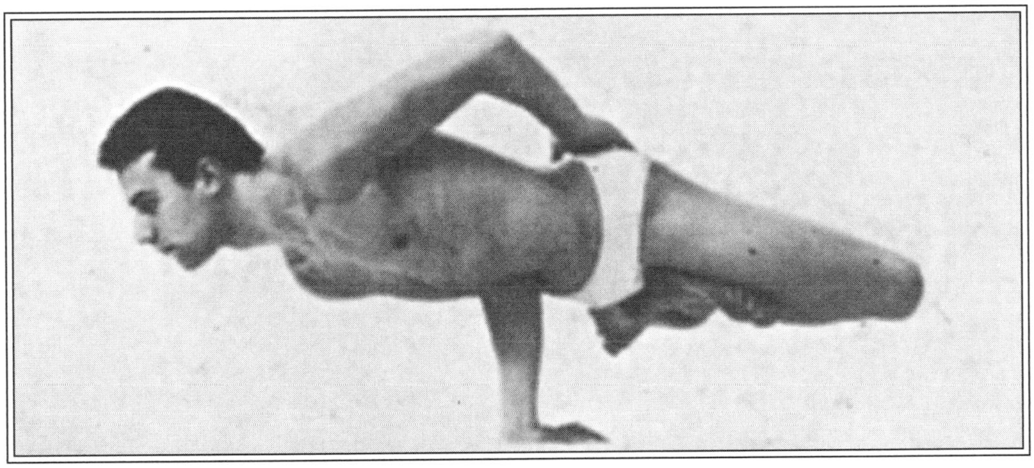

Fig. 18.12. One-Arm Rolling Posture (Ekahasta Lolāsana)

Arm-Stand Posture

1. Stand erect, the arms by the sides.
2. Bend your body forward and downward, place the palms on the floor in front of you, one upon the other, and raise the legs and the trunk with some force upward, making the body stand inversely in a straight line with the head down and the legs stretched straight up, the heels together, the arms straight. Maintain the position for a few seconds (fig. 18.13 on page 202).
3. Return to step 1.

Breathing: Normal.
Dynamic Application: Steps 2 and 3 should be alternately executed.

Static Application: Maintain the final attitude (step 2) as per instruction.

Relaxation: In Standing Posture, after completion of the exercise.

Single Arm-Stand Posture

1. Assume Arm-Stand Posture (fig. 18.13).
2. Lean slowly on the right side, transferring the body weight gradually to the right hand.
3. Raise the left hand off the floor and place the left arm by the side of the body, standing on the right arm only (fig. 18.14).

Breathing: Normal.

Dynamic Application: Steps 1, 2, and 3 should be repeated.

Static Application: Maintain the final attitude (step 3) as long as you can.

Relaxation: In Standing Posture, after completion of the exercise.

Points of Note: This is an advanced balance posture exercise. It should also be practiced with the left arm.

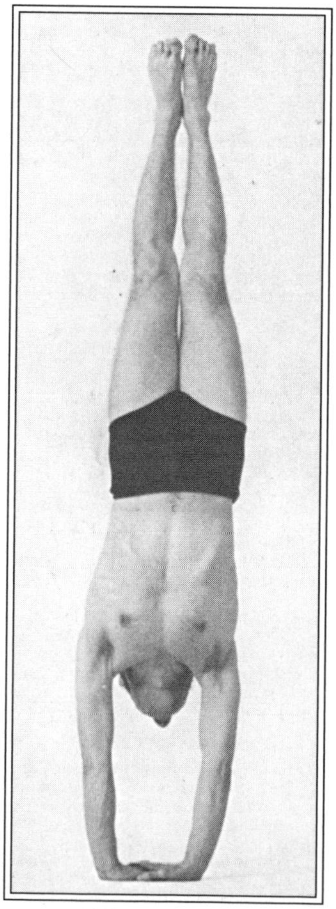

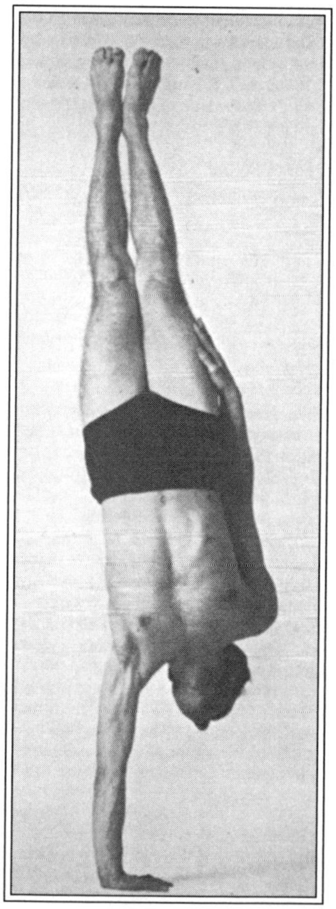

Left: Fig. 18.13. Arm-Stand Posture (Hasta Vṛiksāsana)

Right: Fig. 18.14. Single Arm-Stand Posture (Ekahasta Vṛiksāsana)

Scorpion Posture

1. Assume Head Posture (fig. 19.3) and then slowly move the forearms away from the head and keep them by the sides of the head with the fingers directed forward.
2. Bend the legs downward, bending at the knees and arching the spine to the maximum extent. Now raise the head from the floor upward as much as possible by supporting the body on the forearms and place the soles on your elevated head. Maintain the final attitude for a few seconds (fig. 18.15).
3. Return to step 1.

Breathing: Normal.

Dynamic Application: Steps 2 and 3 should be alternately executed.

Static Application: Maintain the final attitude (step 2) as per instruction.

Relaxation: In a sitting position with the legs extended forward and the arms by the sides, after completion of the exercise.

Points of Note: It is also an excellent posterior trunk-bend posture exercise. It requires great spinal flexibility and well-controlled balance. Beginners are advised to first practice Modified Scorpion Posture, in which the feet are brought near the elevated head.

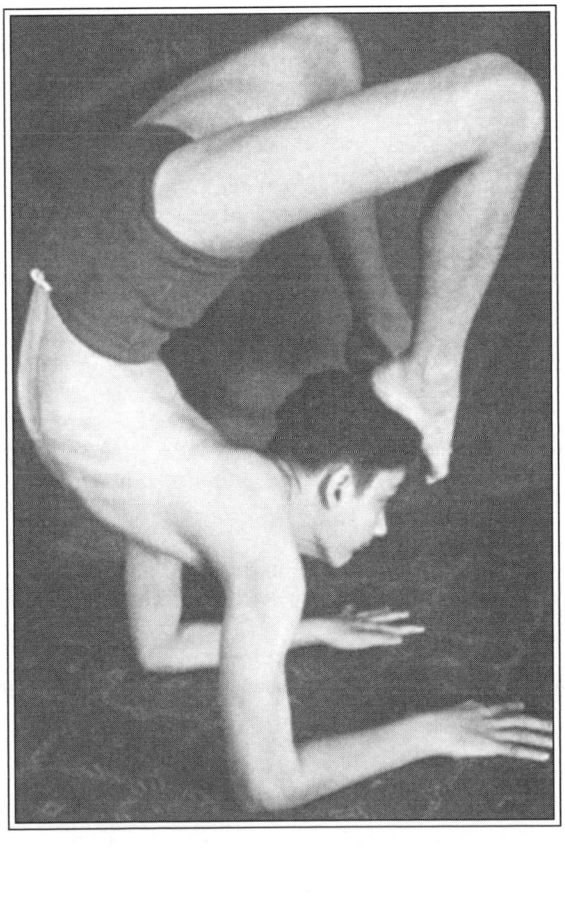

Fig. 18.15. Scorpion Posture (Vṛiścikāsana)

Supplementary Balance Posture Exercise

Dynamic Peacock Posture Exercises

1. Assume Peacock Posture with the legs close together. Extend the legs out to the sides to the maximum extent.
2. Curl the legs on the thighs, keeping the thighs horizontal in Peacock Posture.
3. Curl the legs on the thighs in Peacock Posture and then extend the knees out to the sides as much as possible, keeping the thighs horizontal.
4. Raise one leg as high as possible from the horizontal position in Peacock Posture.
5. Raise both legs upward from the horizontal position in Peacock Posture.
6. Practice Anal Exercise in Peacock Posture.
7. Practice Anal Lock in Peacock Posture.

Head-Stand Posture

1. Assume Head Posture (fig. 19.3).
2. Gradually raise the hands off the floor and place the arms by the sides of the body, standing on the head (fig. 18.16).

Breathing: Normal.

Dynamic Application: Steps 1 and 2 should be alternately executed.

Static Application: Maintain the final attitude (step 2) as long as you can.

Relaxation: In a sitting position with the legs extended forward and the hands resting on the thighs, after completion of the exercise.

Points of Note: This is an advanced balance posture exercise. Students are advised to first practice the Modified Head-Stand Posture, in which only one arm is placed by the body instead of both.

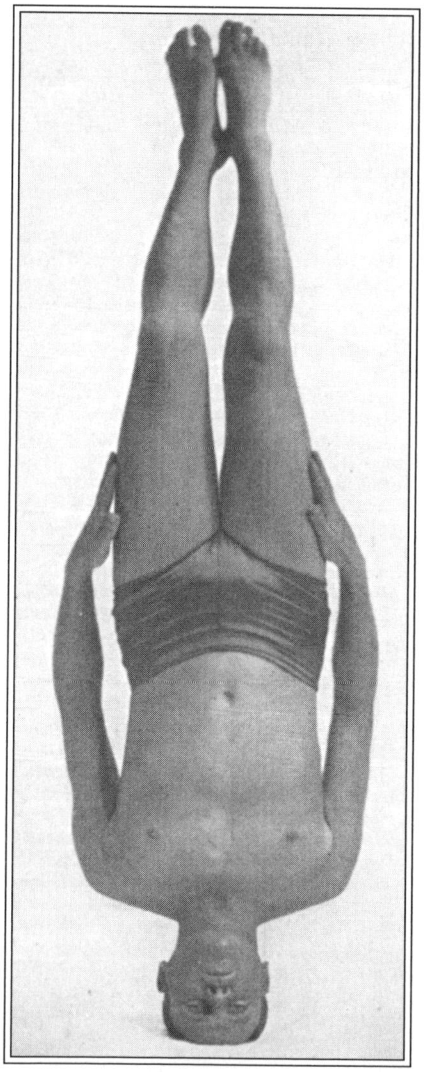

Fig. 18.16. Head-Stand Posture (Śirāsana)

19

Inverse Body Posture Exercise

Inverse body posture exercise has been evolved in Yoga to counteract the evil effects of the biped position, to achieve a healthful circulatory, respiratory, alimentary, eliminative, glandular, and nervous readjustment in the organism, and to increase the power of concentration.

The most palpable effect of the inverse body posture is the acceleration of venous circulation. The blood flow through all the veins that finally pours into the inferior vena cava is hastened. Therefore it is helpful in relieving congestion in the abdominal-pelvic viscera. It is a unique form of venous exercise that is also beneficial to the heart and the arteries.

The changed position of the abdominal and pelvic organs and the altered pressure seem to have a healthful influence on these organs. Inverse body posture exercise is also an excellent diaphragmatic exercise, which can help to correct the downward displacement of the diaphragm due to habitual wrong posture, if other correct exercises are done and the posture itself is corrected. It improves the diaphragmatic pump and facilitates deep breathing.

Inverse posture exercise causes an increased blood supply to the brain, which seems to be very favorable for the efficient functioning of the brain. It has been experienced that clear thinking and concentration are developed. It is also very helpful and healthful for those who sit upright in a motionless posture for concentration for a prolonged period.

The efficiency of inverse body posture exercise becomes pronounced when it is applied statically and the posture maintained for a long period. In the majority of cases the normal systolic pressure goes up when the posture is assumed and remains high during its maintenance. After some time a second rise of the systolic pressure occurs. The posture should be discontinued before the second rise of blood pressure. In other words, when a feeling of discomfort arises, the posture should be discontinued. The duration of time should be very gradually increased.

The static form of inverse body posture exercise is not a heavy form of exercise and may be applied with proper modifications to practically all health conditions. Middle-aged persons can practice it with great advantage. It can be adopted by people with a tendency to have high blood pressure, although it is contraindicated when the blood pressure is very high. Persons who are mentally calm will have little rise in blood pressure in this type of exercise. Those who are not calm can become so while doing this posture exercise, as it has a decidedly sedative influence on the nervous system. It is very good for those who lead a sedentary life, devoting most of their time to intellectual work, and also for those who are leading a life of worry and hurry. Static Head-Stand or Shoulder-Stand postures are also used with japa in a spiritual context.

No harmful results will ever be experienced, if the duration of time for inverse body posture exercise is cautiously increased and internal cleanliness is maintained by right diet, internal baths, and other yogic measures. On the contrary, it will prove physically invigorating and healthful, and will provide calmness, joy, and meditative power. From the reports of the writer's pupils practicing Head-Stand Posture regularly and for prolonged periods certain interesting facts may be pointed out here:

- It improves general health.
- It cures certain types of headaches.
- It relieves pain in the back.
- It relieves fatigue.
- It increases the power of resistance to cold.
- It prevents hair loss and in certain cases keeps the hair from turning grey.
- It provides a feeling of well-being.
- It increases digestive power.
- It provides increased lucidity, brain power, and mental calmness.

The blood pressure experiments done on persons practicing Head Posture show that in the majority of cases the normal systolic pressure suddenly rises high when the posture is assumed and remains high during its maintenance. When the second rise of the systolic pressure takes place the posture is discontinued and the subject lies on his back. At this stage the pressure becomes normal or a little subnormal. The rise of the systolic pressure above the normal is from 15 to 45 mmHg. The highest rise noted was 175 mmHg from the normal 130 mmHg.

There is a little increase of pulse rate during Head Posture. It is about three to ten per minute. The pulse rate becomes a little subnormal immediately after the discontinuance of the posture and the assuming of a supine posture. It becomes normal when the upright position is resumed. In certain cases of complete relaxation it does not increase at all during Head Posture but becomes subnormal. It again becomes normal after the resumption of the upright posture. There is also an increase in the rate of respiration during Head Posture, from two to eight per minute. In certain cases it remains constant.

There are also exceptional cases. It was found in one healthy male subject, aged forty-two, who had been practicing under the writer's guidance for over a year, and with a normal pressure of 120 mmHg, that the rise was very little, about 4 or 5 mmHg after the assumption of Head Posture; it gradually went higher and reached 140 mmHg after five minutes. When the posture was discontinued, the blood pressure returned to the normal level.

In another case a female, forty-nine years of age, had been practicing the posture under the guidance of the writer for more than a year. It was found that there was a gradual fall of blood pressure during Head Posture from 145 to 120 and then 115 occurring at the twenty-fifth minute, and then it gradually rose a little above 125 at the fortieth minute. After the discontinuance (after 40 minutes) the blood pressure went down to 110 in a horizontal position and remained at 135 in an upright position. By the regular practice of this posture the subject became much healthier, stronger, and fitter. Moreover, she is able to make herself more serene and to be contemplative while in this posture.

Inverse Body Posture Exercise

We are presenting here four important inverse body posture exercises, and of the four, Head Posture is the most important. For all of them, it is advisable to practice at least four hours after the last meal has been ingested.

Inversion Posture

1. Assume a supine position with the legs extended, the feet close together, the arms by the sides, the palms downward.
2. Raise the legs and then the pelvis and the lower part of the trunk from the floor until the trunk assumes a slanting position with the legs in a perpendicular position by pressing the arms strongly against the floor. Now support this attitude of the trunk by placing the hands on the hip-bones, bending the forearms at the elbows. The body is now supported on the back of the head, neck, and scapular region of the trunk and arms. The chin is kept away from the chest. Maintain the final attitude (fig. 19.1 on page 208).
3. Return to step 1.

Breathing: Normal.

Dynamic Application: Not necessary.

Static Application: Maintain the final attitude (step 2) as per instruction.

Relaxation: In Corpse Posture, after completion of the exercise.

Points of Note: The best time for this exercise is in the morning (after evacuation and oral cleansing). The next best time is in the evening, before dinner and allowing about four hours after lunch. It should never be practiced when the stomach is full. Concentration is per a qualified Yoga teacher's specific instruction.

Shoulder-Stand Posture

1. Assume a supine position with the legs extended, the feet close together, the arms extended by the sides, the palms downward.
2. Raise the legs, then the pelvis, and finally the trunk upward until the trunk and the legs become perpendicular and in a straight line, by pressing the arms strongly against the floor. The body now stands on the shoulders. Now bring the chest close to the chin and support the body with the hands. Finally, perform Chin Lock. Pushing the trunk toward the head with the hands may be helpful in the execution of Chin Lock. Maintain the final attitude (fig. 19.2).
3. Return to step 1.

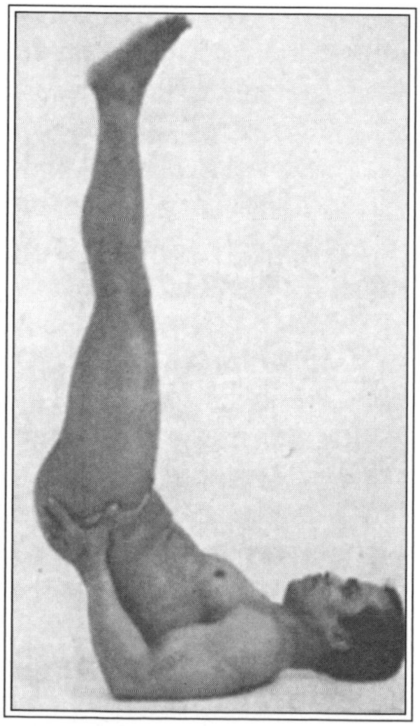

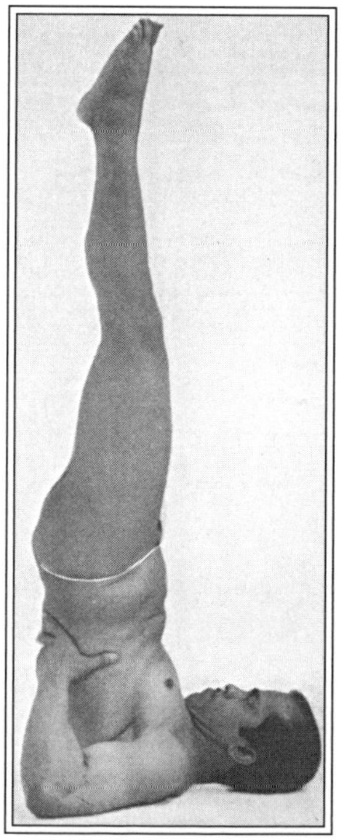

Right: Fig. 19.1. Inversion Posture (Viparīta-karanī-mudrā)

Left: Fig. 19.2. Shoulder-Stand Posture (Sarvāngāsana)

Breathing: Normal.

Dynamic Application: Not necessary.

Static Application: Maintain the final attitude (step 2) as per instruction.

Relaxation: In Corpse Posture, after completion of the exercise.

Points of Note: As for Inversion Posture. It is supposed that Shoulder-Stand Posture improves the functional activities of the thyroid gland by causing an increased blood supply to this organ through the superior thyroid arteries. Concentration is per specific instruction of a qualified Yoga teacher.

Head Posture

1. Kneel on the floor with heels raised, bend the body forward, place the ulnar side of the forearms on the floor in front of you, interlock the fingers of both hands, and place the head on the floor between the forearms in such a way that the back of the head will fit in between the hollows of the interlocked hands. Now, supporting the body on the forearms and head, raise the trunk and hips upward until they are almost perpendicular to the floor with the legs stretched and the toes still remaining on the floor.
2. Slowly raise the legs upward from the floor until they are perpendicular and in a straight line with the raised trunk and the head. If the beginner is not able to raise the legs slowly in this manner, he can first bend his thighs on the trunk with the knees drawn to his chest and from this position slowly extend the legs upward. Maintain the final attitude (fig. 19.3).
3. Return to step 1.

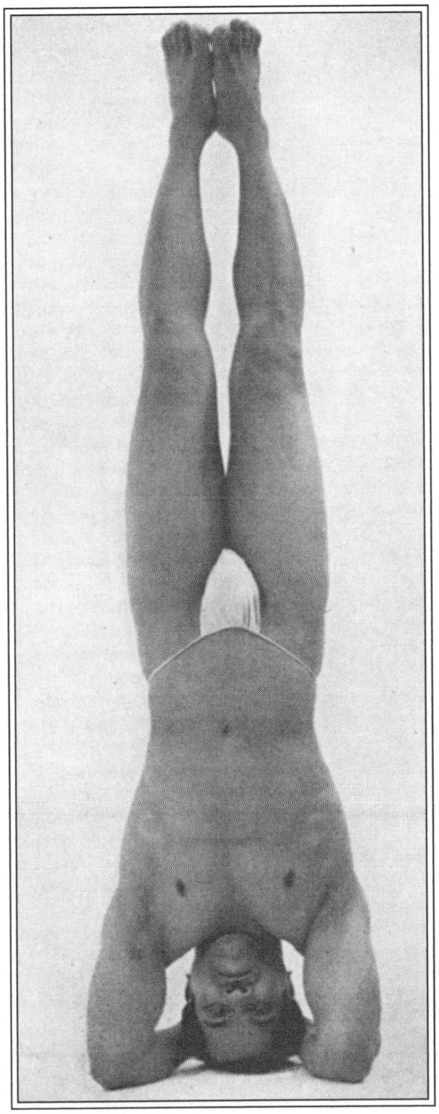

Fig. 19.3. Head Posture (Śīrṣāsana)

Breathing: Normal.

Dynamic Application: Not necessary.

Static Application: Maintain the final attitude (step 2) as per instruction.

Relaxation: In a sitting position with the legs extended forward, after completion of the exercise.

Points of Note: As for Inversion Posture. It is desirable to place a soft cushion under the head when doing Head Posture. Concentration is per specific instruction of a qualified Yoga teacher.

Inverse Lotus Posture

1. Assume Head Posture (fig. 19.3).
2. Perform Lotus Posture (fig. 20.2). Maintain the final attitude (fig. 19.4).
3. Return to step 1.

Breathing: Normal.

Dynamic Application: Not necessary.

Static Application: Maintain the final attitude (step 2) as per instruction.

Relaxation: In a sitting position with the legs extended forward, after completion of the exercise.

Points of Note: As for Inversion Posture. Concentration is per specific instruction of a qualified Yoga teacher.

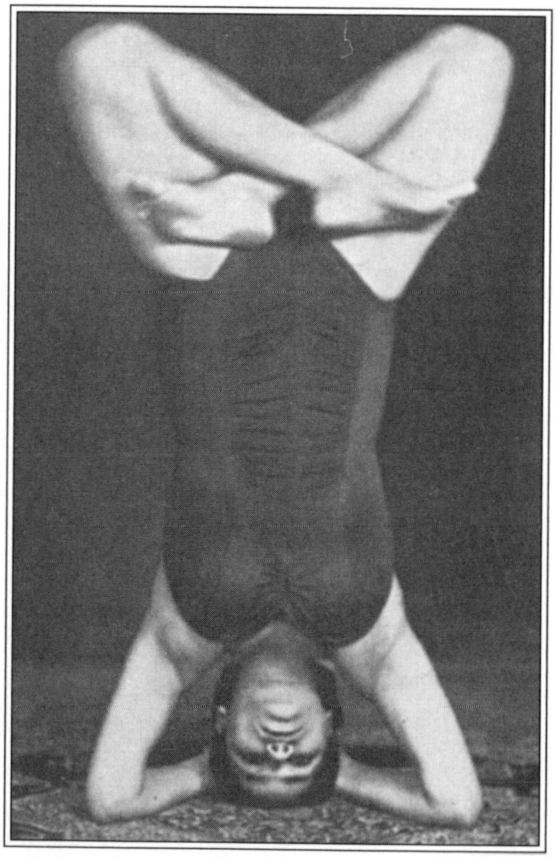

Fig. 19.4. Inverse Lotus Posture (Ūrdhva Padmāsana)

Supplementary Inverse Body Posture Exercise

Certain leg and trunk motion exercises have been evolved in Head Posture. These may be called Head Posture exercises. The movements themselves are valuable, especially for the pelvic and perineal muscles. Another important point is that these exercises make the student maintain the posture for a longer period. Therefore, these exercises help to prolong the duration of time of this posture.

Dynamic Head Posture Exercises

1. Lower both legs sideward and downward simultaneously until they are almost horizontal. Return to the original position. Exhale when lowering the legs, inhale when raising them. Repeat.
2. Lower one leg forward and downward until it is horizontal. Return to the original position. Exhale when lowering the leg, inhale when raising it. Repeat with other leg.
3. The same movement as step 2 with both legs simultaneously.
4. Bend the legs at the knees inward with the soles together, bringing the heels as close to the perineum as possible, exhaling. Return, inhaling. Repeat.
5. Bring the heels as close to the perineum as possible as in step 4. Now bring the knees close together in front, inhaling. Return to the starting position, exhaling.
6. Bend one leg forward and downward until the toes touch the floor. Return to the original position. Breathing normal. Repeat with other leg.
7. The same movement as in step 6 with both legs simultaneously.
8. Bend both legs sideward and a bit forward until the toes touch the floor. Return to the original position. Breathing normal. Repeat.
9. Bend one leg forward and downward and the other leg backward and downward as much as possible. Reverse. Repeat.
10. Bend one leg forward and downward and the other leg backward and downward as in step 9. Now twist the pelvis to the right and left to the fullest extent. Breathing normal. Reverse. Repeat.

20

Folded-Leg Postures

It is the empirical conclusion of Yoga practitioners that folded-leg postures are most suitable for deep concentration and breath control. These postures, when perfected and mastered, create a most favorable condition for breath suspension and mental concentration.

Folded-leg posture is a sitting posture with the legs bent at the knees and placed in a definite manner, the body erect. There are many such postures. We are presenting here four important postures, which will serve our purpose. The real effectiveness of these postures lies in their static application. These postures are also used in connection with contraction exercise, Abdominal Retraction, Straight Muscle Exercise, and other processes and exercises of Yoga. By repeated practice in the right manner, these postures should be perfected and mastered. Then they will give a sense of ease and comfort instead of uneasiness and pain.

The following processes may be adopted for concentration in these postures:

Japa (repeating in a definite manner) of "AUM" or other *mantras*
Concentration on specific objects
Mantra japa with concentration
Breath control with *mantra japa* and concentration

Accomplished Posture

1. Sit with the body erect, the legs extended in front and the arms by the sides.
2. Bend the left leg at the knee and fold it upon itself with the heel tightly set against the perineum and the sole in contact with the upper part of the right thigh. Then bend the right leg at the knee and fold it upon itself with the heel placed against the pubic bone just

above the genitals, the foot within the depression formed by the left thigh and calf. Keep the trunk straight. Either the hands may be placed one upon the other at the center of the body or the arms extended with the hands placed on the knees. Maintain the attitude as instructed by a qualified Yoga teacher (fig. 20.1).

3. After completion of the exercise, return to step 1.

Breathing: Normal. The following breathing exercises may be practiced in this posture:

- Modified Lingual Breath-Control Exercise
- Modified Alternate-Nostril Breath-Control Exercise
- Modified Both-Nostrils Breath-Control Exercise with Abdomen Relaxed
- Modified Both-Nostrils Breath-Control Exercise with Abdomen Retracted
- Modified Both-Nostrils Breath-Control Exercise with Breath Suspension

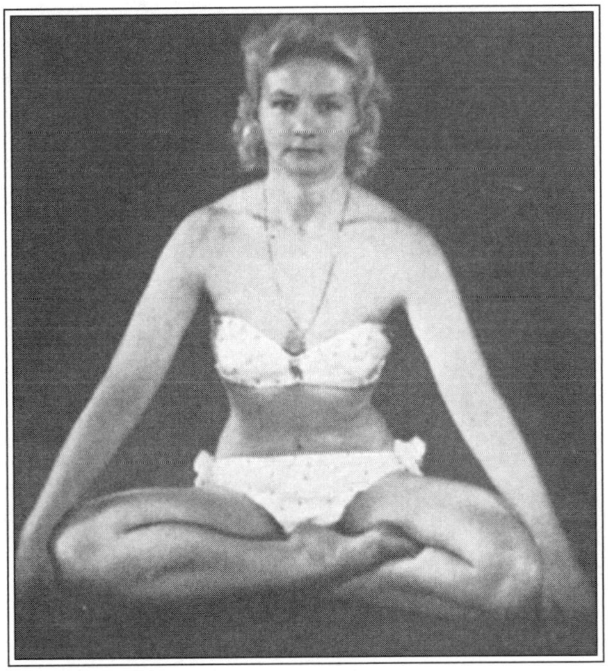

Fig. 20.1. Accomplished Posture (Siddhāsana)

Lotus Posture

1. Sit erect, the legs extended in front and the arms by the sides.
2. Place the right foot on the left groin by bending the right leg at the knee. Place the left foot on the right groin in a similar manner. The feet should be so placed that the heels should be at the center of and in close contact with the abdomen. Either the hands may be placed one upon the other at the center of the body or the arms extended with the hands placed on the knees. Maintain the attitude as instructed by a qualified Yoga teacher (fig. 20.2).
3. After completion of the exercise, return to step 1.

Breathing: Normal. The following breathing exercises may be practiced in Lotus Posture:

- Abdominal Short-Quick Breathing
- Modified Lingual Breath-Control Exercise
- Modified Alternate-Nostril Breath-Control Exercise
- Modified Both-Nostrils Breath-Control Exercise with Abdomen Relaxed
- Modified Both-Nostrils Breath-Control Exercise with Abdomen Retracted
- Modified Both-Nostrils Breath-Control Exercise with Breath Suspension

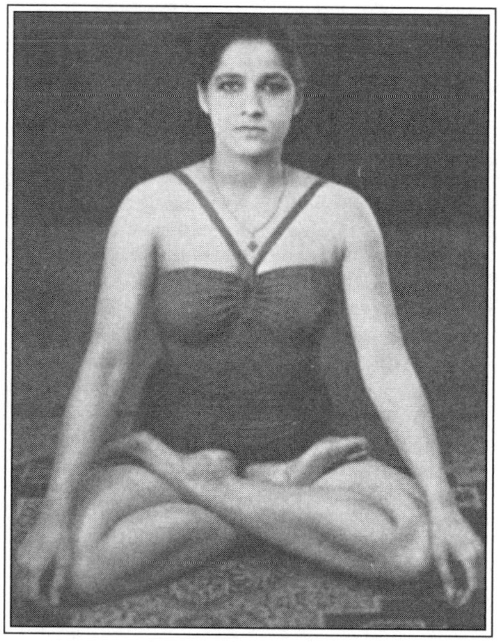

Fig. 20.2. Lotus Posture (Padmāsana)

Pleasant Posture

1. Sit erect with the legs extended in front and the arms by the sides.
2. Bend the left leg at the knee and place it close to the left thigh with the left heel close to the center of the body or in contact with the upper part of the right thigh. Then place the right leg close to the outer side of the folded left leg, bending at the knee. Keep the body erect. Either the hands may be placed one upon the other at the center of the body or the arms may be extended with the hands placed on the knees. Maintain the attitude as instructed by a qualified Yoga teacher (fig. 20.3).
3. After completion of the exercise, return to step 1.

Breathing: Normal. The following breathing exercises may be practiced while in this posture:

- Abdominal Short-Quick Breathing
- Modified Lingual Breath-Control Exercise
- Modified Alternate-Nostril Breath-Control Exercise
- Modified Both-Nostrils Breath-Control Exercise with Abdomen Relaxed
- Modified Both-Nostrils Breath-Control Exercise with Abdomen Retracted
- Modified Both-Nostrils Breath-Control Exercise with Breath Suspension

Points of Note: There are different techniques for this posture. One of them is described above. Another technique is: Sit erect with the left leg bent at the knee and the left heel placed close to and under the upper part of the right thigh, and the outer side (fibular) of the right foot placed in the depression formed by the folding of the left leg on the left thigh. This form may fit many persons.

Toe-Hold Lotus Posture

1. Assume Lotus Posture (fig. 20.2).
2. Bring the right arm to the left side and the left one to the right side, making them cross each other behind the back. Now grasp the left big toe with the right hand and the right big toe with the left hand. Keep the trunk erect. Maintain the attitude as instructed by a qualified Yoga teacher (fig. 20.4).
3. Return to step 1 after completion of the exercise and then to step 4.
4. Sit with the legs extended in front and the arms by the sides.

Breathing: Normal.

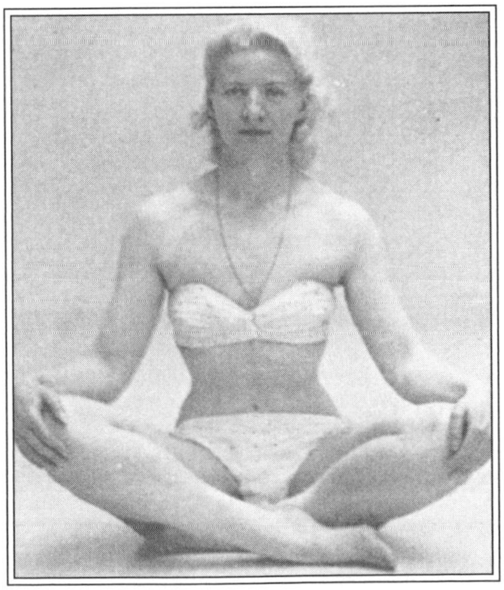

Fig. 20.3. Pleasant Posture (Sukhāsana)

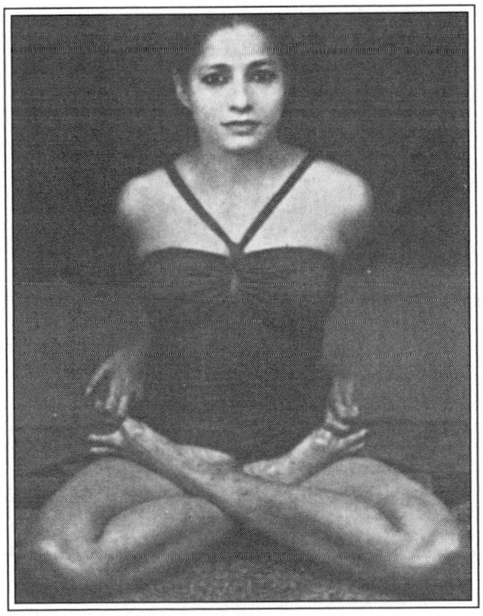

Fig. 20.4. Toe-Hold Lotus Posture (Baddha Padmāsana)

21

Prāṇāyāma—Breath-Control Exercise

In its pulmonary aspect, breathing is composed of air movements through the airways by which the gas exchange is upheld. But breathing is much more than mere pulmonary function. It is an expression of vital-force-motions that occur in the body to promote life; it is also associated with mental life, characterized by both mental outwardness expressed as conscious awareness and an unconscious "recoil" of consciousness.

In its suprapulmonary aspect, breathing is *prāṇāyāmic* breathing. Through the perfection of Sahita (Alternate-Nostril Breath Control with Breath Suspension), an automatic supernormal suspension occurs in which inhalation and exhalation have naturally ceased. Known as *kevala kumbhaka,* natural breath suspension, this causes a static mode of existence, one that is anerobic (metabolism without oxygen), which is associated with the supermental life in which consciousness is in a state of superconcentration.

In order to understand how this takes place, it is helpful to first understand the basics of the anatomy and physiology of breathing.

Ventilation

As pulmonary function, breathing consists of ventilation (lung circulation) and gas exchange. Ventilation is the air movement within the airways of the lungs, which has an inward and an outward flow, carried out alternately. The inward flow is the act of inhalation in which the outside air, under atmospheric pressure, enters the pulmonary airways through the nostrils (or mouth), and passes through the pharynx, larynx, trachea, bronchi, bronchioli, respiratory bronchioles, alveolar ducts, atria, and air sacs and finally reaches the alveoli. The outward flow is the act of exhalation in which the reverse movement of air takes place in the airways; the air, which is under pressure exceeding atmospheric pressure, is expelled from the lungs through the nostrils (or mouth).

The lung is an elastic, highly compliant structure containing within it an intricately arranged air space. The air space consists of airways, which are a unique tubal system, starting with a larger tube that gradually divides and subdivides into smaller and smaller descending tubes. The lungs are encased within an elastic case, called the thorax. It contains the ribs, twenty in number (omitting the four floating ribs), their cartilage, the sternum, and the thoracic vertebrae, twelve in number. Each lung is covered with a part of a delicate serous membrane, called the visceral pleura; the rest of the membrane lines the inner surface of the corresponding half of the thorax, termed the parietal pleura. These two pleurae are continuous with each other and form a cavity between them, termed the pleural cavity, which is only a potential one.

The space between the visceral and the parietal pleurae, or, in other words, between the lung and the inner wall of the thorax, is called the intrapleural space. The elastic force of the lung is continually trying to pull away from the thoracic wall and to decrease its size. The elasticity of the lungs is counteracted by that of the thorax. The action of these two opposing forces creates a negative intrapleural pressure.

At the end of normal exhalation, the inspiratory muscles are in a relaxed state and a balance is created between the elastic force of the lung, which tends to decrease its size, and that of the thorax, which opposes it. This normal end-expiratory opposition is the resting position of the thorax. In this position the lung is slightly stretched, and the thorax is compressed somewhat. The pressure in the intrapleural space is subatmospheric.

From the normal end-expiratory position, the thorax can either be enlarged or further compressed. The enlargement of the thorax from its resting position is caused by the contraction of the inspiratory muscles. During contraction, the inspiratory muscles have to overcome elastic resistance caused by the lung and the thorax, the inelastic resistance of the tissues, and the airway resistance. The inspiratory movement is resisted by lung elasticity but supported by thoracic elasticity up to a lung volume of 70 percent of the vital capacity. The inelastic tissue and airway resistance oppose the inspiratory movement. In inhalation, the venous pressure becomes more negative, from 10 to 15 mmHg.

At the end of inhalation, the inspiratory muscles relax and the expiratory movement starts. In normal, quiet breathing, exhalation is mainly a passive act, which is effected by thoracic and pulmonary elasticity. Exhalation is supported by the lung elasticity and opposed by both the inelastic tissues and the airway resistance. When the lung volume is above 70 percent, the elasticity of the thorax supports exhalation. In exhalation, the negative intrapleural pressure is from -5 to -8 mmHg.

The expiratory muscles remain inactive during normal, quiet exhalation. Under forced exhalation, the expiratory muscles contract during the later state of exhalation. If an expiratory effort is very great, venous pressure may become positive. The negative venous pressure facilitates the return of blood to the heart and helps to maintain the dome-like position of the diaphragm. The positive venous pressure increases the output of blood from the left heart. The pulmonary pressure changes to positive and negative pressures alternately during breathing. At end-expiration and end-inspiration, the intrapulmonary pressure is equal to atmospheric pressure.

Inhalation starts from the end-expiration position. The capacity of the alveoli is much greater than that of the airways (the airways contain 150 mL compared to 3 liters in the alveoli). The thoracic enlargement due to the contraction of the inspiratory muscles creates a negative alveolar pressure. As a result, atmospheric air is sucked into the tubes through the nostrils (or mouth) and passes toward the alveoli, where the major part of it enters. This process is called inhalation.

The inflow of air stops at the end-inspiratory position when alveolar pressure becomes equal to atmospheric pressure. Now, the relaxation of the inspiratory muscles (the intercostal muscles and the diaphragm) allow the elastic recoil forces of the thoracic wall and the alveolar walls to increase alveolar pressure; this causes the alveolar air to be expelled via the airways, through the nose (or mouth). This process is exhalation.

In normal inhalation, the alveolar pressure is about -3 mmHg. During a maximal inspiratory effort, the alveolar pressure may fall to -30 to -147 mmHg. During normal exhalation the alveolar pressure is about +3 mmHg. During maximal exhalation, both pleural and alveolar pressure can be raised from +30 to +250 mmHg.

During inhalation, all of the airways become lengthened and expanded. During exhalation they become shortened and narrowed. The smooth muscles of the intrapulmonary bronchi, bronchioli, respiratory bronchioles, and alveolar ducts may play an important role in the dilating and narrowing of the tubes. When the rate of breathing is very rapid, bronchial "smooth" muscles may have a modulating role. This is because they function more slowly than the skeletal muscle. If the alternate lengthening-expanding and shortening-narrowing are the effects of the action of the inspiratory muscles and elastic recoil respectively, then smooth muscle, which is also highly elastic, may assume a passive role. It may be that the contraction of the bronchial smooth muscle controls the inspiratory expansion of the air tubes, when the latter exceed a certain limit. In this way, the bronchial smooth muscle may function as a restraining influence to prevent excessive expression of the bronchial tubes, thus helping the flow of air into the nonmuscular tubes in a more efficient and controlled manner. The bronchial smooth muscle may also function to maintain a normal-size dead space.

Respiratory Volumes

As the size of the bronchial tubes and alveoli is constantly changing, so the amount of air within them is also varying. The volume of air inhaled or exhaled automatically in each respiration is called the *tidal volume*. It is about 500 mL (resting). The volume of air that can be inhaled from an end-tidal inspiration is termed the *inspiratory reserve volume*. It is 2000–3200 mL. The amount of air that can be exhaled from an end-tidal expiration is called the *expiratory reserve volume*. It is about 750–1000 mL. The volume of air that remains in the alveoli and airways at the end of a maximum exhalation is termed the *residual volume*. It is about 2000 mL. This figure and the following presented here are mean values and there is a large variation around them.

The volume of air that remains in the lungs and airways at the end of maximum inhalation is called *total lung capacity*. It is about 6,500 mL. The maximal volume of air that can be expelled from the lungs by a forceful expiratory effort after a maximal inhalation is called *vital capacity*. It is about 4,500 mL. The volume of air that can be inhaled from the end of a normal exhalation is termed *inspiratory capacity*. It is about 3,500 mL. The volume of gas that remains in the lungs and airways at the end of a normal exhalation is called *functional residual capacity*. It is about 3,000 mL.

Dead space is the volume of air of the conducting airways, which are not provided with alveoli; consequently, this volume of air does not take any part in gas exchange. The conducting airways and their dead space volume consists of the nostrils, mouth, nasal cavities, pharynx, larynx, trachea, extrapulmonary bronchi, intrapulmonary bronchi, and bronchioli. This is what is called *anatomical dead space*. *Physiological dead space* is the anatomical dead space plus the volume of inspired air ventilating those alveoli that have no pulmonary blood flow, plus the volume of inspired air, flowing into some alveoli, exceeding that which can be arterialized. However, the volumes of the anatomical and physiological dead spaces in healthy persons are practically the same.

The volume of dead space varies according to age, sex, and physical condition. In an average healthy person it may be about 150 mL, or slightly more or less. Dead space can be 230–260 mL after maximal inhalation, and 110–180 mL after maximal exhalation. Of the total dead space the intrathoracic volume is almost equal to or slightly less than the extrathoracic. However, in inhalation the whole tidal volume does not reach the alveoli because of the dead space. In each inhalation the tidal volume minus the dead space enters the alveoli.

Suppose that the dead space is 150 mL and the tidal volume 500 mL. At the end of exhalation, the conducting airways are filled with alveolar gas that amounts to 150 mL. In inhalation, 500 mL of outside air gradually enter the airways. The inhaled air will first push down the alveolar gas, which has occupied the airways during the last exhalation, and fresh air thereafter will enter the alveoli. This means that 500 mL of inhaled air minus 150 of dead space air, that is, 350 mL, will enter the alveoli in each inhalation. In each inhalation, the alveoli will first receive 150 mL of gas, which is alveolar gas from the conducting airways, and then 350 mL of fresh air from the inhaled 500 mL; the remaining 150 mL will occupy the airways during the last phase of inhalation. The alveolar gas is mixed with 350 mL of fresh air in each inhalation. So, at the end of normal inhalation, the dead space volume is 150 mL of inhaled fresh air; the remaining 350 mL of inhaled fresh air are in the alveoli. When exhalation starts, first the dead space fresh air is expelled and then the 350 mL of alveolar air are exhaled, and the remaining 150 mL of alveolar air occupy the conducting airways and form the dead space volume.

At the end-expiration, dead space volume consists of alveolar air (150 mL). In the next inhalation, 150 mL of alveolar air, which formed the dead space volume, is rushed back into the alveoli by the inhaled air, and then 350 mL of the inhaled fresh air pass into alveoli, and the remaining 150 mL (of inhaled air) remain at the dead space volume. In this manner, in each respiration, the alveolar gas is mixed with 350 mL of fresh air and the dead space volume is alternately changing from fresh air to alveolar gas and vice versa.

Respiratory Muscles

The respiratory muscles are divided into two groups: inspiratory and expiratory. The inspiratory muscles can be subdivided into two: principal and accessory. The principal muscles of inhalation are diaphragm and intercostals.

Enlargement of the thorax is effected by the upward and outward movements of the upper ribs and the lateral movements of the lower ribs. These costal movements are essentially due to the contraction of the intercostals, especially the external intercostals and probably the intercartilaginous internal intercostals. In inhalation, the most important movement is effected via the diaphragm, the largest of all inspiratory muscles. The contraction of the diaphragm increases the vertical diameter and the expansion of the base of the thorax. They are usually contracted in forced inhalation.

The abdominal muscles, namely the external oblique, the internal oblique, the transversus abdominis, and the rectus abdominis, are the chief muscles of exhalation. They are practically inactive in quiet exhalation, but they contract in forced exhalation.

To summarize:

- Quiet inhalation: Contraction of diaphragm and intercostals.
- Quiet exhalation: Effected by the elastic recoil of the lungs. The expiratory muscles are inactive. During the early phase of exhalation, the inspiratory muscles do not relax completely.
- Forced inhalation: Contraction of diaphragm and intercostals; contraction of scaleni, sternomastoids, and other accessory muscles of inhalation; contraction of the abdominal muscles occurring at the end of maximum inspiratory effort.
- Forced exhalation: Contraction of the abdominal muscles; contraction of scaleni and sacrospinalis.

Respiratory Gas Exchange

Carbon dioxide, oxygen, and hydrogen ion concentration are the three chemical constituents of the blood that are involved in breathing. The alveolocapillary gas exchange consists of the transfer of oxygen from the alveolar gas into the pulmonary capillary blood, and from there the transfer of carbon dioxide into the alveolar gas. At the end of each respiration, the volume of air remaining in the alveoli is equal to the expiratory reserve volume plus the residual volume. This volume of air is diluted with 350 mL of the fresh air inspired with each breath.

The partial pressure of oxygen in the inhaled air is about 150 mmHg and that of carbon dioxide is 0.3 mmHg. The partial pressures of oxygen and carbon dioxide in the alveolar gas after inhalation are 104 and 40 mmHg, respectively. In a healthy young subject the pressures of oxygen and carbon dioxide in the arterial blood are 100 and 40 mmHg respectively, and in the mixed venous blood they are 40 and 46 mmHg respectively.

The full oxygen value of the inhaled air is decreased when it mixes with the alveolar gas. But the oxygen tension of the alveolar gas still remains much higher than that of the pulmonary capillary blood. The higher partial pressure of oxygen causes it (oxygen) to pass from the alveoli into the pulmonary capillary blood where there is a lower tension of oxygen. Oxygen passes through the extremely thin alveolar capillary membrane and blood plasma to reach the erythrocytes of the capillary blood. In a similar manner, carbon dioxide passes into the alveolar gas from the pulmonary capillaries. The total surface of the alveoli is said to be between 80 and 100 square meters, and that of the pulmonary capillaries 75 to 150 square meters. Such large surfaces facilitate the interchange of gases. The pulmonary capillaries are extremely thin and completely unsupported, making them compliant and easy to deform or dilate; it is the dilation that makes possible increased blood flow with little or moderate increase in vascular pressure. All this shows that a great increase in blood flow through these vessels can easily occur and that this amount of blood can be arterialized.

In the pulmonary capillaries venous blood changes into arterial blood by exchange and then passes through the pulmonary veins, left auricle, and left ventricle into the systemic circulation. At the capillary level, oxygen from the erythrocytes passes to the blood plasma and then diffuses into tissue fluids through the capillary wall. On the other hand, carbon dioxide from the tissues passes into capillary blood that goes back to the heart (venous blood). The venous blood returns into the right auricle through the inferior and superior vena cava. Then it passes into the right ventricle, which pumps it into the pulmonary artery. It is then carried into the pulmonary capillaries where oxygenation of blood takes place.

The lung also has the capacity to remove leukocytes and platelets from circulation, store them, and return them when needed.

Both neural control and chemical regulation are involved in breathing. The medullary and pontine centers are very important. The cerebrum or other parts of the brain are supposed to control the respiratory centers.

Automatic Relaxation Breathing

In addition to the normal forms of automatic breathing, Yoga employs the possibilities of what is known as relaxation breathing or *hangsa* breathing, a particular form of conscious automatic breathing. First of all, a *prāṇāyāmic* posture is to be assumed. The fundamental feature of such a posture is the leg-lock done by folding the legs in a particular manner. For this purpose two main postures are advised: Accomplished Posture (Siddhāsana) and Lotus Posture (Padmāsana). In Lotus Posture, there is an additional lock, the foot-lock. The folded legs are in a static state in which some muscles are stretched and others are shortened. In this state, the muscles are merely holding a position, but no movements are made. So the muscles are only in a state of tension. As this tension is not high, it can be maintained for a long time. This is a passive posture—there is no voluntary contraction or voluntary tension of the muscles. In this form of static work, probably a small number of muscle fibers at a time are involved, which contract rhythmically with different rhythms and different frequencies. The expenditure of energy in this posture appears to be negligible.

In a folded-leg posture, there is a partial block of the circulation in the legs, which reduces the oxygen intake of the leg muscles. This reduced circulation is not expected to create an anaerobic process of energy supply, as the demand is minimum. In this state, if a little more oxygen is needed at any time, the oxygen stores in the capillary blood and muscles might prove sufficient. We think that this static folded-leg posture causes a general reduction of circulation, which is helpful in maintaining the body in a more relaxed and restful manner, and the mind more calm and restful.

The second point in the folded-leg posture is the keeping up of the arm-lock. Here the arms are loose by the sides, with the hands resting on the knees or one on the other on the lap. The arm-lock is not so secure as the leg-lock, but serves its purpose. The muscles of the shoulders, arms, and forearms are in a static state without tension, as the muscles are relaxed.

The third point is the maintenance of the straight trunk. The sacrospinalis muscles are mainly involved in keeping the vertebral column in a normal straight position. These muscles are in static tension. This tension, however, is very slight, and by training, it can be maintained for a very long time. When the trunk is kept straight, the muscles of the back, chest, and abdomen are relaxed, and the thorax is in neither an expiratory nor an inspiratory position but at a midlevel. It might be that a slight inhalation can reach a resting level for the thoracic wall position. In this position, the smooth action of the diaphragmatic pump is enough to maintain the smooth venous flow to the right heart. Moreover, the heart functions smoothly under these conditions.

The folded-leg posture, therefore, is a posture in which the muscles of the thighs and legs are in a state of low static tension; all the other muscles are kept in a state of general relaxation, and the body is completely motionless. This is a state of relaxation and rest, with the mind calm. In this resting position, all the activities of the body are at a minimum level, which is expressed by the rate of breathing. The normal breathing rate in which volition does not take any part in a resting position amounts to 12–16 breaths per minute. So, in a folded-leg resting posture, the normal automatic breathing rate may be assumed to be 15 respirations a minute. Supposing that the tidal volume is 500 mL and the dead space volume 150 mL, in each breath the alveolar gas is mixed with fresh air, that is 500 – 150 = 350 mL, or 5250 mL of fresh air in a minute.

There are three possibilities of altering the automatic breathing rate in a resting position. First, it can be increased by voluntarily contracting the inactive muscles; second, it can be further decreased by a voluntary relaxation of the body; and third, by a voluntary alteration of the breathing rate. In all these three factors, volition plays a predominant role. The resting muscles that can be dynamically contracted by volition in the folded-leg resting posture are the muscles of the shoulders, arms, forearms, hands, chest, abdomen, neck, and back.

Generally, the dynamic contraction of muscles during exercise has two phases: shortening, by which positive work is done, and lengthening, which effects negative work. The muscle fibers contract rhythmically with different rhythms and with different frequencies. At the beginning of muscular contraction, breathing is accelerated and, along with it, circulation. The rate of increase in breathing depends on the type and intensity of the muscular exercise. In exercise that requires great speed, such as short sprinting, or great muscular strength, such as heavy weightlifting, breathing may be stopped during the muscular activity. Breath suspension is followed by hyperpnoea after the cessation of the exercise.

In exercise hyperpnoea, two changes occur in breathing: increased frequency and increased depth. The increase in frequency may be as high as two or three times the normal resting rate. Similarly, the depth of respiration is also very high. The increase in depth is the most efficient means of meeting the greater oxygen need of the body, and this is shown in well-trained athletes. The tidal volume may reach up to about 2,400 mL or more (half the vital capacity) during heavy exercise. With the increase in depth of respiration, the dead space volume is also increased. It may be doubled. During exercise the respiratory frequency also increases from the resting level (15 to 40–50 breaths in a minute).

In speed exercise, the increase is maximum. If the tidal volume is 2,000 mL, the respiratory frequency 40 breaths a minute, and the dead space 300 mL, then the total ventilation per minute will be 80,000 mL, and the alveolar ventilation per minute will be 68,000 mL. This is clearly shown in table 1.

In a folded-leg posture the legs are blocked, so they cannot take part in the exercise. The muscles of the neck, arms, and trunk can be moderately exercised. The best exercise in folded-leg postures is the voluntary full contraction method in which the important skeletal muscles are contracted to their full extent without any external load. In this form of exercise the muscles undergo shortening

TABLE I. COMPARISON OF BREATHING RATES AND VOLUME—RESTING AND SPEED EXERCISE

	Breathing (automatic)		Dead space (mL)	Total ventilation (mL)		Alveolar ventilation (mL)	
	Depth mL	*Frequency per min*		*each breath*	*per min*	*each breath*	*per min*
Resting	500	15	150	500	7,500	350	5,250
Exercise	2,000	40	300	2,000	80,000	1,700	68,000

and lengthening, and the degree of contraction is controlled by volition. That the volitional contraction is effective is shown by two factors: one is that the muscles, when shortened, are as hard as wood; the other is that there is full mental control over the contraction of the muscles. This voluntary full contraction is termed *cāraṇā,* an important part of Haṭha Yoga. Both respiratory depth and frequency increase only slightly or moderately in this form of exercise.

On the other hand, all the muscles can be fully relaxed by the voluntary full relaxation method in the folded-leg posture. After attaining general relaxation of the body, all the muscles can be more and more relaxed volitionally by applying the "let go" principle and a sort of detachment from the body, together with conscious passivity. In this manner, all the muscles will gradually undergo full relaxation. At this stage, respiratory frequency decreases, and, most probably, the tidal volume is also reduced. It can be observed that the respiratory frequency decreases from the resting position (15 times) to 10 times or less. This is *hangsa* breathing (relaxation breathing). Here, breathing is also automatic.

When relaxation is fully mastered and the body entirely established in *hangsa* breathing, the yogi begins to be unconscious of his body. Consciousness starts to be elevated, stage by stage, from the sensory level. In time, consciousness becomes superconsciousness, which is a state of deep concentration (*dhyāna*). Breathing frequency is still further reduced, and automatic suspension develops between inhalation and exhalation. Suspension becomes normally prolonged; then inhalation and exhalation are very slight. Breathing goes on in this way: inhalation, followed by prolonged automatic suspension, then exhalation. This is called *dhyāna* breathing or concentration breathing. Ultimately *dhyāna* breathing develops into *kevala kumbhaka* (noninspiratory-nonexpiratory suspension). At this stage, concentration develops into superconcentration at its highest level.

Thus, on the one hand, automatic breathing can be increased in depth and frequency from its resting level by exercise; on the other hand, it can be decreased in depth and frequency in full relaxation. Finally, the inspiratory and expiratory phases of breathing can be reduced to a nominal point and ultimately disappear, being replaced by automatic breath-suspension.

Voluntary Breathing

Voluntary breathing is that in which inhalation or exhalation or both can be lengthened or shortened by volition, and breath can be voluntarily suspended. In Yoga, voluntary breathing has been classified under three forms: short-quick breathing, long-slow breathing, and breath suspension, which in fact is the integral part of long-slow breathing. Let us assume that in a folded-leg resting posture respiratory frequency is 15 breaths per minute, tidal volume 500 mL, and dead space volume 150 mL. In this resting position, it is possible to volitionally reduce respiratory frequency from 15 to 1 breath per minute or to increase it from 15 to 240 or over per minute. When the respiratory frequency has been decreased from the normal resting level, it comes under long-slow breathing. On the other hand, when the respiratory frequency has been accelerated by volition from its resting value, the breathing becomes of a short-quick type.

As mentioned earlier, in Yoga, there are two forms of short-quick breathing: Kapālabhātī (Abdominal Short-Quick Breathing) and Bhastrikā (Thoracic Short-Quick Breathing). The speed rate in both the abdominal and the thoracic type of voluntary short-quick breathing can be classified into three forms—low, medium, and high. When the breathing frequency reaches 60 breaths per minute, that is, 1 per second, it is low speed. When the frequency reaches 120 breaths per minute, that is, 2 per second, it is medium speed, and when 240 breaths per minute, that is, 4 per second, it is high speed. Any rate above this is very high speed. The Lotus Posture is generally assumed in Kapālabhātī and Bhastrikā. Other folded-leg postures can also be adopted.

In Kapālabhātī, exhalation is very rapid due to quick retraction of the front abdominal wall. In the retraction phase, the antero-lateral abdominal muscles are contracted. The retraction can be made one of low order by practice. Quick exhalation is followed by quick inhalation in which automatic retraction and descent of the diaphragm takes place. At the end of exhalation, the front abdominal wall is released from its retracted state and relaxed. Therefore, in Kapālabhātī, the diaphragm is, alternately, retracting while it is descending and relaxing when ascending. Retractions and relaxation are performed very quickly. The intercostals contract during inhalation. But inhalation is so quick that the contraction of the intercostals may persist in quick exhalation. During this breathing, the anterior abdominal wall, especially the upper part, including a small portion of the lateral abdominal wall, lower aspect of the anterior and lateral parts of the thorax, and a small, upper, anterior part of the thorax, undergo shaking movements. In Kapālabhātī, one of the author's pupils has reached the high rate of 345 respirations per minute, that is, close to 6 breaths per second! The same pupil is also able to continue this breathing for about thirty minutes.*

In Bhastrikā the repetitive exhalations-inhalations are also very quickly done. In this breathing, the front abdominal wall is kept relaxed, so it does not participate in exhalation. It appears, however, that exhalation is mainly effected by the utilization of the intercostals and the automatic relaxation of the diaphragm. In inhalation, the diaphragm and the intercostals contract. Keeping the front abdomen in a relaxed state, only the upper part of the thorax will be moving down toward the arms with the hands resting on knees. The rate of 310 respirations per minute in this form of breathing has been demonstrated by another pupil. This indicates that voluntarily increased respiratory frequency

*That yogic hyperventilation can be maintained uninterruptedly during more than one hour was demonstrated by one of the writer's disciples at the University Hospital Huddinge, Sweden. See C. Frostell, J. N. Pande, and G. Hedenstierna, "Effects of High-Frequency Breathing on Pulmonary Ventilation and Gas Exchange," The American Physiological Society, publication number 0161-7567/83, 1983.

is much greater than the automatic hyperpnoea of aerobic exercise.

The tables below compare a resting rate of 15 breaths per minute to variations in short-quick breathing at different speed rates while the body is kept in a folded-leg resting posture. Table 2 assumes a dead space of 150 mL and a tidal volume of 500 mL, while Table 3 assumes a dead space of 150 mL and a tidal volume of 250 mL.

Now the question arises as to whether the normal, resting tidal volume and the dead space volume remain the same in short-quick breathing. It has been assumed that a smaller tidal volume will cause an increase in total ventilation to maintain the alveolar ventilation. It has also been stated that alveolar ventilation increases with a greater tidal volume and decreased respiratory frequency. We have seen that both respiratory depth and frequency are increased in automatic hyperventilation caused by exercise. The increased depth may amount to about 50 percent of the individual's vital capacity, and frequency may reach 50 breaths a minute. But in short-quick breathing the frequency is still higher.

In fact, ventilatory response is greater in maximum voluntary ventilation (in which one breathes as hard and as fast as possible) than in exercise. The respiratory frequency in yogic short-quick breathing is about four times that caused by exercise in which respiratory depth and frequency are increased simultaneously. Another significant difference is the fact that yogic short-quick breathing is not done

TABLE 2. COMPARISON OF BREATHING RATES—RESTING AND SHORT-QUICK BREATHING

(Assuming a dead space of 150 mL and a tidal volume of 500 mL)

	Frequency per min	Type of breathing	Total ventilation per minute in mL	Alveolar ventilation per minute in mL
Resting	15	Automatic	7,500 (7,5 L)	5,250 (5,25 L)
Short-Quick	60	Voluntary	30,000 (30 L)	21,000 (21 L)
Short-Quick	120	Voluntary	60,000 (60 L)	42,000 (42 L)
Short-Quick	240	Voluntary	120,000 (120 L)	84,000 (84 L)
Short-Quick	300	Voluntary	150,000 (150 L)	105,000 (105 L)

TABLE 3. COMPARISON OF BREATHING RATES—SHORT-QUICK BREATHING

(Assuming a dead space of 150 mL and a tidal volume of 250 mL)

	Frequency per min	Type of breathing	Total ventilation per min in mL	Alveolar ventilation per min in mL
Short-Quick	60	Voluntary	15,000 (15 L)	6,000 (6 L)
Short-Quick	120	Voluntary	30,000 (30 L)	12,000 (12 L)
Short-Quick	240	Voluntary	60,000 (60 L)	24,000 (24 L)
Short-Quick	300	Voluntary	75,000 (75 L)	30,000 (30 L)

in a physically strenuous manner, but in a relaxed attitude.

One of our experiments on *prāṇāyāmic* breathing has disclosed certain important facts. Our object was to observe the difference between voluntary long-slow and short-quick breathing. The subject who was tested was a healthy young man aged twenty-nine who had been practicing Yoga exercises for about eight years. The results are shown in table 4 below.

Tidal volume is the highest in one breath per minute in long-slow breathing. Then it begins to fall step by step as the frequency is increased. The tidal volume in short-quick breathing is generally less than in long-slow breathing. The total ventilation is greater, however, in short-quick breathing than in long-slow breathing. The absorption of oxygen and the elimination of carbon dioxide are also greater in short-quick breathing than in long-slow breathing. We do not know if the increased oxygen consumption in short-quick breathing is due to excessive activities of the respiratory muscles. It would seem, thus, that the respiratory action is large enough to cause the increase in oxygen uptake/consumption. The probable oxygen storage increase in the body, in hemoglobin in red blood cells and in myoglobin in muscle cells, may be related to an increase in oxygen tension or possibly to a right shift of the oxygen-hemo/myoglobin curve.

There is no reason to suppose that all of the increased amount of oxygen has been solely utilized by the respiratory muscles. We have reason to believe that the increased oxygen consumption represents both metabolic oxygen and a storage of oxygen and this storage oxygen helps in prolonging breath suspension during the first stage. The washing out of carbon dioxide indicated by an increased elimination of this gas is favorable for breath suspension and

TABLE 4. COMPARISON OF BREATHING RATES AND VOLUME—NORMAL, LONG-SLOW, AND SHORT-QUICK BREATHING

	Normal Breathing			Long-Slow Breathing						Short-Quick breathing		
								Kapālabhātī			*Bhastrikā*	
Duration in minutes	5	10	10	5	5	2	2	2	5	2	2	2
Number of respirations per minute	16	1	2	4	8	16	32	64	128	248	256	230
Volume of inhaled air in liters per minute	10.1	4.7	5.3	6.9	7.6	15.5	22.3	40.3	40.2	71.7	51.2	65
Tidal volume per respiration in mL	631	4,690	2,635	1,725	948	967	698	630	314	289	200	283
Absorption of O_2 per minute in mL	342	329	293	301	341	313	428	573	411	816	554	954
Absorption of O_2 per inhalation in mL	21.4	329	146.5	75.3	42.6	19.6	13.4	9	3.2	3.3	2.2	4.1
Elimination of CO_2 per minute in mL	229	237	226	243	241	309	397	716	471	752	344	799
Elimination of CO_2 per exhalation in mL	14.3	237	113	60.6	30.1	19.3	12.4	11.2	3.7	3	1.3	3.5

for a new, lower, level of organic functioning, which is helpful in concentration. However, this increased carbon dioxide elimination never gives rise to acapnial alkalosis nor does it cause an abnormal reduction in cerebral circulation.

On the basis of the data presented in the above table, we can approximately calculate the rate of alveolar ventilation in relation to total ventilation, if we assume that the dead space volume is 150 mL and is maintained throughout the changes in the respiratory frequency as shown in table 5.

TABLE 5: COMPARISON OF ALVEOLAR VENTILATION TO TOTAL VENTILATION—DIFFERENT BREATHING RATES

(Assuming a dead space of 150 mL)

Respiratory frequency per minute in liters	Total ventilation per minute in liters	Alveolar ventilation per minute
16 (normal)	10.1	7.7
1	4.7	4.5
2	5.3	5
4	6.9	6.3
8	7.6	6.4
16	15.5	13.1
32	22.3	17.5
64	40.3	30.7
128	40.2	21
230	65	30.5
248	71.7	34.5

Voluntary Long-Slow Breathing

There are several forms of long-slow breathing in Yoga, from which Ujjāyī has been selected here. Ujjāyī breathing consists of both-nostrils inhalation–breath-suspension–left-nostril exhalation or both-nostrils exhalation. It can be divided into three main forms—mild, medium, and heavy.

The mild form consists of (in seconds):

a) Inhaling 10 – exhaling 10
b) Inhaling 10 – exhaling 20
c) Inhaling 10 – suspending 20 – exhaling 20
d) Inhaling 10 – suspending 40 – exhaling 20

The medium form consists of (in seconds):

a) Inhaling 30 – exhaling 30
b) Inhaling 30 – exhaling 60
c) Inhaling 30 – suspending 60 – exhaling 120
d) Inhaling 60 – suspending 120 – exhaling 60

The heavy form consists of (in seconds):

a) Inhaling 60 – exhaling 60
b) Inhaling 60 – exhaling 120
c) Inhaling 60 – suspending 120 – exhaling 120
d) Inhaling 60 – suspending 240 – exhaling 120

It requires prolonged practice to reach this last stage.

Let us consider the medium form of Ujjāyī. Inhalation lasts for a period of 30 seconds, with the possibility of prolonging it still farther up to the heavy type. During the first part of inhalation, the dead space air, which is the alveolar gas, is pushed back into the alveoli, causing the maximum concentration of carbon dioxide with a minimum of oxygen in the alveolar gas. As the alveolar gas moves downward, inhaled fresh air begins to occupy the dead space. When all the alveolar gas has left the dead space, it is filled with fresh air. This is the first phase. During the second phase of inhalation, inhaled fresh air begins to enter through the dead space into the alveoli. As more and more fresh air enters the alveoli, carbon dioxide concentration is reduced and oxygen concentration increased in the alveolar gas. In normal respiration, the alveoli are ventilated 16 times (if the frequency is 16 times) in a minute. But in half-minute inhalation, they are continuously ventilated with fresh air for half a minute. This prolonged inhalation increases the absorption of oxygen from the normal 21.4 mL to 329 mL per inhalation, that is, more per minute than in normal breathing.

In normal exhalation, the partial pressure of carbon dioxide rises and that of oxygen falls. At the respiratory frequency of 16 breaths a minute, the elimination of carbon dioxide per minute is 229 mL, almost the same as in half-minute exhalation (about 237 mL); in half-minute the total ventilation is 4.7 L, and alveolar ventilation 4.5 L (assuming a dead space volume of 150 mL), whereas in normal exhalation (frequency 16 breaths a minute) they are 10.1 L and 7.7 L respectively. But the tidal volume in half-minute exhalation is 4,690 mL against the normal tidal volume (frequency 16 breaths per minute) of 631 mL. However, in yogic breathing, the usual ratio between inhalation and exhalation is 1 to 2, so that a half-minute inhalation is followed by a one minute exhalation. Moreover, between the phases of inhalation (*pūraka*) and exhalation (*recaka*), measured suspension (*kumbhaka*) becomes a part of the breathing.

The natural momentary breath suspension at end-inspiration and pre-expiration and end-expiration and pre-inspiration has a zero value. Although certain actions, such as swallowing, may cause momentary suspension, effective suspension is voluntary. Voluntary suspension has two phases: Easy Breath Suspension (Sahaja Kumbhaka)—in which breath can be held without any discomfort—and Difficult Breath Suspension—in which there is discomfort. That discomfort finally develops to a point, called the breaking point, when it is almost impossible to suspend the breath any longer.

The suspension time depends on many factors, the most important of which are chemical and volitional. Any condition that decreases carbon dioxide pressure in the arterial blood and increases oxygen pressure in the alveolar gas prolongs suspension. Voluntary hyperventilation on air and especially on oxygen prolongs suspension. With preliminary hyperventilation on oxygen, breath can be suspended over ten minutes. Hyperventilation on air while the body is at rest prolongs suspension, though not to the extent caused by hyperventilation on oxygen. Suspension can be prolonged by volition and when volition is forcefully applied, breath can be held up to 15 to 20 minutes, even to the point of being unconscious. Yogic short-quick breathing on air also helps to prolong suspension. We have observed that suspension is prolonged up to two or three minutes or even more after short-quick breathing.

We may assume that at a certain state of breath suspension, the only source of oxygen is the oxygen stored up in the body. The main oxygen stores are the alveolar gas, the arterial blood, and the venous blood. To these may be added myoglobin. However, it is said that these stores can maintain life only for a short time—not more than five minutes. But the writer has observed *prāṇāyāmic* breath suspension for up to sixty minutes, done in a folded-leg posture. How was life maintained? These facts demonstrate that there is a possibility of maintaining life anaerobically under certain conditions. Life can be maintained for a couple of hours by apnoic oxygenation via the mouth when gas is sucked down to the alveoli by continuous uptake of oxygen via the lung capillary blood.

Long inhalation, as is done in long-slow breathing, allows the continuous flow of fresh air to penetrate deep into the alveoli. This prolonged inspiratory flow causes the full expansion and stretching of the alveoli; uneven ventilation is equalized and, in this way, the inactive alveoli are made active. The lungs are maintained in a lengthened and widened state during inspiratory suspension. Suspension causes more thorough diffusion. As the external source of oxygen supply is completely stopped during suspension, the body is trained to endure an oxygen lack under these conditions, when the cardiac activity is also decreased and the body develops its uncommon power. Suspension also deepens respiration when it is insufficiently deep.

There is another far-reaching effect of breath suspension. It raises pressure in the cerebrospinal fluid in the ventricle of the brain, the central canal, and the subarachnoid space. The increased pressure in the cerebrospinal fluid produces compression on the nerve matter of the brain and the spinal cord, both from outside and inside. This compression may be an important factor, especially when applied with a measured dose, in improving the vital activities of the nerve cells and in arousing their dormant power.

Suspension is followed by long exhalation. The alveoli, now squeezed of air, become narrow and short. The alternate inspiratory fillings and expiratory emptyings exercise the alveoli and the respiratory muscles to a remarkable degree. The diaphragm is fully contracted in inhalation and fully relaxed in exhalation. All the respiratory muscles are adequately exercised by long inhalation and exhalation, and their fatigue-resisting power is increased. In a word, Ujjāyī turns out to be an excellent means of most efficiently exercising the alveolar and the pulmonary capillary systems and the respiratory muscles.

Sahita (Alternate-Nostril Breath Control with Breath Suspension)

Sahita consists of left inhalation–suspension–right exhalation–right inhalation–suspension–left exhalation. The ratio of inhalation, suspension, and exhalation is 1–4–2. Sahita has three versions: Nāḍī Śuddhi, Bhūta Śuddhi, and suspension breathing. Suspensive breathing ultimately leads to *kevala* suspension. Here we shall consider only the first two forms of Sahita.

Nāḍī Śuddhi

When the inhalation ratio for inhalation, suspension, and exhalation is gradually developed to 16–64–32, Sahita becomes Nāḍī Śuddhi breathing. The *nāḍīs* are the force-motion lines created by the motional directions of *vāyu,* the manifested life-force. *Vāyu* has five principal forms: *prāṇā*-force, *apāna* force, *samāna* force, *udāna* force, and *vyāna* force.

The flows of the five life-forces create a complex *nāḍī* system; in that system, three *nāḍīs,* known as *idā, pingalā,* and *suṣumnā,* are the most important. The *nāḍī* system is connected to the mind by *idā* and to the body by *pingalā.*

Suṣumnā is the central force-motion line created by five life-forces in their specific forms expressing five types of control in suspension. When *idā-pingalā* is brought under the control of *suṣumnā,* the body is vitalized, purified, and controlled from within; the mind is also rarefied and energized and exhibits its control power from within.

In relation to the body, the principal operational center of the *prāṇā*-force (*prāṇā-vāyu*) is the thorax, where the heart and lungs are located. As we have no volitional control over the heart, it is not possible to utilize it as the center of pranic operation. The best pranic center is the lung, which is nearly under volitional control.

In both inhalation (*pūraka*) and exhalation (*recaka*), *kumbhaka* (suspension) indicates a stop of an action that emerges from our latent action principle or *prāṇā*. That action is composed of plus (+) inhalation, plus (+) exhalation, and zero (0) pause. In the flow of plus inhalation, plus exhalation, and zero pause, the *prāṇā*-force operates without *suṣumnā* control. Under this condition the general functions of the life-forces are exhibited, but their specific control aspect remains hidden. When the "0 pause" is made a "+ pause," and the value of the pause is made greater than that of inhalation and exhalation combined, through volitional control of ventilation, the intrinsic aspect of pranic force is reached. In this form of Sahita *suṣumnā* control is developed and made to operate on pranic and other life-forces.

When suspension is mastered in Sahita, and becomes like a mode of being by long practice, a point is reached when the pranic force begins to radiate a red color, which finally changes to deep green, thus indicating the *suṣumnā* control over the *prāṇā*-force. When this control is fully established in suspension, *prāṇā* exhibits its well-controlled activities in the body (when it is functioning in a normal state with normal ventilation). At this stage the intrinsic contraction system of the heart operates on a higher level; the ventilatory and alveocapillary functions improve to a great extent; the alimentary canal's muscular activities become more efficient; the process of oxidative release of energy is normalized; the hemoglobin content of the blood is improved; sweat becomes fragrant and urine and feces are free from too much unpleasant odor; voice becomes sweet; the whole body is vitalized; and the faculties of perception are developed. All these effects are due to the controlling influence of the *prāṇā*-force.

The *samāna* force is brought under *suṣumnā* control through pranic force in respiratory harmonization occurring in Sahita suspension. When *samāna* is under control, it becomes white. *Samāna* control has the following effects:

1. Perfecting gastrointestinal digestion
2. Perfecting metabolism
3. Improved heart action through blood supply
4. Improved blood circulation
5. Promotion of growth
6. Perfecting oxidative removal of waste

The *udāna*-force can also be controlled through the *prāṇā*-force in suspension, as *udāna* plays a role in the nervous regulation of respiration. The *udāna* energy is related to pranic energy in the vitalization process of the body. The *suṣumnā*-controlled *udāna* emits smoke-colored energy and produces the following effects:

1. Improved sensory-mental function
2. Improved function of conation
3. Improved concentration through inactivation of sense-mind
4. Improved nervous control

As *vyāna* has the same center of operation, the *vyāna*-force is under *suṣumnā* control through pranic force in Sahita suspension. *Vyāna* emits golden-colored rays. When controlled, *vyāna* results in:

1. Improved nervous functions
2. Well-developed strength and agility
3. Improved muscular functions
4. Promotion of growth
5. Improved natural immunity of the body

Apāna force is controlled through the process of Yoni Mudrā, which is a specific sexual-control process, in combination with Sahita suspension. The fully controlled *apāna* emits red rays and causes the following effects:

1. Promotion of growth
2. Improved elimination
3. Effective sexual control

All these effects in the body and mind are due to the influence of Nāḍī Śuddhi, the process of bringing the five forms of the life-force under under *suṣumnā* control, which is effected through Sahita suspension. To summarize, the body becomes normally healthy and efficient, and natural immunity develops to its highest level. All unpleasant body odors disappear and the power of the senses increase. The mind becomes calm and well-controlled, and exhibits constructive and clear thinking. To make Sahita suspension most effective, the body should be purified and vitalized by fasting, frugal diet, internal cleansing, and muscular exercise.

Bhūta Śuddhi

The yogic breathing method of Bhūta Śuddhi is a combined form of breathing that includes *mantras* and thoughts. It consists of left inhalation–suspension–right exhalation; right inhalation–suspension–left exhalation; left inhalation–suspension–right exhalation. The measures of inhalation, suspension, exhalation are 16–64–32 seconds. In this breathing, appropriate *mantras* are used and, along with them, specific thoughts are maintained.

Five *mahābhūtas* (the "essentials") and five *tanmātras* (thatness) are the basic elements. In combination with the life-forces and the mind, they constitute the subtle body, the gross manifestation of which is the organized material body. The *mahābhūtas* are five forms of subtle energy, termed supermatter, which are reducible to *tanmātras*. The phenomena of mass, waves, and radiation arise from *prithivi mahābhūta* (mass principle), *ap mahābhūta* (wave principle), and *tejas mahābhūta* (radiation principle). At the background of these energies is *vāyu mahābhūta* (pure-energy principle); all these are unified into a coordinated functioning whole, by *ākāsha mahābhūta* (void factor).

There is a constant interaction between the subtle and the gross body, which is effected through the life-forces. The latter not only impart life to the gross body, but its pattern is shaped by *mahābhūta* energies through the instrumentation of the life forces. The changes in the physical body may be an expression of the *mahābhūta-prāṇā* force activities at a particular level or, alternatively, the effects of the physical changes are conducted to the inner body through an energy transformation that causes an alteration of the inner force-motions. The transfer of influences from one to the other occurs through the *idā-pingalā* lines. Unless *idā-pingalā* power flows are under *suṣumnā* control, they are disturbed in the course of their functions, and the disturbances are then reflected in the subtle and the material bodies.

The *suṣumnā* control is brought about by *mantras*. The functioning power of *mahābhūtas* and *tanmātras* is the nature of sound emission caused by force motion with which pranic operation is fused. Each *mahābhūta-tanmātra* has its particular *mantra* form. When the *mantras* are worked upon in Sahita, the *mantra* force is aroused in *suṣumnā* and exercises its control over *idā-pingalā* flows. *Mahābhūta-tanmātra* energies can be controlled and made to exhibit their specific actions by the *mantras*. The inner aspect of the control is the harmonious development of the power system of the subtle body. When this is done, the physical body undergoes a change that causes its superpurification and super-vitalization. This is the outer aspect of the control. However, when *mantra* is worked upon, it is more fruitful if, at the same time, the body is purified through diet-exercise-cleansing processes, because of the interactions of the subtle body and the gross body. Moreover, as *mantra* is aroused when worked upon in conjunction with breathing, physical purification also is necessary for effective breathing, especially in its suspensive aspect.

The *mahābhūta-tanmātra mantras* are "Lang," "Wang," "Rang," "Yang," and "Hang." Each has a specific color and exhibits a specific action. These specific actions are: drying (*ṣoṣana*) caused by the *mantra* "Yang;" burning (*dahana*) and elimination (*protsārana*) by "Rang;" irradiation (*plāvana*) by either the white-colored water germ "Wang" or the whitish-colored moon germ *mantra* "Thang;" construction (*dehagāthana*) by "Wang;" and firming (*dridhikārana*) by "Lang." "Hang" is concerned with organization (*vyuhikārana*). These processes are for the deep purification of the subtle body and the effects extend to the material body.

Drying is the process of reduction. In the subtle body, "impurities" are caused by the sensory-mental impression of purposiveness aroused in relation to sensory objects of mental choice. *Mahābhūta* energies are directed to give distinct sensory forms, which are imaged in consciousness. The affective aspect of the mind is aroused and attachment to the chosen object is established. Under this condition, life forces deviate from the central *suṣumnā* line and flow as *idā-pingalā* force-motion lines. In this way the subtle body gets an "ungodly" character. The impurities are made inactive by the drying process and yet the germ remains. This unspiritual potential is destroyed via the burning process. The burning process has two phases: residual destruction and its evaporation. What is unspiritually radiated in the subtle body becomes divinely purified from within by the processes of drying and burning. This is achieved by the *mantras* "Yang" and "Hang." This deep internal purification is only possible through *mantra*.

Vaikhari is an aspect of *mantra* in which the inaudible sound (*madhyama*) becomes audible. The audible sound of the *mantra* is given a conscious form by *japa* (repetition of the *mantra*) when done with measured inhalation, suspension, and exhalation, in conjunction with a specific thought form. In fact, the sound process (*japa*) is an intrinsic part of Sahita, and its effect is more pronounced in thought. The combination of sound process, breathing, and thought, when practiced regularly and continuously under the direction of a guru, makes the audible sound living in consciousness with the development of holding-concentration (*dhāraṇā*); gradually the inner power of the *mantra* is released and *mantra* becomes really effective.

Breathing is not mere pulmonary ventilation but a focus of the sum of all force-motion-activities through which a power-concentration is possible when the sound-forms, as *vaikhari-mantras* of the subtle forces, are fused in its suspensive aspect. Here lies the immense value of Bhūta Śuddhi breathing. The deep internal purification becomes a reality through breathing infused with *mantra*.

Following the purification of the subtle body by the processes of drying and burning, the life infusion into the subtle body is performed by the process of irradiation with the *mantra* "Thang." The *mantra* is effective when *japa* (sound process) is done in conjunction with left-inhalation. The life-forces become activated by this process. Then the process of construction should be applied via the *mantra* wang in suspension, in conjunction with specific thought. Through this process the pranic forces are caught in the *mātrikā,* or primary sound units, which become the building units, and a new subtle body is thereby constructed. After this, the newly constructed subtle body of *mātrikā* is strengthened by the process of firming, which is effected by the *mantra* "Lang," done in right exhalation with thought form. During *japa,* the *mantra* should be thought of in its appropriate color, together with its specific effectiveness.

All these processes—the processes of drying, burning, irradiating, constructing, and firming—are constantly operating in the physical body to maintain life and exhibit functions associated with its being alive. The body has been functionally organized to maintain its vitality, and associated with it is the manifestation of mental life. At the highest level, the organization is under the control of the sound *tanmātra* (*shabda-mantra*), the power of which is concentrated in the *mantra* "Hang." On one side of the organization lies the germ factor, called *cell,* which is a living organized unit, exhibiting all life activities; on the other side is the detailed manifestation of life activities through different cell-made organs.

Growth and Metabolism

The life activities at the material level are expressed as chemical changes occurring in the body, causing two fundamental phenomena—energy storage in the form of proteins, fats, carbohydrates, and special energy-rich compounds, and energy release by the catabolism of food in the body. The liberated energy appears as heat and work and also causes energy storage. However, when energy storage is a predominating factor, growth and development are promoted; on the other hand, when energy expenditure is higher, the body undergoes decline.

The normal growth of the body means a proportionate growth of different parts and organs of the body occurring at different periods. The growth capacity is best developed by eating the right food, getting appropriate exercise, and fostering positive endocrine influence. Interrupted nutrition and lack of exercise inhibit the growth impulse. The growth of the body as a whole is based on cellular growth, which is comprised of three processes: cellular enlargement, cell proliferation, and an accumulation of intracellular and intercellular substance.

In normal growth, all these processes work harmoniously. Under unfavorable conditions, growth is retarded and may even stop, as in inanition, but is not destroyed. Growth starts again when favorable conditions are reestablished. Growth appears to maintain a certain mass of an organ, which is necessary for its functional efficiency. In glands and many other tissues, when a part from the necessary bulk has been removed, cells multiply to form the removed part. Muscle proliferation stops at a certain stage of growth, but cell growth continues. On the other hand, it is supposed that neurons do not proliferate at all during an individual's lifetime.

Protein plays a most important role in cellular growth. Amino acids, the end products of protein digestion, are absorbed into the blood and then diffused throughout the body fluids. The larger quantities of amino acids are transported through the cell membrane to the cells by carrier mechanisms. Then almost all the amino acids are conjugated into cellular proteins by the intracellular enzymatic processes. In this way, amino acids become an essential part of the cells. On other hand, some proteins of the cells, except the genes of the nucleus and structural proteins, are continually undergoing disintegration into amino acids and are released into the extracellular fluid. There is no distinction between amino acids released by the cells and those from food. The surplus amino acids, that is the amino acids that are not utilized, undergo oxidative deamination in the liver to form ammonia, which is converted into urea by the liver, leaving the non-nitrogenous residues, which are either catabolized or converted into glucose, fat, or other amino acids.

Monosaccharides (glucose, fructose, and galactose), the final products of carbohydrate digestion, are first brought to the liver. From the liver, they are carried by the blood to the interstitial fluid; they are then transported through the cell membrane by a carrier mechanism into the cytoplasm of the cell. Glucose forms the largest part of the monosaccharides. Both galactose and fructose can be converted into glucose in the liver. Fructose is also converted into glucose in the muscles. However, the absorbed glucose in the cell is used in two forms: converted into glycogen, it is stored by the cells (in larger quantities by the liver and muscle cells); it is also dissimilated for the release of energy to be utilized by the cell. Glycogen is again broken down to form glucose in the cells when needed. The main function of glucose is to supply energy, which is essential for cellular functions. Glucose is first split into smaller hydrocarbons, which are catabolized into carbon dioxide and water, giving rise in the process to a large amount of energy. The surplus glucose, that is the amount of glucose that is not metabolized for energy and cannot be stored as glycogen, is converted into fat and stored in the fat depots.

The main source of fats in the organism is the fats derived from food, which are absorbed into the lymph to finally enter the venous blood through the thoracic duct. The food fats consist of neutral fats (triglycerides) and small quantities of phospholipids and cholesterol. Fats in the organism may also arise from the conversion of carbohydrate and protein into fats. Phospholipids become integral parts of the cells. They combine with structural proteins to form membranous structures of the cells. Cells also contain neutral fat and cholesterol. Neutral fat is either oxidized to release energy for the functional activities of the cells, or is stored in the fat cells in the fat depots. Fat is also absorbed into the liver where it is either used for energy or converted and deposited. Water, minerals, and water are absorbed into the cells. Water and minerals are constituents of protoplasm. Vitamins are also absorbed in the cells to a slight extent.

So we find that a living cell absorbs amino acids, monosaccharides, fats, minerals, vitamins, and water. Of all these substances, amino acids being conjugated into cellular proteins become an essential part of the cells, phospholipids become constituents of the cells; minerals and water form parts of the cells; vitamins, which play an essential role in metabolism, are stored in the cells; glucose is catabolized for energy, and also converted into glycogen and stored for future use; and neutral fat is also catabolized for energy.

In the cells, the processes of construction as well as drying, burning, and elimination are constantly going on. The breaking down of the cell proteins by cellular activities and the ejection of amino acids into extracellular fluid, water elimination, consumption of glycogen—all these are the drying process. The absorption of amino acids into the cell and their conversion into cellular proteins is the process of construction by which cell growth is promoted. The catabolism of glucose, fats, and proteins for the release of energy is the process of burning; the process of elimination by which the end-protects of catabolism are discharged from the body is associated with burning. Those amino acids that are not used for the growth of the cell are converted into urea, which is then eliminated. The absorption and utilization of phospholipids for building purposes form the process of construction. The storing of neutral fat by the fat cells is also a process of construction. The mobilization and utilization of storage fats for energy are the processes of burning and elimination.

The body is constantly undergoing the processes of building up and breaking down in all its stages. The former are the processes of construction and the breaking-down processes are those of drying, burning, and elimination. At a certain period of life the process of construction predominates, and, as a result, the organism grows normally. The normal growth impulse can be helped by appropriate diet and exercise when growth is promoted to a high level. Normal growth is associated with development, which is the unfoldment of powers of the organism. The developmental process is the process of firming. On the other hand, when the processes of drying and burning predominate, the organism begins to decline, as in old age.

There is also a biological plateau, a period between these two when growth and development are sustained, and decline is prevented. By diet, exercise, and internal cleansing that plateau can be prolonged. However, in periods of growth, sustainability, and decline, something may develop in the organism that interrupts the body's normal functioning. In the normal growth period, it has a high degree of vitality. When growth and development are enhanced by physical culture, vitality is still higher. During the course of growth and development, it is experienced that vitality ebbs temporarily with the symptoms of constipation, loss of appetite, coated tongue, and foul breath. If this condition is allowed to persist, disease symptoms develop.

What is it that develops when the organism is at its highest stage of efficiency, and that causes a decrease of the normal immunizing power of the body? It appears that it is a substance (or substances) formed within the body or introduced into the body that does not promote the vital vigor of the body but rather causes its diminution. This substance may be called an "impurity" or a "poison." That it is a real substance is proved by the fact that fasting causes its burning and elimination, and as a result the organism again becomes free from failing vitality and disease symptoms. This impure substance, when developed to an extent to cause the appearance of subvitality symptoms, may be eliminated by blood purification, through fasting, special diet, special exercise, and internal cleansing. However, the formation of this substance cannot be prevented.

The impure substance is the material form of the subtle impurity that slowly develops in the organism, mainly caused by disharmonious *iḍā-piṅgalā* pranic flows. The physical processes of Haṭha Yoga can control the formation of the impure substance in the body partially, but not completely. When the growth impulse in the cells becomes sluggish, this can be remedied by fasting. But when the vital activities of the cell go to a very low level, it requires prolonged fasting to invigorate the cells so they again exhibit their youthful activities. In many cases this is impossible, because of very low general vitality, caused by the influence of this substance.

The pranic forces exercise their control influences on all the processes and functions of the gross body. Deep internal purification for the evaporation and prevention of the formation of the impure substance is effected via Bhūta Śuddhi. But if the pranic forces are not under *suṣumnā*-control, their control influence on the functions of the body will not be fully effective; though subvitality and disease symptoms can be controlled, their reappearance cannot altogether be prevented.

Pranic Control

Life-infusion into the body as a whole and into the cells constitutes the basic activities of the pranic forces. A cell can be regarded as a minute, organized living structure, which is the gross vehicle of pranic forces—or the latter being metamorphosed into cells. The whole organism represents the detailed manifestation of pranic forces in which a cell is playing its role as a part of the whole. This vitalization process is mainly controlled by pranic force; it is supported by *udāna*-force and a subordinate pranic force called *dhanañjaya*. When *udāna* force ceases its function, the activities of the senses and the mind are stopped, and the death of the body occurs. The specific function of *dhañanjaya* force is to keep the cells alive after the death of the body. The cell life can be maintained indefinitely in a suitable fluid medium under the influence of this force.

The life process is intrinsically associated with the vital activities of the cells and organic functioning of the entire organism. The cells require oxygen, amino acids, lipids, minerals, vitamins, and water to maintain their vital activities. These substances have to be transported to the extracellular fluid in order to enter the cells. It requires the coordinated functional activities of the different organs and systems of the body. Oxygen is absorbed from the atmospheric air into the alveoli by pulmonary ventilation and is transferred to the pulmonary capillary blood by alveolocapillary gas exchange. Then the oxygen is transported to the cells by the extracellular fluid. Pulmonary ventilation and gas exchange are controlled by pranic force, in which *samāna* force is also involved. Oxygen transport from the lungs to the cells is controlled by *samāna* force in conjunction with pranic force.

Proteins, fats, carbohydrates, minerals, and vitamins are substances contained in food. Food is first masticated and mixed with saliva. Mastication is under the control of pranic force, while *vyāna* force controls the secretion of saliva. The masticated food is then swallowed, and enters the pharynx, and then passes through the esophagus to the stomach by peristalsis (primary). There is a secondary peristalsis, which helps to propel the food into the stomach. Swallowing is controlled by pranic force. Peristalsis in the esophagus is under the control of *apāna* force. Then the food undergoes digestion in the stomach. At first the food is stored in the body of the stomach and then it begins to be mixed with gastric juices by mixing wave movements until it becomes a thick semifluid called chyme. The food is gradually pushed toward the antrum of the stomach by the mixing waves. Here, the mixing is helped by strong peristalsis, by which chyme is taken into the small intestine. The gastric secretions are under the control of *samāna* force. *Prāṇa* controls the mixing wave movements while *apāna* controls antral peristalsis.

In the small intestine, food undergoes intestinal digestion and absorption. Chyme is kneaded and mixed with intestinal and pancreatic juices and bile and is kept in contact with the mucosa which facilitate absorption by segmentation contractions. The mixing with the digestive juices is also helped by pendular movements by which chyme is moved back and forth. Chyme is pushed onward and forced into the cecum by peristalsis. Segmentation contractions and pendular movements are controlled by *prāṇa* and peristalsis by *apāna*. The intestinal and pancreatic secretions and the secretions of bile are under the control of *samāna*.

By intestinal digestion proteins are broken down to amino acids; fats (neutral) are split into fatty acids and glycerol or monoglycerides which are resynthesized into chylomicrons; carbohydrates are broken down into monosaccharides (glucose, fructose, and galactose). Amino acids are absorbed into the intestinal capillaries and pass through the portal vein and the liver to the general circulation. Fats are absorbed by the intestinal mucosa and resynthesized and pass into the lymph and finally the venous blood. Monosaccharides are absorbed into the portal blood and pass through the liver into the general circulation. Minerals, vitamins, and water are absorbed from the small intestine into the general circulation. Absorption is essentially controlled by *prāna*. In absorption, *samāna* plays a specific role. *Samāna* retains the end products of digestion until their absorption is complete, and thereafter it allows the undigested portion to be transported into the cecum by peristalsis, which is controlled by *apāna*.

All food elements are carried by the blood and are concentrated in the extracellular fluid around the cells. The nutrients are absorbed into the cells according to their needs. The carrying of the nutrients by the blood and their concentration in the extracellular fluid are effected by *samāna*. *Prāṇa* helps the action of *samāna* by controlling the contraction of the heart. The nutrients are absorbed into the cells from the extracellular fluid through the cell members by the processes of diffusion and active transport. These processes are controlled by *vyāna*. Water metabolism is controlled, by *prāṇa*. *Samāna* also plays a role in the water distribution. The utilization of the absorbed nutrients by the cells is under the control of *samāna*. *Vyāna* controls cellular growth. The general growth of the body is controlled by *apāna*, *samāna,* and *vyāna*. The catabolism of glucose, neutral fat, and amino acids for the liberation of energy is controlled by *prāṇa*. The elimination of carbon dioxide, water, urea, and other wastes of metabolism is controlled by *apāna*.

There are two main types of movements in the colon: haustral contractions, by which the fluid portion of the colon contents is absorbed, and mass peristalsis, which starts in the transverse colon and passes onward, thus pushing the colon contents toward the anus. The haustral contractions are controlled by *prāṇa* and mass peristalsis by *apāna*. Defecation consists of strong mass peristaltic contractions of the rectum and relaxation of the internal and external anal sphincters. The process is helped by the simultaneous contraction of the diaphragm and abdominal and perineal muscles. Defecation is controlled by *apāna*. Formation of urine is controlled by *prāṇa*. Urination is controlled by *apāna*. The circulatory removal of wastes of metabolism is under the control of *samāna*. The skin elimination is controlled by *vyāna*.

The inflow of atmospheric air to the alveoli, transfer of oxygen from the alveoli to the blood; the transport of nutrients and oxygen by the blood to the interstitial fluid; the transport of these substances into the cells, and cell growth—all these belong to the construction process as well as to oxidation, which is the burning process. The removal from the body of carbon dioxide, urea, excess water, and other wastes of metabolism is the elimination process, and cellular development is the firming process. The reduction of mass of the cells and body, and rendering impure substances inactive and attenuated, are the drying process. In all these processes pranic forces are involved. But if the pranic forces are not controlled in their *idā-pingalā* flow by *suṣumnā,* these processes are incomplete and inadequate. To make these processes fully effective, pranic forces are aroused and controlled by appropriate *mantras* in conjunction with breathing. In this manner, deep internal purificatory effects are achieved by Bhūta Śuddhi and the body becomes superpurified.

An Experiment with Sahita

The author conducted an experiment to ascertain the effects of Sahita (Alternate-Nostril Breath Control with Breath Suspension) when combined with a heavy form of developmental exercise. The subjects did a vigorous form of muscular exercise including weightlifting thrice a week, in the evening, and the time devoted to it was from two to three hours. Sahita Breath Control was practiced thrice a day: morning, noon, and evening. On the exercise days, the breath exercise was performed about two hours after the muscular exercise was over.

The diet consisted of raw and cooked vegetables, fruits, small quantities of cereals, and plenty of milk and butter; no meat, fish, or eggs. Three meals were served. Once a week only raw vegetables, fresh fruits, and sour milk were eaten. The body was kept clean internally by various cleansing processes. Sexual continence was strictly observed.

For the students who continued this program for six months, it was found that the general health was excellent, the body full of energy, and the mind cheerful. The development of the size and strength of the muscles was extraordinary. There were no evil aftereffects.

Sahita breath-control exercise is an excellent way to maintain perfect health and to increase the power of concentration. It should be practiced regularly. The right diet should be observed, carefully avoiding overeating. The body should be kept purified internally.

Practice of Breath-Control Exercise

Yoga breath-control exercises are executed while the body is in a stationary attitude. There are also certain breath-control exercises that are done in conjunction with dynamic muscular exercise.

The morning and the evening are the best times for the practice of breath-control exercise. For special purposes, it may also be performed at midday and midnight. Ordinarily, once or twice will be sufficient. In the morning it should be practiced after normal evacuation, oral cleansing, and other appropriate internal cleansing acts. Oral cleansing and nasal cleansing are important before commencing breath-control exercise in the morning. In the evening, it should be done after normal evacuation and a Colonic Auto-Lavage or enema about twice a week in the evening before the practice, which should be done before dinner.

If breath-control exercise is undertaken mainly for physical education purposes, it should be done outdoors. If the weather does not permit this, a well-ventilated, clean room should be selected for the purpose. If breath-control exercise is undertaken for concentration, a secluded but well-ventilated place, free from all disturbances, should be selected.

A number of postures are suitable for the practice of breath-control exercise, particularly the Accomplished Posture, Lotus Posture, and Pleasant Posture (see chapter 20). Of these three, the Lotus Posture is the most suitable, especially for the short-quick type of breath-control exercise. Pleasant Posture is more suitable for beginners and those who have not mastered the Accomplished Posture or Lotus Posture. The traditional seat used in breath-control exercise consists of a *kuia* grass carpet on which is spread a well-tanned deer hide covered with a piece of clean cloth. A suitable cushion of proper size may be utilized.

In certain breath-control exercises it is necessary to keep one of the nostrils closed with a view to doing inhalation or exhalation with a particular nostril. During the period of breath suspension, both nostrils are to be kept closed. For the purpose of closing the nostrils, the ring finger, the little finger, and the thumb of the right hand are used, with the index and middle fingers folded on the palm. The right thumb is used for the right nostril and the right ring finger and little finger for the left nostril. Ugly facial contortions should be avoided during breath-control exercise.

Breath suspension forms the most important part of the long-slow type of breath control, but it is omitted in the preparatory stages. It is only incorporated after the respiratory organs are strengthened and a certain measure of control over them is gained by the practice of the long-slow and short-quick respiratory exercises. The higher forms of breath-control exercise cannot be learned without the help of a teacher. Here we are presenting the less complicated exercises. They are, of course, of immense value and very suitable both for students of physical education and concentration.

Long-Slow Breath-Control Exercise

Assume any of the three folded-leg postures, with the arms extended and the hands placed on the knees. Relax the body and make the mind calm. This may best be achieved by concentrating the mind on the normal breathing movements for a few minutes. These preparations apply to all breath-control exercises. After completion of the exercise relax completely and breathe normally. This also applies to all of the exercises.

Modified Both-Nostrils Breath-Control Exercise (Laghu Ujjāyī) with Abdomen Relaxed

1. Inhale slowly through both nostrils, keeping the glottis partially closed, which will produce a soft sobbing-like sound.
2. At the end of inhalation, exhale slowly through both nostrils without making any sound.
3. The abdomen should be kept relaxed throughout the exercise.

Concentration: On breathing.

Repetitions, Rounds, and Measures: 5 to 21 rounds. Commence with 5 rounds and increase by 2 rounds each week until 21 rounds are reached.

Modified Both-Nostrils Breath-Control Exercise (Laghu Ujjāyī) with Abdomen Retracted

The technique is the same as the Modified Both-Nostrils Breath-Control Exercise with Abdomen Relaxed, with the following difference: the front abdominal wall should be kept slightly retracted throughout both inhalation and exhalation. In exhalation the abdominal wall will naturally be more retracted than in inhalation.

Concentration: On breathing.

Repetitions, Rounds, and Measures: 5 to 21 rounds.

Both-Nostrils Breath-Control Exercise with Breath Suspension (Ujjāyī)

1. Inhale slowly through both nostrils with the soft sobbing-like sound.
2. Then hold the breath with Chin Lock and raise the head up.
3. Finally exhale through both nostrils very slowly without making any sound but retracting the front abdominal wall slightly.

The relative measures of inhalation, suspension, and exhalation are shown below. The counting should be done mentally and slowly, about 1 count per second.

1. Long inhalation–easy suspension–long exhalation.
2. Inspiration 10 counts–suspension 20 counts–long exhalation.
3. Inspiration 20–suspension 40–long exhalation.
4. Inspiration 20–suspension 40–exhalation 40.

Concentration: On breathing.

Repetitions, Rounds, and Measures: 3 to 11 rounds.

Points of Note: The number of rounds should be increased very slowly and a sufficient length of time should be allowed in each stage.

Modified Lingual Breath-Control Exercise (Laghu Śītalī Prāṇāyāma)

1. Roll the tongue lengthwise into a trough and protrude the rolled tongue a little beyond the lips.
2. Inhale slowly through the rolled tongue until the lungs are filled. No straining should be made in inhalation with the object of taking more air into the lungs.
3. Make a swallowing movement and then exhale slowly through both nostrils.

Concentration: On breathing.

Repetitions, Rounds, and Measures: 10 to 50 times. Commence with 10, and increase by 3 each week until you reach 50.

Modified Alternate-Nostril Breath-Control Exercise (Laghu Sahita)

1. Inhale slowly through the left nostril until the lungs are filled, closing the right nostril with the right thumb.
2. At the end of inhalation, exhale slowly through the right nostril, closing the left one with the right ring and little fingers.
3. Then inhale through the right nostril and exhale through the left one. This is one round.

Concentration: On breathing.

Repetitions, Rounds, and Measures: 3 to 21 rounds. Commence with 3 rounds and increase by 1 round each week until 21 rounds are reached.

Alternate-Nostril Breath Control with Breath Suspension (Sahita)

The best posture to assume for Sahita is the Lotus Posture. If the posture is not fully mastered, either of the other two may be adopted. For ordinary students and students of physical education it is sufficient to practice this breath exercise once or twice a day, morning and evening. Advanced students are advised to practice it four times—morning, midday, evening, and midnight—or thrice, omitting the midnight practice.

1. First inhale slowly through the left nostril, closing the right nostril with the right thumb.
2. At the end of inhalation suspend the breath, closing the nostrils with the right thumb and the little and ring fingers. During suspension make Chin Lock, Abdominal Retraction, and Anal Lock.
3. At the end of suspension, raise the head to its normal position, relax the abdomen and the anal region, release the thumb and very slowly exhale through the right nostril without making any sound, closing the left one with the right ring and little fingers.
4. In this manner again inhale through the right nostril, suspend, and exhale through the left nostril. Repeat. After the exercise is over, relax and breathe normally.

Concentration: Either on a chosen object as instructed, with or without *mantra,* or on the respiratory acts.

Repetitions, Rounds, and Measures: One round consists of one inhalation, one suspension, and one exhalation. From 3 to 20 rounds at one sitting is sufficient for ordinary students. Commence with 3 rounds. Increase the rounds very slowly. The relative measures of inhalation–suspension–exhalation for beginners are 1–2–2 and for advanced pupils 1–4–2. In the first case this means that the period of suspension is twice that of inhalation and the period of exhalation is the same as that of suspension. In the second case this means that the period of suspension is four times that of inhalation and the period of exhalation twice that of inhalation.

Progress can be made by slow increases through the stages shown in the following table.

	Inhalation	Suspension	Exhalation
Stage 1	8	16	16
Stage 2	16	32	32
Stage 3	20	40	40
Stage 4	4	16	8
Stage 5	8	32	16
Stage 6	10	40	20
Stage 7	12	48	24
Stage 8	14	56	28
Stage 9	16	64	32

A student who wants to go beyond 16–64–32 requires personal instruction from a competent teacher.

Short-Quick Breath-Control Exercise

The Lotus Posture is the best posture for this type of exercise. The other two postures may be assumed, if the Lotus Posture is not properly mastered. Whatever posture is assumed, the body should be kept erect and relaxed, and the hands on the knees. An attempt should be made to execute short-quick breathing as quickly as possible without, of course, sacrificing thoroughness.

Abdominal Short-Quick Breathing (Kapālabhātī)

1. First, exhale through both nostrils quickly with an inward abdominal push, that is, a quick retraction of the front abdominal wall.
2. This quick exhalation should be immediately followed by quick inhalation through both nostrils with the relaxation of the front abdominal wall.
3. Exhalation and inhalation should go on in a continuous series without any break or any rest between, until a round is complete.

Concentration: On the respiratory act.

Repetitions, Rounds, and Measures: One expulsion a second, 60 a minute, is the mild type of speed. Two expulsions a second, 120 a minute, is the medium type of speed. The rate of 240 or more a minute is the fast type. The beginner should try to attain a 60 a minute rate. In time the student will be able to increase to a rate of 120 a minute, and finally to the rate of 240 expulsions or more per 1 minute. The ordinary round consists of 120 expulsions. This should be attained in a graduated manner, commencing from 20 or 30 expulsions and adding 10 each week until 120 expulsions are reached. Three rounds should be performed at each sitting. At the end of one round the whole body, especially the abdomen, should be relaxed, and normal breathing assumed.

Points of Note: This exercise always commences with exhalation and ends with inhalation. It can be performed either before or after muscular exercise or both before and after. When done before exercise it serves as an excellent warming-up process and drives the idle blood from the abdominal region into general circulation. It may help to lessen the extent of oxygen debt during muscular exercise within certain limits and hasten the recovery period when performed after exercise is over. It may also be practiced in the morning or evening alone.

Thoracic Short-Quick Breathing (Bhastrikā)

The technique is exactly the same as that of Abdominal Short-Quick Breathing with the following exception: the breathing should be done mainly by the intercostal and other thoracic muscles while keeping the abdomen relaxed and unmoved. The real difference between this breathing exercise and Abdominal Short-Quick Breathing is that this is a thoracic type of breath exercise instead of the abdominal type.

Concentration: On the chest and breathing.

Repetitions, Rounds, and Measures: The same as for Abdominal Short-Quick Breathing.

Points of Note: The same as for Abdominal Short-Quick Breathing.

22
Concentration Exercise

A suitable place should be selected for the practice of concentration. A quiet room is the best for beginners. There should be neither too much light nor any disturbing air currents. It should be clean and comfortable and free from any kind of disturbance.

A soft comfortable cushion should be used as a seat. It should be covered with a clean washable piece of cloth. No other person should be allowed to use it.

It is absolutely necessary to adopt a folded-leg posture for the practice of concentration. Real concentration cannot be developed without it. Accomplished Posture, Lotus Posture, and Pleasant Posture are the best. Of the three, Pleasant Posture is the easiest and most suitable for beginners. The posture should first be fully mastered, otherwise it will not be possible to utilize it for the practice of concentration. In other words, there should not be any uneasiness, discomfort, or pain while assuming the posture; rather, it should give you a calm and pleasurable feeling. The body should be straight and fully relaxed during concentration.

The best time for the practice of concentration is the morning and evening. An advanced practioner may also add midnight.

Physical Preparation for Concentration Exercise

The body should be made clean, internally as well as externally, and vital by internal and external baths, a healthy diet, periodic fasting, muscular and breathing exercises, and other measures prescribed in Yoga. If the body is not vigorous and healthy, you cannot make much progress in concentration. The undisturbed condition of the mind demands a body that is energetic, purified, and free from disease.

Overeating is very disturbing and a great hindrance to concentration. Eating unhealthy foods also is a hindrance. Food should be balanced, nutritious, and laxative. Milk, fruits, and vegetables should form an important part of the diet. Abstemious eating is the best. When the colon is loaded with fecal matter and becomes the breeding place of poison-forming bacteria, progress in concentration is very obstructed. Mental restlessness is closely related to a lack of colonic health. Colonic health should be maintained by a good diet, Colonic Auto-Lavage or enemas, and other measures.

The maintaining of vigorous blood movement through every part of the body by some suitable general muscular exercise, in the right amount, creates a very favorable state for concentration. On the other hand, the exercise should not be too fatiguing. If there is excessive fatigue in the body due to heavy exercise, the mind becomes incapable of concentrating. Haṭha Yoga prescribes measured physical education for the development of concentration.

A Method of Developing Concentration Power

There are various methods in Yoga for developing the power of mental concentration. We are presenting here a simple but efficacious method that a student can practice without much difficulty. The method consists of seven stages. It should be practiced stage by stage.

First Stage

1st Day:

1. After normal evacuation and oral cleansing, perform the Gastric Auto-Lavage. It should be followed by a Colonic Auto-Lavage or enema.
2. Then take some form of steam bath such as sauna or similar, to produce copious perspiration. During the steam bath drink a few glasses of warm water. After this take a cleansing bath.
3. Then rest and take a glass of cool water.
4. Another Colonic Auto-Lavage or enema may be taken in the evening.
5. Observe a fast.

2nd Day:

1. Take a Colonic Auto-Lavage or enema in the morning, followed by Gastric Auto-Lavage.
2. After an hour begin drinking warm water at intervals of 45 minutes, 5 or 6 times, one glass each time.
3. Thereafter take a general bath. Then rest.
4. Now and then drink a cup of cool water. In the evening drink a glass of orange juice.

3rd Day:

1. Take a Colonic Auto-Lavage or enema in the morning.
2. Eat the following three meals:
   - 1st Meal: Fresh fruits.
   - 2nd Meal: Milk or buttermilk, fresh acid fruits.
   - 3rd Meal: Same as 2nd meal.

4th to 9th Days:

1. Take a Colonic Auto-Lavage or enema in the evening.
2. Eat the following three meals a day:
   - 1st Meal: Milk, fresh acid fruits.
   - 2nd Meal: Buttermilk, acid and sweet fruits.
   - 3rd Meal: Milk, acid and sweet fruits.

10th Day and thereafter:

1. Eat a normal diet, with three meals a day. Drink a liberal quantity of milk, and eat plenty of fruits and vegetables. Add laxative food. Drink water freely.
2. Take a Colonic Auto-Lavage or enema once or twice a week, in the evening (before dinner).
3. Do Gastric Auto-Lavage about once a week, in the morning. Nasopharyngeal Water Baths may be taken daily in the morning.
4. General exercise should include neck exercise, spinal exercise, and abdominal exercise, in addition to exercise for the rest of the body. An hour's walking at least four times a week is recommended.

5. Once a month observe a complete or partial fast, fruit diet, fruit and milk diet, or milk diet. Take sunbaths and plenty of fresh air.

Cleansing, dieting, and exercising should be continued in all succeeding stages.

Second Stage

Breathing

1. Abdominal Short-Quick Breathing or Thoracic Short-Quick Breathing.
2. Modified Both-Nostrils Breath-Control Exercise.

Gazing

In preparation for this practice, an eye bath can be taken daily at some convenient time, preferably before the practice.

1. Sit in Accomplished Posture. Keep the body erect, with either the hands on the knees or the palms facing upward in your lap. Relax fully.
2. Select a suitable object for your mental concentration. To facilitate your ability to concentrate, use a light yellow-colored card with a black or deep blue circle about a third of an inch in diameter at the center. Fix this center at a proper height, on a level with the space between your eyebrows. The distance to the card is measured by extending the arm forward with the fingers outstretched to touch it. You may use a suitable stand if needed to place the card at the desired height.
3. Gaze on the card without blinking until tears begin to flow. (At the beginning do not gaze so long that tears begin to flow. Start the exercise with one or two minutes of gazing. Then gradually increase the duration until tears come.)
4. Not only the eyes but also the mind should be fixed on the object. The body should be kept motionless during the entire gazing exercise.
5. At the end of gazing, close the eyes and cover them with your cup-shaped hands to keep them in darkness for some time.

Concentration

1. Sit in Accomplished Posture. If unable to do so, assume Pleasant Posture. Place your palms facing upward in your lap. Keep the body erect. Relax every part of your body. Your mind should be joyous and peaceful. Sit for a few minutes calmly. This attitude should be assumed in every succeeding stage.
2. Make a clear mental picture of the full moon. Now close your eyes and mentally place the picture of the full moon in the space between the eyebrows. Concentrate on the moon. Continue concentration for 5 minutes. Gradually increase the time up to 30 minutes or more. After the concentration is over, or when you find concentration too difficult, do not force your mind to concentrate but commence *mantra japa*.

Japa

1. Any convenient posture may be assumed for *japa*.
2. *Japa*, that is, the saying of *mantra*, may be done either mentally, uttered in a very low voice, or said verbally. Here, you should utter your *mantra* in a very low voice so as not to be heard by others. If you have not been initiated and given a particular *mantra*, you can use "AUM." In *japa* it should be pronounced as "ONG." The right pronunciation should be learned from a teacher.
3. The *mantra* should be repeated a minimum of 108 times. You can thus count 108, 208, 508, 1,008, and so on, up to 5,008 if you have time. For counting the number of repetitions, it is convenient to use a garland of beads, made of some suitable material. It should have 100 beads with a separate string containing 8 beads attached to the main string.

4. The *japa* should be done at a moderate speed, neither too quickly, nor too slowly. In doing *japa* you need not think of the meaning of the *mantra*, nor concentrate on any sensory form. Simply think that "AUM" is the divine power in the form of sound and concentrate on the sound. Regular *japa* practice will gradually increase your power of concentration.

Third Stage

Breathing

1. Abdominal Short-Quick Breathing or Thoracic Short-Quick Breathing.
2. Modified Alternate-Nostril Breath-Control Exercise.

Gazing

1. Gaze as per the instructions for the second stage. Your gazing object should be a small ball of the size of an ordinary playing marble of transparent glass, to be placed on a stand at the level of the space between the eyebrows.
2. Gazing should be continued until tears flow.

Concentration

Follow the instructions for concentration for the second stage. The object of concentration should be the moon between the eyebrows. Here more time should be devoted to concentration than in the second stage.

Japa

Follow the instructions for *japa* for the second stage.

Fourth Stage

Breathing

1. Abdominal Short-Quick Breathing or Thoracic Short-Quick Breathing.
2. Modified Alternate-Nostril Breath-Control Exercise.

Gazing

Follow the gazing instructions for the third stage.

Void Thinking

1. Remain in the same posture as was assumed for gazing. Immediately after the gazing is over, close your eyes, fully relax every part of the body, and try to make your mind completely void by allowing, passively, the flow of thoughts to vanish naturally.
2. Relax your mind, discarding calmly all thoughts, and try to be conscious of nothing. The awareness of ego, of any action or thought—of everything—should be dissolved. Try to forget yourself completely, making yourself as though dead. Remain in this mental state as long as you can.

Concentration

Follow the instructions for concentration for the second stage. The object of your concentration is a clear mental image of the moon between the eyebrows.

Japa

Follow the instructions for *japa* for the second stage.

Fifth Stage

Breathing

1. Abdominal Short-Quick Breathing or Thoracic Short-Quick Breathing.
2. Modified Both-Nostrils Breath-Control Exercise.

Gazing

Follow the instructions for gazing for the third stage.

Void Thinking

Follow the instructions for void thinking for the fourth stage.

Sahita (Alternate-Nostril Breath Control with Breath Suspension) with Concentration

Mantra and concentration are added to the process that has been fully described in chapter 21, in the following manner.

1. During inhalation mentally repeat the *mantra* "Ang" 4, 8, or 16 times; use the thumb against the other fingers to count the repetitions. Along with counting, concentrate on the divine form of your choice. Picture the divine form in red, residing inside you at the navel region.
2. During suspension mentally count the *mantra* "Ung" 16, 32, or 64 times and at the same time concentrate on the divine form in blue color at the region of the heart (inside).
3. During exhalation mentally count the *mantra* "Mang" 8, 16, or 32 times and concentrate on your divine form in white inside yourself at the space between the eyebrows.
4. Concentrate on both the mental picture and the *mantra* at the same time. By constant practice you will be able to do it.

Japa

Follow the instructions for *japa* for the second stage.

Sixth Stage

Breathing

1. Abdominal Short-Quick Breathing or Thoracic Short-Quick Breathing.
2. Modified Both-Nostrils Breath-Control Exercise.

Gazing

1. Gaze here on a lit candle, placed so that the flame will be at the level of the space between the eyebrows. The flame should be still. It should not be allowed to move at all.
2. The gazing should be continued until tears flow.

Void Thinking

1. Follow the instructions for void thinking for the fourth stage.
2. After finishing with closed eyes, open the eyes and try not to see anything. This is an extremely difficult form of void thinking, but by constant practice you will be able to do it. When doing this with the eyes open, make yourself void as completely as possible. This is the practice of conscious thoughtlessness.

Sahita (Alternate-Nostril Breath Control with Breath Suspension) with Concentration

Follow the instructions given for the sixth stage.

Japa

Follow the instructions for *japa* for the second stage.

Seventh Stage

This seventh process of concentration is essentially based on Laya Yoga. A student who is seriously thinking of working on this process is advised to take instructions directly from a guru.

Breathing

1. Abdominal Short-Quick Breathing or Thoracic Short-Quick Breathing.
2. Modified Both-Nostrils Breath-Control Exercise.

Gazing

1. The object of gazing should be a lit candle, placed so that the flame will be at the level of the space between the eyebrows. The flame should be perfectly still.
2. The gazing should be continued until tears flow.

Void Thinking

Follow the instructions from the fifth stage for void thinking with and without closed eyes.

Advanced Concentration

1. Sit in Accomplished Posture (fig. 20.1), with the trunk erect, the whole body relaxed, palms upward in the lap.
2. Think that Kuṇḍalinī, the Grand Spiritual Potential, is in a sleeping state, remaining coiled round the *svayambhū,* the static support, in the subtle *mūlādhāra* center situated within the lowest portion of the filum terminale in the upper part of the coccyx. It is the center of the yellow-colored quadrangular Earth principle. Think of Kuṇḍalinī as a subtle white luminous body remaining in a sleeping state.
3. Now bring your "I" to Kuṇḍalinī. Then mentally say "Yang," the sound symbol of the Air principle, and at the same time think that Kuṇḍalinī is agitated by the force of air. Then mentally say "Rang," the sound symbol of the Fire principle, and at the same time think that Kuṇḍalinī is being heated by the force of fire. Then mentally say "Hung," the sound symbol of strength and think that Kuṇḍalinī is being aroused by the strength of the *mantra*. Now think that "Lang," the sound symbol of the Earth principle, has been dissolved in Kuṇḍalinī.
4. Now say "Hangsah" and think that Kuṇḍalinī is rising upward by the force of the *mantra* from the *mūlādhāra* center and enters the second center named *svādhiṣthāna,* situated within the spine at the level of the root of the genitals. It is the center of the white-colored half-moon Water principle, represented by the sound symbol "Wang." Think that "Wang" sinks into Kuṇḍalinī.
5. From here Kuṇḍalinī ascends and enters the third spinal center named *maṇipūra*, situated at the level of the navel region. It is the center of the red-colored triangular Fire principle, represented by the sound symbol "Rang." Think that "Rang" is absorbed into Kuṇḍalinī.
6. Then think that Kuṇḍalinī rises up and enters into the fourth spinal center, named *anāhata,* situated at the level of the heart. It is the center of the smoke-colored, six-cornered Air principle, represented by the sound "Yang." Think that "Yang" is absorbed in Kuṇḍalinī.
7. Think that Kuṇḍalinī ascends and enters the fifth spinal center named *viśuddha* situated at the base of the throat. It is the center of the white-colored circular Ether principle, represented by "Hang." Think that "Hang" is absorbed into Kuṇḍalinī.
8. Think that Kuṇḍalinī rises up into the sixth white-colored center named *ājñā*, situated within the brain (under the cerebrum) at a level of the space between the eyebrows. Think that the subjective and objective aspects of the mind are absorbed in Kuṇḍalinī.
9. Think that Kuṅḍalinī rises up and enters the moon-white thousand-petalled center in the cerebrum. Here resides the Grand Static Consciousness, named Parama Śiva—the birthless, deathless, changeless, and eternal. Think that Kuṇḍalinī becomes united with and dissolved into the Grand Static Consciousness. Try to be in that mental state as long as you can.
10. Now do the Sahita (Alternate-Nostril Breath Control with Breath Suspension), adding the following method of concentration:
    a. During inhalation through the left nostril, mentally count the *mantra* "Yang" 16 times and at the same time think that "Yang" is the manifested power of the Air principle, smoke-colored, with the power to dry impurities within the body.
    b. The inhalation through the left nostril is

immediately followed by suspension. During suspension mentally count "Yang" 64 times, and at the same time deeply think that the inefficient and impure part of the body is being dried up by the power of the *mantra*.

c. The suspension is followed by exhalation through the right nostril. During exhalation mentally count "Yang" 32 times and think that the wastes of your body have been dried up.
d. Then inhale through the right nostril, and at the same time mentally count the red-colored "Rang," the symbol of the Fire principle, 16 times and deeply think that the *mantra* has the burning power. Now suspend for 64 counts of "Rang" and at the same time think that the dried wastes of the body are being burned by the fire generated from "Rang."
e. Then exhale through the left nostril, counting "Rang" 32 times, and at the same time think that the burning of the wastes has been complete.
f. Again inhale through the left nostril, counting the moon-colored *mantra* "Thang" 16 times, and at the same time think that nectar is flowing from the thousand-petalled lotus to all parts of the body.
g. Suspend, counting the white-colored "Wang" 64 times, and at the same time think that a new vital body has been constructed.
h. Then exhale through the right nostril, counting the yellow-colored "Lang" 32 times, and at the same time think that the newly reconstructed body has become firm by the power of "Lang."
i. Now think that your body has become vital, healthy, vigorous, strong, refined, and divine. If you like, you can do a few more rounds of Sahita without *mantras*.
j. Now think that the Grand Static Consciousness lying in the thousand-petalled center and Kuṇḍalinī become one and manifest as the Great Creative Consciousness, the Lord of Known and Unknown. Now give the Lord a human form, that which is most appealing to you and which excites in you a divine feeling, a sacredness, bliss, and peace. Bring that form to the region of your heart, worship it mentally, and mentally do *japa* of the specific *mūlā-mantra* if initiated, otherwise "Oṇg," for 1,008 or 508 times. The minimum is 108 times. You can do more if you feel like it. During the time of *japa* think that the form of the Lord is the Manifested Consciousness, having two aspects—the *mantra* and the form (human shape), and that they are inseparably related to each other. It may be noted here that there are particular forms associated with particular *mūlā-mantras*, which are given to the students by the *guru* (spiritual teacher) during initiation.
k. Now fully concentrate your mind on the Lord without *japa,* and try to be in that state as long as you can, increasing the time of concentration.
l. After finishing the concentration bring the form of the Lord to the thousand-petalled center. Think that Kuṇḍalinī has been separated from the Grand Static Consciousness. Bring Kuṇḍalinī (by thinking) to the *ājñā* center and think that the mind, being purified, comes out from Kuṇḍalinī, and is placed in the center.
m. Then bring Kuṇḍalinī to the *viśuddha* center and replace the purified Ether principle (emerging

from Kuṇḍalinī) there. Next bring Kuṇḍalinī to the *anāhata* center and replace the purified Air principle there. Then bring Kuṅḍalinī to the *maṇipūra* center and replace the purified Fire principle. Now bring Kuṇḍalinī to the *svādhiṡṫhāna* center and replace the purified Water principle there. Finally bring Kuṇḍalinī to the *mūlādhāra* center and replace the purified Earth principle there.

n. Now think that Kuṇḍalinī again goes to her sleeping state. Bring back your "I principle" from Kuṇḍalinī.

Japa

If you have the inclination and time you can do *japa* as in the second stage.

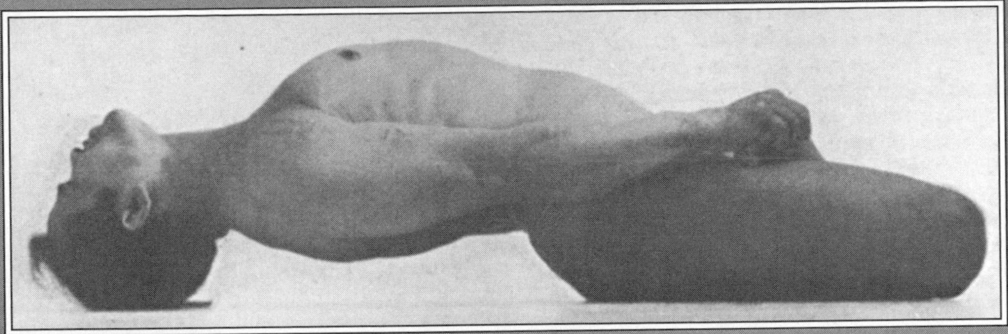

PART THREE

EXERCISE PLANS

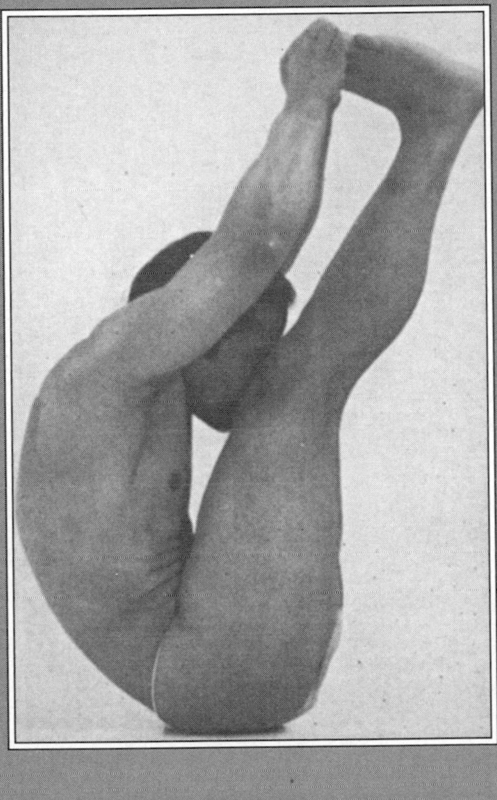

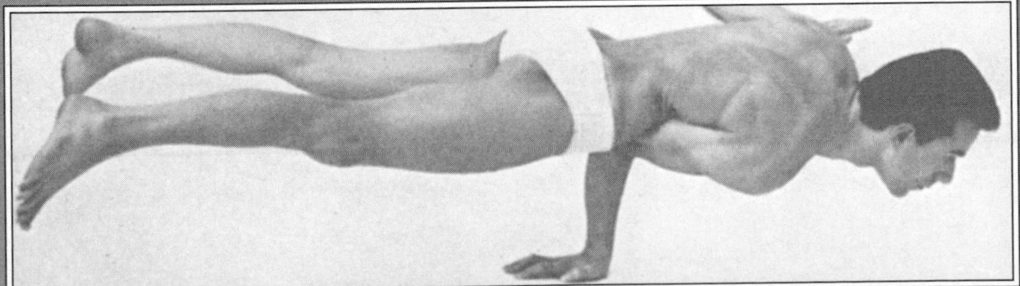

23

General Exercise Plans

The efficacy of exercise greatly depends on the right combination and order. The following exercise plan represents a light, medium, or heavy form of exercise. The exercises may also be made lighter or heavier by the adoptions of low, medium, or high repetition methods. In each plan there should be a definite order of exercise.

To simplify matters, we are here presenting three forms of exercise, with two plans for each form. A suitable plan should be selected, based on your age, gender, health, capacity, previous training, and requirements. Generally speaking, it is always desirable to commence with a light plan of exercise and gradually work toward the heavier plans.

Light Form of Exercise

PLAN 1

Order	Figure	Exercise Name
1	—	Modified Both-Nostrils Breath-Control Exercise with Abdomen Relaxed (5–20 times)
2	—	Neck Flexion-Extension
3	—	Neck Rotation
4	17.7	Toe Posture
5	17.1	Thigh Posture
6	12.1	Cobra Posture
7	—	Modified Locust Posture
8	12.15	Spinal-Stretch Posture
9	14.1	Spine Posture
10	14.17	Head-Knee Spine Posture
11	15.1	Pelvis-Raise Posture
12	18.1	Eagle Posture
13	—	Modified Lingual Breath-Control Exercise (10 to 30 times)

Relaxation in Corpse Posture

PLAN 2

Order	Figure	Exercise Name
1	—	Modified Both-Nostrils Breath-Control Exercise with Abdomen Relaxed (20 times)
2	14.23	Abdominal Retraction
3	—	Neck Flexion-Extension
4	—	Neck Rotation
5	17.7	Toe Posture
6	17.1	Thigh Posture
7	12.1	Cobra Posture

8	12.2	Snake Posture
9	12.4	Locust Posture
10	12.5	Bow Posture
11	12.15	Spinal-Stretch Posture
12	12.25	Twist Posture
13	12.22	Half-Moon Posture
14	14.2	Spine Posture with Hands Clasped behind Head
15	14.5	Oblique Spine Posture
16	14.9	Plow Posture
17	12.9	Cuckoo Posture
18	16.1	Risen Lotus Posture
19	16.9	Arm Motion
20	16.4	Four-Point Posture
21	15.3	Single Foot-Head Posture
22	18.9	Peacock Posture
23	—	Modified Lingual Breath-Control Exercise (30 times)

Relaxation in Corpse Posture

Medium Form of Exercise

PLAN 1

Order	Figure	Exercise Name
1	—	Modified Both-Nostrils Breath-Control Exercise with Abdomen Retracted (20 times)
2	14.23	Abdominal Retraction
3	—	Neck Flexion-Extension
4	—	Neck Rotation
5	17.7	Toe Posture
6	17.1	Thigh Posture
7	17.3	Feet-Extending Thigh Posture
8	12.2	Snake Posture
9	12.7	Swing Posture
10	12.15	Spinal-Stretch Posture
11	12.23	Hip-Bend Posture
12	12.26	Modified Spinal-Twist Posture
13	14.18	Knee-Touching Spine Posture
14	14.6	Oblique Spine Posture with Hands Clasped behind Head
15	14.10	Plow Posture with Forearms Locked behind Head
16	16.2	Cock Posture
17	15.5	Single Foot-Head Head-Knee Posture
18	18.3	Wing Posture
19	—	Modified Lingual Breath-Control Exercise (30 times)

Relaxation in Corpse Posture

PLAN 2

Order	Figure	Exercise Name
1	—	Modified Both-Nostrils Breath-Control Exercise with Abdomen Retracted or Relaxed (20 times)
2	14.23	Abdominal Retraction
3	14.24	Straight Muscle Exercise
4	—	Neck Flexion-Extension
5	13.1	Neck Posture
6	17.7	Toe Posture
7	17.5	Leg-Raise Thigh Posture
8	12.11	Bent-Head Adamantine Posture
9	12.15	Spinal-Stretch Posture
10	12.17	Forward Head-Bend Posture
11	12.3	Back-Raise Posture with Forearms Locked behind Head
12	12.27	Ankle-Hold Modified Spinal-Twist Posture
13	14.3	Spine Posture with Forearms Locked behind Head
14	14.7	Oblique Spine Posture with Forearms Locked behind Head
15	14.14	Risen Leg Posture
16	16.4	Four-Point Posture
17	16.6	Arm-Leg Posture
18	15.7	Pillar Posture
19	15.5	Single Foot-Head Head-Knee Posture
20	18.8	Mountain Posture
21	18.7	Standing Leg-Stretch Posture
22	—	Abdominal Short-Quick Breathing
23	—	Modified Lingual Breath-Control Exercise (30 times)

Relaxation in Corpse Posture

Heavy Form of Exercise

PLAN 1

Order	Figure	Exercise Name
1	—	Modified Both-Nostrils Breath-Control Exercise
2	14.23	Abdominal Retraction
3	14.24	Straight Muscle Exercise
4	—	Neck Flexion-Extension
5	13.2	Neck-Bridge Posture
6	17.8	One-Legged Toe Posture
7	17.5	Leg-Raise Thigh Posture
8	12.3	Back-Raise Posture with Forearms Locked behind Head
9	12.13	Back Posture
10	12.21a	Foot-Hand Posture
11	12.18	Head-Bend Posture
12	12.31	Sideward Head-Bend Posture
13	14.12	Risen Back Posture
14	14.19	Pillow Posture
15	16.6	Arm-Leg Posture
16	16.7	Opposite Arm-Leg Posture
17	15.4	Double Foot-Head Posture
18	18.15	Scorpion Posture
19	—	Abdominal Short-Quick Breathing
20	—	Modified Lingual Breath-Control Exercise (30 times)

Relaxation in Corpse Posture

PLAN 2

Order	Figure	Exercise Name
1	—	Modified Both-Nostrils Breath-Control Exercise with Abdomen Retracted or Relaxed (20 times)
2	14.23	Abdominal Retraction
3	14.24	Straight Muscle Exercise
4	—	Neck Flexion-Extension
5	13.2	Neck-Bridge Posture
6	17.8	One-Legged Toe Posture
7	17.6	One-Legged Squat Posture
8	12.8	King-Cobra Posture
9	12.14	Wheel Posture
10	12.21a	Foot-Hand Posture
11	12.24	Moon Posture
12	12.29	Spinal-Twist Posture
13	14.4	Risen Balance Posture
14	14.20	Toe-Hold Lateral Spine Posture
15	14.7	Oblique Spine Posture with Forearms Locked behind Head
16	16.1	Risen Lotus Posture
17	16.7	Opposite Arm-Leg Posture
18	16.8	Arm Posture
19	15.8	Noose Posture
20	18.12	One-Arm Rolling Posture
21	18.15	Scorpion Posture
22	—	Abdominal Short-Quick Breathing
23	—	Modified Lingual Breath-Control Exercise (30 times)

Relaxation in Corpse Posture

24

Specific Dynamic Exercise Plans and Daily Schedules

Specific exercise is mainly intended for developing a particular part of the body to a high standard and for specific results. For the best results specific exercise should be combined with general exercise. Specific exercise may either be incorporated into the general exercise plan or done separately, according to individual requirements.

Specific exercise is classified as spinal posture exercise, neck posture exercise, abdominal posture exercise, pelvic posture exercise, pectoral limb posture exercise, and pelvic limb posture exercise. When specific exercise is combined with general exercise and practiced at the same time, the exercises that are in the specific group may be omitted from the general group. But if specific exercises are practiced separately, at some other time, it is not necessary to eliminate them from the general exercise plans. As with the general plans, each type given below has two plans of increasing difficulty.

Dynamic Spinal Posture Exercise

PLAN 1

Order	Figure	Exercise Name	Repetition
1	—	Modified Both-Nostrils Breath-Control Exercise with Abdomen Retracted or Relaxed	10–20 times
2	12.1	Cobra Posture	10–20 times
3	12.4	Locust Posture	8–16 times
4	12.5	Bow Posture	10–20 times
5	12.21a	Foot-Hand Posture	10–20 times
6	12.15	Spinal-Stretch Posture	10–20 times
7	12.22	Half-Moon Posture	10–20 times
8	12.25	Twist Posture	10–20 times
9	12.26	Modified Spinal-Twist Posture	6–12 times
10	—	Modified Lingual Breath-Control Exercise	15–30 times

Relaxation in Corpse Posture

PLAN 2

Order	Figure	Exercise Name	Repetition
1	—	Modified Both-Nostrils Breath-Control Exercise with Abdomen Retracted or Relaxed	10–20 times
2	12.1	Cobra Posture	5–10 times
3	12.2	Snake Posture	5–10 times
4	12.4	Locust Posture	3–5 times
5	12.11	Bent-Head Adamantine Posture	3–5 times
6	12.17	Forward Head-Bend Posture	3–5 times
7	12.12	Modified Wheel Posture	3–5 times
8	12.13	Back Posture	3–5 times
9	12.14	Wheel Posture	3–5 times
10	12.21a	Foot-Hand Posture	5–10 times
11	12.18	Head-Bend Posture	3–5 times
12	12.20	Forward Body-Bend Posture	3–5 times
13	12.22	Half-Moon Posture	3–5 times
14	12.23	Hip-Bend Posture	3–5 times
15	12.24	Moon Posture	3–5 times
16	12.31	Sideward Head-Bend Posture	3–5 times
17	12.27	Ankle-Hold Modified Spinal-Twist Posture	3–5 times
18	12.29	Spinal-Twist Posture	3–5 times
19	—	Modified Lingual Breath-Control Exercise	15–30 times

Relaxation in Corpse Posture

Dynamic Neck Posture Exercise

PLAN 1

Order	Figure	Exercise Name	Repetition
1	—	Modified Both-Nostrils Breath-Control Exercise with Abdomen Retracted or Relaxed	10–20 times
2	—	Neck Flexion-Extension	10–20 times
3	—	Neck Rotation	10–20 times
4	—	Lateral Neck Flexion	10–20 times
5	—	Modified Lingual Breath-Control Exercise	15–30 times

Relaxation in Corpse Posture

PLAN 2

Order	Figure	Exercise Name	Repetition
1	—	Modified Both-Nostrils Breath-Control Exercise with Abdomen Retracted or Relaxed	10–20 times
2	—	Neck Flexion-Extension	25–50 times
3	—	Neck Rotation	25–50 times
4	—	Lateral Neck Flexion	25–50 times
5	13.1	Neck Posture	10–20 times
6	13.2	Neck-Bridge Posture	10–20 times
7	—	Modified Lingual Breath-Control Exercise	15–30 times

Relaxation in Corpse Posture

Dynamic Abdominal Posture Exercise

PLAN 1

Order	Figure	Exercise Name	Repetition
1	—	Modified Both-Nostrils Breath-Control Exercise with Abdomen Retracted or Relaxed	10–20 times
2	14.1	Spine Posture	10–20 times
3	14.2	Spine Posture with Hands Clasped behind Head	10–20 times
4	14.5	Oblique Spine Posture	10–20 times
5	14.9	Plow Posture	10–20 times
6	14.15	Sideward Leg-Motion Posture	10–20 times
7	14.17	Head-Knee Spine Posture	10–20 times
8	14.18	Knee-Touching Spine Posture	10–20 times
9	12.5	Bow Posture	10–20 times
10	12.6	Boat Posture	10–20 times
11	—	Modified Lingual Breath-Control Exercise	15–30 times

Relaxation in Corpse Posture

PLAN 2

Order	Figure	Exercise Name	Repetition
1	—	Modified Both-Nostrils Breath-Control Exercise with Abdomen Retracted or Relaxed	15–30 times
2	14.23	Abdominal Retraction	50–100 times
3	14.24	Straight Muscle Exercise	50–100 times
4	14.2	Spine Posture with Hands Clasped behind Head	3–6 times
5	14.3	Spine Posture with Forearms Locked behind Head	3–6 times
6	14.4	Risen Balance Posture	3–6 times
7	14.6	Oblique Spine Posture with Hands Clasped behind Head	3–6 times
8	14.7	Oblique Spine Posture with Forearms Locked behind Head	3–6 times
9	14.9	Plow Posture	3–6 times
10	14.10	Plow Posture with Forearms Locked behind Head	3–6 times
11	14.12	Risen Back Posture	3–6 times
12	14.14	Risen Leg Posture	3–6 times
13	14.13	Lotus-Plow Posture	3–6 times
14	14.18	Knee-Touching Spine Posture	3–6 times
15	14.19	Pillow Posture	3–6 times
16	14.8	Lateral Spine Posture	3–6 times
17	14.20	Toe-Hold Lateral Spine Posture	3–6 times
18	12.5	Bow Posture	5–10 times
19	12.14	Wheel Posture	3–6 times
20	—	Modified Lingual Breath-Control Exercise	15–30 times

Relaxation in Corpse Posture

Dynamic Pelvic Posture Exercise

PLAN 1

Order	Figure	Exercise Name	Repetition
1	—	Modified Both-Nostrils Breath-Control Exercise with Abdomen Retracted or Relaxed	10–20 times
2	15.1	Pelvis-Raise Posture	15–30 times
3	15.2	Arm-Head Posture	10–20 times
4	15.3	Single Foot-Head Posture	10–20 times
5	15.6	One-Leg Pillar Posture	10–20 times
6	15.7	Pillar Posture	10–20 times
7	—	Modified Lingual Breath-Control Exercise	15–30 times

Relaxation in Corpse Posture

PLAN 2

Order	Figure	Exercise Name	Repetition
1	—	Modified Both-Nostrils Breath-Control Exercise with Abdomen Retracted or Relaxed	10–20 times
2	15.1	Pelvis-Raise Posture	10–20 times
3	15.3	Single Foot-Head Posture	3–6 times
4	15.5	Single Foot-Head Head-Knee Posture	3–6 times
5	15.4	Double Foot-Head Posture	3–6 times
6	15.6	One-Leg Pillar Posture	3–6 times
7	15.7	Pillar Posture	3–6 times
8	15.8	Noose Posture	3–6 times
9	—	Anal Exercise	250–500 times
10	—	Modified Lingual Breath-Control Exercise	15–30 times

Relaxation in Corpse Posture

Dynamic Pectoral Limb Posture Exercise

PLAN 1

Order	Figure	Exercise Name	Repetition
1	—	Modified Both-Nostrils Breath-Control Exercise with Abdomen Retracted or Relaxed	10–20 times
2	16.1	Risen Lotus Posture	10–20 times
3	16.2	Cock Posture	10–20 times
4	16.9	Arm Motion	15–30 times
5	16.4	Four-Point Posture	15–30 times
6	16.5	Three-Footed Posture	10–20 times
7	—	Modified Lingual Breath-Control Exercise	15–30 times

Relaxation in Corpse Posture

PLAN 2

Order	Figure	Exercise Name	Repetition
1	—	Modified Both-Nostrils Breath-Control Exercise with Abdomen Retracted or Relaxed	10–20 times
2	16.1	Risen Lotus Posture	10–20 times
3	16.2	Cock Posture	10–20 times
4	16.3	One-Arm Cock Posture	5–10 times
5	16.9	Arm Motion	10–20 times
6	16.4	Four-Point Posture	30–50 times
7	16.5	Three-Footed Posture	15–30 times
8	16.6	Arm-Leg Posture	15–30 times
9	16.7	Opposite Arm-Leg Posture	15–30 times
10	16.8	Arm Posture	10–20 times
11	—	Modified Lingual Breath-Control Exercise	15–30 times

Relaxation in Corpse Posture

Dynamic Pelvic Limb Posture Exercise

PLAN 1

Order	Figure	Exercise Name	Repetition
1	—	Modified Both-Nostrils Breath-Control Exercise with Abdomen Retracted or Relaxed	10–20 times
2	17.1	Thigh Posture	30–50 times
3	17.2	Knee-Touching Thigh Posture	10–20 times
4	17.3	Feet-Extending Thigh Posture	10–20 times
5	17.4	Sideward Feet-Extending Thigh Posture	10–20 times
6	17.7	Toe Posture	20–40 times
7	—	Modified Lingual Breath-Control Exercise	15–30 times

Relaxation in Corpse Posture

PLAN 2

Order	Figure	Exercise Name	Repetition
1	—	Modified Both-Nostrils Breath-Control Exercise with Abdomen Retracted or Relaxed	10–20 times
2	17.1	Thigh Posture	25–50 times
3	17.3	Feet-Extending Thigh Posture	15–30 times
4	17.4	Sideward Feet-Extending Thigh Posture	15–30 times
5	17.5	Leg-Raise Thigh Posture	10–20 times
6	17.6	One-Legged Squat Posture	10–20 times
7	17.7	Toe Posture	20–40 times
8	17.8	One-Legged Toe Posture	10–20 times
9	—	Modified Lingual Breath-Control Exercise	15–30 times

Relaxation in Corpse Posture

Daily Schedule

According to general physical condition, previous training, the extent of muscular development, individual requirements, age, and sex, a suitable schedule may be selected and followed.

SCHEDULE 1

Day	Morning	Evening
Monday	Breath-Control Exercise	General Posture Exercise (Light Form)
Tuesday	Breath-Control Exercise	General Posture Exercise (Light Form)
Wednesday	Breath-Control Exercise	Walking or other Constitutional Exercise
Thursday	Breath-Control Exercise	General Posture Exercise (Light Form)
Friday	Breath-Control Exercise	General Posture Exercise (Light Form)
Saturday	Breath-Control Exercise	Distance Walking
Sunday	Breath-Control Exercise	Rest

SCHEDULE 2

Day	Morning	Evening
Monday	Breath-Control Exercise	General Posture Exercise (Medium Form)
Tuesday	Breath-Control Exercise	General Posture Exercise (Medium Form)
Wednesday	Breath-Control Exercise	Walking or other Constitutional Exercise
Thursday	Breath-Control Exercise	General Posture Exercise (Medium Form)
Friday	Breath-Control Exercise	General Posture Exercise (Medium Form)
Saturday	Breath-Control Exercise	Distance Walking or Swimming
Sunday	Breath-Control Exercise	Rest

SCHEDULE 3

Day	Morning	Evening
Monday	Breath-Control Exercise	General Posture Exercise (Heavy Form)
Tuesday	Breath-Control Exercise	General Posture Exercise (Heavy Form)
Wednesday	Breath-Control Exercise	Walking or other Constitutional Exercise
Thursday	Breath-Control Exercise	General Posture Exercise (Heavy Form)
Friday	Breath-Control Exercise	General Posture Exercise (Heavy Form)
Saturday	Breath-Control Exercise	Distance Walking or Swimming
Sunday	Breath-Control Exercise	Rest

SCHEDULE 4

Day	Morning	Evening
Monday	Breath-Control Exercise, Abdominal Retraction, Straight Muscle Exercise	General Posture Exercise (Light, Medium, or Heavy Form according to necessity, and so on)
Tuesday	Breath-Control Exercise, Abdominal Retraction, Straight Muscle Exercise	General Posture Exercise (Light, Medium, or Heavy Form according to necessity, and so on)
Wednesday	Breath-Control Exercise, Abdominal Retraction, Straight Muscle Exercise	Walking or other Constitutional Exercise
Thursday	Breath-Control Exercise, Abdominal Retraction, Straight Muscle Exercise	General Posture Exercise (Light, Medium, or Heavy Form according to necessity, and so on)

Friday	Breath-Control Exercise, Abdominal Retraction, Straight Muscle Exercise	General Posture Exercise (Light, Medium, or Heavy Form according to necessity, and so on)
Saturday	Breath-Control Exercise, Abdominal Retraction, Straight Muscle Exercise	Distance Walking or Swimming
Sunday	Breath-Control Exercise	Rest

SCHEDULE 5

Day	Morning	Evening
Monday	Breath-Control Exercise, Abdominal Retraction, Straight Muscle Exercise	General Posture Exercise (Heavy Form)
Tuesday	Breath-Control Exercise, Abdominal Retraction, Straight Muscle Exercise	General Posture Exercise (Medium Form)
Wednesday	Breath-Control Exercise, Abdominal Retraction, Straight Muscle Exercise	Walking or other Constitutional Exercise
Thursday	Breath-Control Exercise, Abdominal Retraction, Straight Muscle Exercise	General Posture Exercise (Light Form)
Friday	Breath-Control Exercise, Abdominal Retraction, Straight Muscle Exercise	General Posture Exercise (Light, Medium, or Heavy Form according to necessity, and so on)
Saturday	Breath-Control Exercise, Abdominal Retraction, Straight Muscle Exercise	Distance Walking, Running, or Swimming
Sunday	Breath-Control Exercise	Rest

SCHEDULE 6

Day	Morning	Evening
Monday	Breath-Control Exercise, Abdominal Retraction, Straight Muscle Exercise	General Posture Exercise and Specific Posture Exercise
Tuesday	Breath-Control Exercise, Abdominal Retraction, Straight Muscle Exercise	General Posture Exercise
Wednesday	Breath-Control Exercise, Abdominal Retraction, Straight Muscle Exercise	Walking or other Constitutional Exercise
Thursday	Breath-Control Exercise, Abdominal Retraction, Straight Muscle Exercise	General Posture Exercise
Friday	Breath-Control Exercise, Abdominal Retraction, Straight Muscle Exercise	General Posture Exercise and Specific Posture Exercise
Saturday	Breath-Control Exercise, Abdominal Retraction, Straight Muscle Exercise	Distance Walking, Running, or Swimming
Sunday	Breath-Control Exercise	Rest

SCHEDULE 7

Day	Morning	Evening
Monday	Specific Posture Exercise	General Posture Exercise
Tuesday	Specific Posture Exercise	General Posture Exercise
Wednesday	Breath-Control Exercise	Walking or other Constitutional Exercise
Thursday	Specific Posture Exercise	General Posture Exercise
Friday	Specific Posture Exercise	General Posture Exercise
Saturday	Breath-Control Exercise	Distance Walking, Running, or Swimming
Sunday	Breath-Control Exercise	Rest

SCHEDULE 8

Day	Morning	Evening
Monday	Specific Posture Exercise	General Posture Exercise
Tuesday	Breath-Control Exercise	General Posture Exercise
Wednesday	Specific Posture Exercise	Walking or other Constitutional Exercise
Thursday	Breath-Control Exercise	General Posture Exercise
Friday	Specific Posture Exercise	General Posture Exercise
Saturday	Breath-Control Exercise	Distance Walking, Running, or Swimming
Sunday	Breath-Control Exercise	Rest

SCHEDULE 9

Day	Evening
Monday	General Posture Exercise
Tuesday	General Posture Exercise
Wednesday	General Posture Exercise
Thursday	General Posture Exercise
Friday	General Posture Exercise
Saturday	Distance Walking
Sunday	Complete Rest

Points of Note: Constitutional exercise may be taken 3 or 4 times a week in the morning or any other suitable time.

SCHEDULE 10

Day	Evening
Monday	General Posture Exercise
Tuesday	Constitutional Exercise
Wednesday	General Posture Exercise
Thursday	Constitutional Exercise
Friday	General Posture Exercise
Saturday	Distance Walking
Sunday	Complete Rest

25

Static Exercise Plans and Daily Schedules

Static exercise plans may be divided into light, medium, and heavy forms. Here two plans are given for each form. You are advised to practice static exercise in a graduated manner, from the light to the heavy forms. In selecting a plan, the individual's age, sex, general health, capacity, previous training, and requirements should be carefully considered. It is always desirable to begin with a lighter plan and gradually work toward a heavier one. The repetition method may be adopted according to the individual condition and requirements.

For your convenience, the maximum time period for holding each posture in these plans is given in exact minutes. You may go still higher if you wish and are well prepared. See chapter 6.

It is an advantage if you first perform certain dynamic exercises before commencing static exercises. The following is a group of dynamic exercises that should be done before static exercises are commenced. This group, termed "fundamental dynamic exercises," is included in each plan.

FUNDAMENTAL DYNAMIC EXERCISES

Order	Figure	Exercise Name
1	14.23	Abdominal Retraction
2	14.24	Straight Muscle Exercise
3	—	Neck Flexion-Extension
4	17.7	Toe Posture
5	17.1	Thigh Posture
6	14.18	Knee-Touching Spine Posture
7	12.6	Boat Posture

Light Form of Exercise

PLAN 1

Order	Figure	Exercise Name	Time Period
1	—	Modified Both-Nostrils Breath-Control Exercise with Abdomen Retracted or Relaxed	10–20 times
2	—	Fundamental Dynamic Exercises	—
3	—	Modified Lingual Breath-Control Exercise	15–30 times

4	—	Relaxation in Corpse Posture	10 mins.
5	12.1	Cobra Posture	Up to 2 mins.
6	12.2	Snake Posture	Up to 2 mins.
7	12.15	Spinal-Stretch Posture	Up to 3 mins.
8	12.21a	Foot-Hand Posture	Up to 1 min.
9	12.26	Modified Spinal-Twist Posture	Up to 2 mins.
10	14.1	Spine Posture	Up to 1 min.
11	14.9	Plow Posture	Up to 3 mins.
12	15.1	Pelvis-Raise Posture	Up to 2 mins.
13	18.1	Eagle Posture	Up to 1 min.
14	19.1	Inversion Posture	Up to 6 mins.
15	—	Abdominal Short-Quick Breathing	—
16	—	Relaxation in Corpse Posture	10 mins.
17	20.3	Concentration in Pleasant Posture	—

PLAN 2

Order	Figure	Exercise Name	Time Period
1	—	Modified Both-Nostrils Breath-Control Exercise with Abdomen Retracted or Relaxed	Rep. 10–20 times
2	—	Fundamental Dynamic Exercises	—
3	—	Modified Lingual Breath-Control Exercise	Rep. 15–30 times
4	—	Relaxation in Corpse Posture	10 mins.
5	12.1	Cobra Posture	Up to 2 mins.
6	12.9	Cuckoo Posture	Up to 2 mins.
7	12.5	Bow Posture	Up to 2 mins.
8	12.19	Head-Bend Lotus Posture	Up to 1 min.
9	12.15	Spinal-Stretch Posture	Up to 3 mins.
10	12.27	Ankle-Hold Modified Spinal-Twist Posture	Up to 3 mins.
11	14.9	Plow Posture	Up to 4 mins.
12	14.22	Bent-Knee Inverse Lotus Posture	Up to 1 min.
13	15.5	Single Foot-Head Head-Knee Posture	Up to 1 min.
14	16.2	Cock Posture	Up to 2 mins.
15	17.2	Knee-Touching Thigh Posture	Up to 1 min.
16	18.4	Bent-Head Wing Posture	Up to 1 min.
17	18.5	Knee-Heel Posture	Up to 1 min.
18	19.4	Inverse Lotus Posture	Up to 6 mins.
19	—	Abdominal Short-Quick Breathing	—
20	—	Relaxation in Corpse Posture	10 mins.
21	20.1	Concentration in Accomplished Posture	—

Medium Form of Exercise

PLAN 1

Order	Figure	Exercise Name	Time Period
1	—	Modified Both-Nostrils Breath-Control Exercise with Abdomen Retracted or Relaxed	Rep. 10–20 times
2	—	Fundamental Dynamic Exercises	—
3	—	Modified Lingual Breath-Control Exercise	Rep. 15–30 times
4	—	Relaxation in Corpse Posture	10 mins.
5	12.1	Cobra Posture	Up to 3 mins.
6	12.3	Back-Raise Posture with Forearms Locked behind Head	Up to 2 mins.
7	12.15	Spinal-Stretch Posture	Up to 5 mins.
8	12.17	Forward Head-Bend Posture	Up to 2 mins.

9	12.23	Hip-Bend Posture	Up to 2 mins.
10	12.32	Fish Posture	Up to 2 mins.
11	13.2	Neck-Bridge Posture	Up to 2 mins.
12	14.3	Spine Posture with Forearms Locked behind Head	Up to 2 mins.
13	14.10	Plow Posture with Forearms Locked behind Head	Up to 3 mins.
14	17.5	Leg-Raise Thigh Posture	Up to 2 mins.
15	18.6	Standing Single Foot-Head Posture	Up to 1 min.
16	18.8	Mountain Posture	Up to 2 mins.
17	15.9	Happy Posture	Up to 2 mins.
18	19.1	Inversion Posture	Up to 15 mins.
19	—	Abdominal Short-Quick Breathing	—
20	—	Relaxation in Corpse Posture	10 mins.
21	20.2	Concentration in Lotus Posture	—

PLAN 2

Order	Figure	Exercise Name	Time Period
1	—	Modified Both-Nostrils Breath-Control Exercise with Abdomen Retracted or Relaxed	—
2	—	Fundamental Dynamic Exercises	—
3	—	Modified Lingual Breath-Control Exercise	—
4	—	Relaxation in Corpse Posture	—
5	12.1	Cobra Posture	Up to 4 mins.
6	12.4	Locust Posture	Up to 1 min.
7	12.5	Bow Posture	Up to 3 mins.
8	12.15	Spinal-Stretch Posture	Up to 6 mins.
9	12.17	Forward Head-Bend Posture	Up to 3 mins.
10	12.27	Ankle-Hold Modified Spinal-Twist Posture	Up to 4 mins.
11	14.10	Plow Posture with Forearms Locked behind Head	Up to 4 mins.
12	16.2	Cock Posture	Up to 3 mins.
13	18.11	Rolling Posture	Up to 2 mins.
14	18.15	Scorpion Posture	Up to 1 min.
15	15.9	Happy Posture	Up to 4 mins.
16	—	Anal Lock	Up to 1 min. each, 12 times
17	19.1	Inversion Posture or	Up to 15 mins.
	19.3	Head Posture	Up to 20 mins.
18	—	Modified Alternate-Nostril Breath-Control Exercise	—
19	—	Abdominal Short-Quick Breathing	—
20	—	Relaxation in Corpse Posture	10 mins.
21	20.2	Concentration in Lotus Posture or	—
	20.1	Accomplished Posture	—

Heavy Form of Exercise

PLAN 1

Order	Figure	Exercise Name	Time Period
1	—	Modified Both-Nostrils Breath-Control Exercise with Abdomen Retracted or Relaxed	Rep. 10–20 times
2	—	Fundamental Dynamic Exercises	—
3	—	Modified Lingual Breath-Control Exercise	Rep. 15–30 times
4	—	Relaxation in Corpse Posture	10 mins.

5	12.1	Cobra Posture	Up to 6 mins.
6	12.8	King-Cobra Posture	Up to 3 mins.
7	12.15	Spinal-Stretch Posture	Up to 6 mins.
8	12.18	Head-Bend Posture	Up to 3 mins.
9	12.24	Moon Posture	Up to 3 mins.
10	12.29	Spinal-Twist Posture	Up to 2 mins.
11	14.12	Risen Back Posture	Up to 2 mins.
12	14.19	Pillow Posture	Up to 2 mins.
13	15.4	Double Foot-Head Posture	Up to 2 mins.
14	—	Anal Lock	Up to 1 min. each, 12 times
15	18.12	One-Arm Rolling Posture	Up to 2 mins.
16	19.1	Inversion Posture	Up to 30 mins.
17	—	Abdominal Short-Quick Breathing	—
18	—	Modified Both-Nostrils Breath-Control Exercise with Breath Suspension	—
19	—	Relaxation in Corpse Posture	10 mins.
20	20.4	Concentration in Toe-Hold Lotus Posture	—

PLAN 2

Order	Figure	Exercise Name	Time Period
1	—	Modified Both-Nostrils Breath-Control Exercise with Abdomen Retracted or Relaxed	—
2	—	Fundamental Dynamic Exercises	—
3	—	Modified Lingual Breath-Control Exercise	—
4	—	Relaxation in Corpse Posture	—
5	—	Chin Lock	Up to 2 mins.
6	12.32	Fish Posture	Up to 6 mins.
7	12.1	Cobra Posture	Up to 6 mins.
8	12.8	King-Cobra Posture	Up to 3 mins.
9	12.15	Spinal-Stretch Posture	Up to 6 mins.
10	12.20	Forward Body-Bend Posture	Up to 3 mins.
11	12.24	Moon Posture	Up to 3 mins.
12	12.29	Spinal-Twist Posture	Up to 3 mins.
13	14.3	Spine Posture with Forearms Locked behind Head	Up to 2 mins.
14	14.10	Plow Posture with Forearms Locked behind Head	Up to 6 mins.
15	14.19	Pillow Posture	Up to 3 mins.
16	15.4	Double Foot-Head Posture	Up to 3 mins.
17	15.9	Happy Posture	Up to 6 mins.
18	—	Anal Lock	Up to 1 min. each, 12 times
19	16.2	Cock Posture	Up to 3 mins.
20	18.11	Rolling Posture	Up to 3 mins.
21	19.3	Head Posture	Up to 30 mins.
22	—	Abdominal Short-Quick Breathing	—
23	—	Modified Both-Nostrils Breath-Control Exercise with Breath Suspension	—
24	—	Relaxation in Corpse Posture	10 mins.
25	20.1	Concentration in Accomplished Posture	—
		or	
	20.2	Lotus Posture	—
		or	
	20.4	Toe-Hold Lotus Posture	—

Daily Schedule

You may follow a suitable training schedule according to your general physical condition, previous training, extent of muscular development, personal requirements, age, and gender. With the regular practice of dynamic exercises some of the exercises from the fundamental dynamic group may be found superfluous.

SCHEDULE 1

Day	Morning	Evening
Monday	Static Exercise	Dynamic Exercise (general)
Tuesday	Static Exercise	Dynamic Exercise (general)
Wednesday	Static Exercise	Walking or other Constitutional Exercise
Thursday	Static Exercise	Dynamic Exercise (general)
Friday	Static Exercise	Dynamic Exercise (general)
Saturday	Static Exercise	Distance Walking, Swimming, and so on
Sunday	Breath-Control Exercise	Rest

SCHEDULE 2

Day	Morning	Evening
Monday	Static Exercise	Dynamic Exercise (general and specific)
Tuesday	Static Exercise	Dynamic Exercise (general)
Wednesday	Static Exercise	Walking or other Constitutional Exercise
Thursday	Static Exercise	Dynamic Exercise (general and specific)
Friday	Static Exercise	Dynamic Exercise (general)
Saturday	Static Exercise	Distance Walking, Swimming, and so on
Sunday	Breath-Control Exercise	Rest

SCHEDULE 3

Day	Morning	Evening
Monday	Static Exercise	Dynamic Exercise (general)
Tuesday	Static Exercise	Dynamic Exercise (general)
Wednesday	Breath-Control Exercise	Walking or other Constitutional Exercise
Thursday	Static Exercise	Dynamic Exercise (general)
Friday	Static Exercise	Dynamic Exercise (general)
Saturday	Static Exercise	Distance Walking, Swimming, and so on
Sunday	Breath-Control Exercise	Rest

SCHEDULE 4

Day	Morning	Evening
Monday	Static Exercise	Dynamic Exercise (general and specific)
Tuesday	Static Exercise	Dynamic Exercise (general)
Wednesday	Breath-Control Exercise	Walking or other Constitutional Exercise
Thursday	Static Exercise	Dynamic Exercise (general and specific)
Friday	Static Exercise	Dynamic Exercise (general)
Saturday	Static Exercise	Distance Walking, Swimming, and so on
Sunday	Breath-Control Exercise	Rest

SCHEDULE 5

Day	Morning	Evening
Monday	Static Exercise	Dynamic Exercise (general)
Tuesday	Static Exercise	Dynamic Exercise (specific)
Wednesday	Static Exercise	Walking or other Constitutional Exercise
Thursday	Static Exercise	Dynamic Exercise (general)
Friday	Static Exercise	Dynamic Exercise (specific)
Saturday	Breath-Control Exercise	Distance Walking, Swimming, and so on
Sunday	Breath-Control Exercise	Rest

SCHEDULE 6

Day	Morning	Evening
Monday	Static Exercise	Walking
Tuesday	Breath-Control Exercise	Dynamic Exercise
Wednesday	Static Exercise	Walking or other Constitutional Exercise
Thursday	Breath-Control Exercise	Dynamic Exercise
Friday	Static Exercise	Walking
Saturday	Breath-Control Exercise	Distance Walking, Swimming, and so on
Sunday	Breath-Control Exercise	Rest

SCHEDULE 7

Day	Morning	Evening
Monday	Breath-Control Exercise	Static Exercise
Tuesday	Breath-Control Exercise	Dynamic Exercise
Wednesday	Breath-Control Exercise	Static Exercise
Thursday	Breath-Control Exercise	Dynamic Exercise
Friday	Breath-Control Exercise	Static Exercise
Saturday	Breath-Control Exercise	Distance Walking, Swimming, and so on
Sunday	Breath-Control Exercise	Rest

SCHEDULE 8

Day	Morning	Evening
Monday	Breath-Control Exercise	Static Exercise
Tuesday	Breath-Control Exercise	Dynamic Exercise
Wednesday	Breath-Control Exercise	Walking or other Constitutional Exercise
Thursday	Breath-Control Exercise	Static Exercise
Friday	Breath-Control Exercise	Dynamic Exercise
Saturday	Breath-Control Exercise	Static Exercise
Sunday	Breath-Control Exercise	Distance Walking, Swimming, and so on

Yoga Demonstrations

Given by the author and his pupil Dinabandhu Pramanick at medical, educational, physical culture, and other institutions in India, Japan, U.S.A., and Europe.

In India

- Assembly Chambers, Shillong
- Bowring Hospital, Bangalore
- British Legation, Nepal
- British Medical Association (Hyderabad Branch)
- British Medical Association (South Indian Branch)
- Government House, Shillong
- His Highness the Maharaja of Benares' palace, Benares
- His Highness the Maharaja of Jammu and Kashmir, Srinagar
- His Highness the Maharaja of Mysore's palace, Bangalore
- His Highness the Maharaja of Patiala's palace
- Hyderabad Medical Association
- King George Hospital, Vizagapatam
- Madras Medical Association
- Nizam Club, Hyderabad (Deccan)
- Singha Durbar (His Highness' palace), Nepal

In Japan

- Physiological Department, Imperial University, Tokyo
- St. Luke's International Medical Center, Tokyo

In the U.S.A.

- American Physiotherapy Association, New York
- Chicago Osteopathic Association
- 43rd Congress of the American Naturopathic Association
- Macfadden's Physical Culture Institute, New York
- New York Athletic Club
- 1939 New York World's Fair
- Physicians' Square Club of Greater New York
- St. Luke's Hospital, Chicago

In Europe

- Comité France-Inde, Paris, 1950
- L'Hôpital de la Salpétrière, Paris, 1950
- India House, London, 1950
- International Club, Stockholm, 1949
- Karolinska Sjukhuset, Stockholm, 1949
- Musée Guimet, Paris, 1950
- Physical Therapy Department, Zurich University, 1950

Société de Kinésitherapie, Paris, 1950
Société de Morpho-Physiologie Humaine, Paris, 1950
Sorbonne (University of Paris), Paris, 1950
UNESCO (United Nation's Educational, Scientific and Cultural Organization), Paris, 1951
Uppsala University, Uppsala, 1949
World Physical Education Congress, in connection with the Lingiad in Stockholm, 1949

Note on the Pronunciation of Transliterated Sanskrit Words

The following are the approximate English equivalents together with the symbols adopted by the International Phonetic Association:

a	has the sound of a	in all (c:)
ā	has the sound of a	in father (a:)
i	has the sound of i	in it(iɔ
ī	has the sound of ee	in see (i:)
u	has the sound of u	in full (u)
ū	has the sound of oo	in moon (u:)
ṛi	has the sound of ri	in river (ri)
e	has the sound of ey	in prey (ei)
ai	has the sound of oy	in boy (oi)
o	has the sound of o	in molest (o)
au	has the sound of o	in go (ɔu)
k	has the sound of k	in kind (k)
kh	has the sound of kh	in inkhorn (kh)
g	has the sound of g	in go (g)
gh	has the sound of gh	in log hut (gh)
ṅ	has the sound of ng	in king (ŋ)
c	has the sound of ch	in chapter (tʃ)
ch	has the sound of ch	in chop-house (tʃh)
j	has the sound of j	in job (d3)
jh	has the sound of dgeh	in hedgehog (d3h)
ñ	has the sound of ny	in canyon (nj)
ṭ	has the sound of t	in tie (t)
ṭh	has the sound of th	in anthill (th)
ḍ	has the sound of d	in do (d)
ḍh	has the sound of dh	in red-haired (dh)
ṇ	has the sound of n	in not (n)
t	has the sound almost of t (t)	
th	has the sound of th	in three (þ)
d	has the sound of th	in there (ð)
dh	has the sound of dh	in adhere (dh)
n	has the sound of n	in no (n)
p	has the sound of p	in pan (p)
ph	has the sound of ph	in philosophy (f)
b	has the sound of b	in bar (b)
bh	has the sound of v	in vanish (v)
m	has the sound of m	in mother (m)
y	has the sound of y	in yet (j)
r	has the sound of r	in ram (r)
l	has the sound of l	in lady (l)
v	has the sound of w	in walk (w)
ś	has the sound of sh	in shade (ʃ)
ṣ	has the sound of sh	in shade (ʃ)
s	has the sound of s	in saint (s)
h	has the sound of h	in hot (h)
ṉ	has the sound almost of ṅ (ŋ)	
ṃ	has the sound almost of m (m)	

Bibliography

Original Unpublished Works on Yoga

Manuscripts

Bhavadeva: *Yoga-sāra-samgraha*

Dattatreya: *Dattātreya-samhītā*

Deva, Sundara: *Haṭha-samketa-candrikā*

——— *Haṭha-tattva-kaumudī*

Gorakṣa: *Gorakṣa-śataka*

Śiva: *Yoga-bīja*

Amṛita-siddhi

Khecarī-vidyā

Tattva Yoga-bindu

Yoga-kalpa-latikā

Yoga-prakriyā

Yoga-vacana-samgraha

Books

Dattātreya: *Yoga-rahasya*

Gheraṇḍa: *Gheraṇḍa-samhītā*

Gorakṣa: *Gorakṣa-samhītā*

Patañjali: *Yoga-sūtra*

Śiva: *Śiva-samhītā*

Svātmārāma: *Haṭha-dīpikā*

Vyāsa: *Bhagavadgītā*

Yājñāvalkya: *Yogi-yajñāvalkya*

Other Original Works

Vedas

Atharvaveda

Ṛigveda

Sāmaveda

Yajurveda

Brāhmaṇas

Aitareya Brāhmaṇa

Kauṣītaki Brāhmaṇa

Satapatha Brāhmaṇa

Upaniṣads

Amritānandopaniṣad

Dhyānabindupaniṣad

Śandilyopaniṣad

Yogacuḍāmanyupaniṣad

Yogakuṇḍalyupaniṣad

Yogaśikhopaniṣad

Itihasas

Vyāsa: *Mahābhārata*

Purāṇas

Vyāsa: *Agni-purāṇa*

——— *Bhāgavata-purāṇa*
——— *Garuḍa-purāṇa*
——— *Linga-purāṇa*
——— *Mārkaṇḍeya-purāṇa*
——— *Padma-purāṇa*
——— *Śiva-purāṇa*
——— *Skanda-purāṇa*

Other Selected Works

Alvarez, Walter C. *An Introduction to Gastroenterology.* 4th ed. New York: Paul B. Hoeber, Medical Book Department of Harper and Brothers, 1948.

Burrows, Harold. *Biological Actions of Sex Hormones.* 2nd ed. Cambridge, U.K.: The University Press, 1949.

Corner, George W. *The Hormones in Human Reproduction.* Princeton, N.J.: Princeton University Press, 1947.

Fulton, John F. *A Textbook of Physiology.* 16th ed. Philadelphia and London: S. B. Saunders Company, 1949.

Goldthwait, Joel E., Lloyd T. Brown, Loring T. Swaim, and John G. Kuhns. *Essentials of Body Mechanics in Health and Disease.* 5th ed. Philadelphia, London, Montreal: J. B. Lippincott Company, 1952.

Goswami, Shyam Sundar. *Layayoga: The Definitive Guide to the Chakras and Kundalini.* Rochester, Vt.: Inner Traditions, 1998. (Orig. pub 1988.)

Harris, Leslie J. *Vitamins: A Digest of Current Knowledge.* London: J. and A. Churchill Ltd., 1951.

Hawley, Gertrude. *The Kinesiology of Corrective Exercise.* Philadelphia: Lea and Febiger, 1949.

Johnston, T. B., and J. Whillis. *Gray's Anatomy, Descriptive and Applied.* 30th ed. London, New York, Toronto: Longmans, Green & Co., 1949.

Kendall, Henry O., and Florence P. Kendall. *Muscles, Testing and Function.* Baltimore: The Williams and Wilkins Company, 1949.

Lockhart, R. D. *Living Anatomy.* London: Faber and Faber Ltd., 1948.

Morehouse, Laurence E., and Augustus T. Miller, Jr. *Physiology and Exercise.* St. Louis: The C. V. Mosby Company, 1948.

Oakley, Kenneth P., and Helen M. Muir-Wood. *The Succession of Life through Geological Time.* 2nd ed. London: British Museum (Natural History), 1949.

Quiring, Daniel P. *The Head, Neck, and Trunk Muscles and Motor Points.* Philadelphia: Lea and Febiger, 1947.

Prosser, C. Ladd, David W. Bishop, Frank A. Brown, Jr., Theodore L. Jahn, and Verner J. Wulif. *Comparative Animal Physiology.* Philadelphia and London: W. B. Saunders Company, 1950.

Robson, J. M. *Recent Advances in Sex and Reproductive Physiology.* 3rd ed. London: J. and A. Churchill Ltd., 1949.

Romer, Alfred Sherwood. *Man and the Vertebrates.* 7th Impression. Chicago: The University of Chicago Press, 1948.

———. *The Vertebrate Body.* Philadelphia and London: W. B. Saunders Company, 1950.

Schneider, Edward C., and Peter V. Karpovich. *Physiology of Muscular Activity.* 3rd ed. Philadelphia and London: W. B. Saunders Company, 1948.

Tuner, G. Donnell. *General Endocrinology.* Philadelphia and London: W. B. Saunders Company, 1949.

Wells, Katharine F. *Kinesiology.* Philadelphia and London: W. B. Saunders Company, 1950.

Wiggers, Carl J.: *Physiology in Health and Disease.* 5th ed. Philadelphia: Lea and Febiger, 1949.

Glossary

ahimsā Abstinence from injury

anāhata Extraphysical sound

ānanda samādhi Fourth stage of *samādhi* where the sensory organs are disconnected from objects, and where the subject-object relation starts to disappear; happiness

aparigraha Abstinence from acceptance of gifts

asamprajñāta samādhi Supreme concentration

āsana Posture, posture exercise

Ashtangha Yoga Yoga doctrine composed of the eight sub-disciplines—*yama, niyama, āsana, prāṇāyāma, pratyāhāra, dhāraṇa, dhyāna,* and *samādhi*

asmitā samādhi Third stage of *samādhi* where the yogi is aware of the self, released of the non-self (non-sensory)

asteya Abstinence from theft

Bhastrikā Thoracic Short-Quick Breathing

Bhūta Śuddhi Combined form of breathing with *mantras* and thoughts

brahmacarya Sexual control in thoughts, emotion, and action

Cakrī Bhanda Wheel-Forming Lock

Cālana (Mani, Meru) Cervical exercises

cāraṇā muscular contraction and muscular control exercise

Daṇḍa Dhautī Esophageal Cleansing

Danta Dhautī Oral Cleansing

deva deha Yogic idealization pattern of human life

dhāraṇā Elementary concentration

dhyāna Unbroken concentration

idā One of the three principal *nādīs* (pranic forces)

īśvarapraṇidhāna Meditation on God

Jālandhara Bandha Chin Lock

Jala Vasti Colonic Auto-Lavage

japa Repetition of a *mantra* according to a special process

jñanendriya The five senses of perception or cognitive faculties for smell, taste, colors and forms, touch sensations, and sound

Kapālabhātī Abdominal Short-Quick Breathing

karmendriyas The five conative senses—speech,

prehension, locomotion, organic activities, and reproduction

kevala kumbhaka Natural breath suspension

Khecarī Mudrā Advanced Breath Suspension

Kumbhaka Controlled breath suspension

Kuṇḍalinī The Grand Spiritual Potential

Laulikī See Naulī

madhyama Inaudible (*mantra*) sound

mahābhūta Nonmaterial subtle energy; "essential"

mantra A particularized form of sound, endowed with the power of awakening conscious radiant energy, residing in it

manas Mind (perceptive)

mātrikā Primary sound units; the letters of the Sanskrit alphabet

mudrā Special posture and control exercise

Mūla Bandha Anal Lock

mūla-mantra The *mantra* received in initiation

nāḍī Pranic force; radiation line created by the motion direction of *vāyu.*

Nāḍī Śuddhi Purficatory breath control with internal contraction to prolong breath suspension

Naulī (Laulikī) Straight Muscle Exercise

Neti; Sutra Neti Nasal thread-cleansing

nirodha The process of elimination of *vṛittis*

niyama Self-regulation with five ethical rules

ojas Vital force derived from prāṇa

pingalā One of the three principle *nāḍīs* (pranic forces)

Plāvaṇī Floating Breath Control

prāṇa Energy entity that connects the body to the mind; one of the five vital breaths moving in the body; the kinetic principle, or life principle at the basis of mind, life, and matter

prāṇāyāma Breath control; breath-control exercise

pratyāhāra Sensory control

rishi Sage, "seer" of ancient India

sādhana The Yoga path or means of accomplishment

Sahita Alternate-Nostril Breath Control with Breath Suspension

samādhi Super concentration

samprajñāta samādhi Super concentration with super knowledge

ṣaṭ karman Six purifications

Śakti Consciousness in the form of will-energy; consciousness in the form of radiant energy (conscious radiant energy)

santoṣa contentment

satya truthfulness

Śankprakṣalana Auto-Lavage of the alimentary canal

śauca cleanliness

Śītali Prāṇayāma Lingual Breath Control

Sītkārī Prāṇāyāma Dental Breath Control

Śītkrama Kapālabhātī Inverted Nasopharyngeal Water Bath

śukra The sexual energy that activates sexual glands in both men and women

Śuṣka Vasti Colonic Auto-Air Bath

suṣumnā one of the three principal *nāḍīs* (pranic forces)

smṛiti Memory

svādhyāya Study

tanmātra Nonmaterial subtlest and most concentrated form of energy; "thatness"

tapas, tapasyā Asceticism; specific energy process

Trāṭaka Gazing exercise

Tunda Cālana Abdominal Control Exercise

Uḍḍīyāna Bandha Abdominal Retraction

Ujjāyī Both-Nostrils Breath Control

Vajrolī Mudrā Gonadal Control or Sexual Control Exercise

Vamana Dhautī Gastric Auto-Lavage

Vāri Sāra Alimentary Canal Auto-Lavage

Vāsa Dhautī Gastric Cloth-Cleansing

Vāta Sāra Alimentary Canal Auto-Air Bath

vāyu The constant motional state of *prāṇa* (the principle of eternal energy embedded in the supreme); its principle forces are *prāṇa, apāna, samāna, udāna,* and *vyāna,* respectively

vicāra samādhi Second stage of *samādhi* where the yogi perceives one *tanmātra* or "thatness" (presensory)

vitarka samādhi First stage of *samādhi* where the yogi perceives one *mahābhūta* or "essential" as a separate element (presensory)

vṛitti Molding of the objective aspect of consciousness into an image

Vyutkrama Kapālabhātī Nasopharyngeal Water Bath

yama self-restraint including five ethical rules

Yoga *yogacittavṛitti nirodha* (Patañjali); "Skill (in modern parlance, efficiency) in action" (Bhagavad Gītā); the Science of Man; a way of life, yoking of the personal self with the Universal Self in cosmic harmony

Yoni Mudrā An advanced sexual-control practice, which, in the yogic tradition, is instructed orally and only to fit practitioners

Index

Page numbers in *italics* reference illustrations.

Books of Related Interest

Layayoga
The Definitive Guide to the Chakras and Kundalini
by Shyam Sundar Goswami

The Heart of Yoga
Developing a Personal Practice
by T. K. V. Desikachar

Weight-Resistance Yoga
Practicing Embodied Spirituality
by Max Popov

Chakras
Energy Centers of Transformation
by Harish Johari

The Wisdom Teachings of Harish Johari on the Mahabharata
Edited by Wil Geraets

Yoga Spandakarika
The Sacred Texts at the Origins of Tantra
by Daniel Odier

INNER TRADITIONS • BEAR & COMPANY
P.O. Box 388
Rochester, VT 05767
1-800-246-8648
www.InnerTraditions.com

Or contact your local bookseller